Fundamental Aspects of Children's and Young People's Nursing Procedures

Note:

While the authors and publishers have made every effort, as far as is possible, to confirm the information in this book complies with the latest standards of practice and legislation, the author and the publishers cannot take any responsibility from any instance arising as a result of errors. Healthcare practice and knowledge are constantly changing and developing. Practitioners are encouraged to seek help where they are not competent to carry out a procedure.

Fundamental Aspects of Children's and Young People's Nursing Procedures

edited by
Alan Glasper, Marion Aylott and Gill Prudhoe

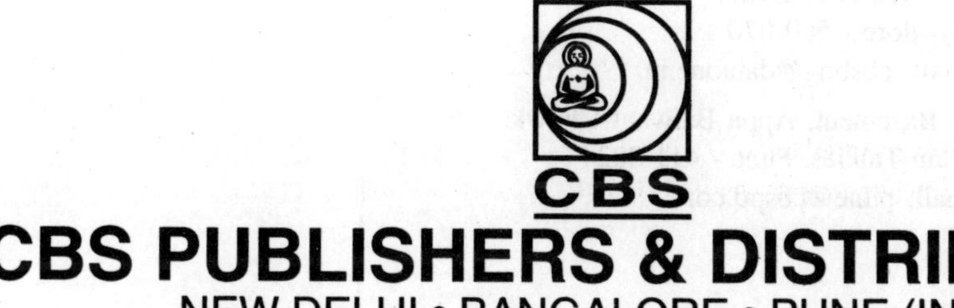

CBS PUBLISHERS & DISTRIBUTORS
NEW DELHI • BANGALORE • PUNE (INDIA)

CBS Publishers ISBN : 978-81-239-1746-7
Quay Books ISBN : 978-1-85642-188-1

First Indian Reprint : 2009

Authorised reprint from the English language edition published by
Quay Books, a division of MA Healthcare, London

Published by Satish Kumar Jain and produced by Vinod K. Jain for
CBS Publishers & Distributors,
4819/XI Prahlad Street, 24 Ansari Road, Daryaganj, New Delhi - 110 002, India.
e-mail: cbspubs@vsnl.com, cbspubs@airtelmail.in
Website: www.cbspd.com

Branches:

- Seema House, 2975, 17th Cross, K.R. Road,
  Bansankari 2nd Stage, Bangalore - 560 070
  Fax: 080-26771680 • e-mail: cbsbng@dataone.in
- Shaan Brahmha Complex, Basement, Appa Balwant Chowk,
  Budhwar Peth, Next to Ratan Talkies, Pune - 411 002
  Fax: 020-24464059 • e-mail: pune@cbspd.com

Printed at :
Chaman Offset, Delhi (India)

Dedication

Mrs Mary Taylor (secretary to the children's and young peoples nursing team at the University of Southampton) for helping to organise the making of this book.

Contents

List of contributors

Dawn Ashbee is a Senior Staff Nurse, Portsmouth Hospitals NHS Trust

Marion Aylott is a Lecturer in Children's and Young People's Nursing, University of Southampton

Dr Gary Barrett is a Lecturer in Children's and Young People's Nursing, University of Southampton

Catherine Bentley is a Senior Staff Nurse, University of Southampton Hospitals NHS Trust

Gemma Blagdon is a Senior Staff Nurse, University of Southampton Hospitals NHS Trust

Louise Butler is a Senior Staff Nurse, University of Southampton Hospitals NHS Trust

Sally Cooke is a Senior Staff Nurse, University of Southampton Hospitals NHS Trust

Karen Dick is a Senior Staff Nurse, University of Southampton Hospitals NHS Trust

Terri Fletcher is a Lecturer in Children's and Young People's Nursing, University of Southampton

Michelle Fuller is a Senior Staff Nurse, University of Southampton Hospitals NHS Trust

Dr Alan Glasper is Professor of Children's and Young People's Nursing, University of Southampton

Diane Gow is a Lecturer in Children's and Young People's Nursing, University of Southampton

Joanna Groves is a Hospital Play Specialist, University of Southampton Hospitals NHS Trust

Maureen Harrison is a Lecturer in Children's and Young People's Nursing, University of Southampton

Jan Heath is Head of Clinical Skills, University of Southampton Hospitals NHS Trust

Laura Ho is a Senior Staff Nurse, University of Southampton Hospitals NHS Trust

Lorraine Ireland is a Lecturer in Children's and Young People's Nursing, University of Southampton

Di Keeton is Paediatric Dermatology Nurse Specialist, University of Southampton Hospitals NHS Trust

Jane McConochie is a Senior Staff Nurse, Portsmouth Hospitals NHS trust

Joanne Miller is a Senior Staff Nurse, University of Southampton Hospitals NHS Trust

Helen Pearson is a Registered Children's Nurse and Student Liaison Coordinator, School of Nursing and Midwifery, University of Southampton

Margaret Porter is a Senior Sister, University of Southampton Hospitals NHS Trust

Gill Prudhoe is a Lecturer in Children's and Young People's Nursing, University of Southampton

Odette Rodda is a Clinical Skills Demonstrator, University of Southampton

Jane Shelswell is a Senior Staff Nurse, University of Southampton Hospitals NHS Trust

Sue Twells is a Staff Nurse, Portsmouth Hospitals NHS Trust

Chrissie Ward is a Senior Sister, Children's Neurological Unit, University of Southampton Hospitals NHS Trust

Katy Weaver is a Hospital Play Specialist, University of Southampton Hospitals NHS Trust

Preface

Fundamental Aspects of Children's and Young People's Nursing Procedures has been adapted from Penny Tremayne and Sam Parboteeah's successful book Fundamental Aspects of Adult Nursing Procedures.

It has been edited and written by children's nurses for children's' nurses in practice. The clear and straightforward descriptions of clinical procedures are an excellent resource for nursing students and newly qualified staff nurses in their everyday working lives within the child field of practice.

The complexities of caring for sick children, and their families, require nurses who are fully conversant with the special needs of this client group, and the first chapter of this book covers in detail the crucial considerations of risk assessment, consent and child safeguarding.

Fundamental Aspects of Children's and Young People's Nursing Procedures has been designed with a specific readership in mind, to give maximum clarity and to be simple to use. Each chapter is structured around the what, how and why of children's nursing procedures, and throughout the text there are helpful exercise activities for readers to practise and hone their skills within the safety of the skills laboratory. The step-by-step approach takes readers through each procedure logically. It is designed to encompass both the knowledge that underpins the skills and the practicalities of carrying them out. Readers will find particularly useful the sections on the equipment needed to carry out each skill and the actions that need to be carried out both before and after each procedure.

As the complexity of children's nursing procedures grows year by year, this timely book, supplemented with important information pertinent to the skills in question, will prove an invaluable text for nurses working in contemporary children's nursing settings.

Alan Glasper
Marion Aylott
Gill Prudhoe

Foreword

So often we hear that children and young people's nursing is changing more now than ever before. It remains a view inextricably linked to even further technological advances. But is this the whole story? And what does it mean to the children's nurse in hospital or the community? Is children and young people's nursing care provision really altering beyond merely learning future aftercare of new treatments? Change is occurring from a variety of angles that clearly impact not only on healthcare provision on the wider scale, but also the grass roots of individual children's nurse practitioners.

This book embodies the knowledge of numerous nurses working with children and young people, and its primary purpose is to provide information on the fundamental aspects and essential requirements of nursing care for children, young people and their family or carer. The child or young person is an integral member of the family. Children and young people's nursing care is most effective when it is integrated with the value and belief that family-centred care is crucial. When a child or young person is healthy, the child's health is enhanced if the family is a fully functioning health-promoting system. The family can be made up of many different structures, each with the potential to provide a caring, supportive environment in which the child and/or young person can grow, mature and maximise his or her potential.

This book is remarkable for its honesty about the essential and fundamental aspects of nursing care of babies, children, young people and their families or carers. There are two main questions which we should ask ourselves as nurses who work with babies, children, young people and their families and carers. The first is, do fundamental aspects of nursing care influence the nursing profession? The second, does this book help babies, children, young people and their families to be prepared and recover more effectively?

Scientific evidence in favour of both of these issues is slowly building up. The broader your knowledge about children and young people's nursing, the more interesting you are as a children's nurse, and this allows you to see babies, children and young people in a different way. In addition, I have seen the growth and increased self-confidence of nurses caring for babies, children, young people and their families or carers; their quality of life during this time is fulfilling for all.

The book is designed to support the learning needs of nurses, not only by virtue of its design, but also by the level of knowledge acquisition it facilitates. It must be noted here that by knowledge acquisition I do not simply mean the supply of relevant and up-to-date information – important though this may be. The claim here is that higher levels of knowledge extend beyond the learning environment to absorb and reproduce information in the same form that it is conveyed. It includes the capacity to understand and apply knowledge to nursing practice with babies, children, young people and their families and carers. These are vitally important aspects of knowledge in children and young people's nursing today.

This book provides a sensible compromise between a lengthy discussion of basic sciences on the one hand, and a didactic handbook on the other. It will be an excellent source of information for nurses learning about caring for babies, children, young people and their families and carers, and a useful reference for experienced nurses working with children and young people.

Rory Farrelly MSc RGN RSCN
Director of Nursing, Children's Services NHS Greater Glasgow, Clyde National Adviser to Chief Nursing Officer for Children, Young People's Nursing for Scotland Scottish Executive Health Department
Yorkhill Royal Hospital for Sick Children
Glasgow

Chapter 1

Fundamental aspects for undertaking nursing procedures with children, young people and their families

Alan Glasper, Diane Gow, Lorraine Ireland and Gill Prudhoe

This chapter identifies areas of practice that must be considered before any procedure can take place to ensure that children and their families receive quality care from competent professional nurses. The areas covered are:

- Consent to treatment
- Risk and child-patient safety
- Dignity and family-centred care
- Privacy
- Comfort
- Safeguarding

All procedures must be accompanied by accurate documentation to demonstrate that the duty of care has been fulfilled, to enable continuity of care, and to show the nurse's professionalism. Part of the preparation for procedures must always be to ensure that health and safety, infection control and local and, if applicable, national policies and procedures are adhered to.

Consent to treatment

The NHS Plan (Department of Health [DH], 2000) identified a need to change the way that patients are asked to give their consent, to ensure that the process is properly focused on the rights of individual patients. Consent is a unifying principle, that represents the legal and ethical expression of the human right to have one's autonomy and self-determination respected (McHale *et al*, 1997). The issue of consent is particularly pertinent to children's and young people's nurses in the wake of the events at Alder Hey Children's Hospital in Liverpool and the children's cardiac unit at the Bristol Royal Infirmary during the 1990s where consent procedures were shown to be less than optimal (Department of Health, 2001a, Kennedy, 2001).

The intention of consent is to protect and respect a patient's autonomy and to promote meaningful decision making (Beauchamp and Childress, 2001; Department of Health, 2001a; Nursing and Midwifery Council [NMC], 2002; Dimond, 2003). The issues of consent and people aged under 16 years were not addressed in the Family Law Reform Act of 1969, but this was tested in the early 1980s in a case where the courts were asked to rule on the rights of parents in respect of their children. The Gillick case, considered to be a watershed legal decision, established that minors under the age of 16 could, if they had capacity, consent to treatment, (Gillick v West Norfolk & Wisbech Area Health Authority 1986, AC11). In this respect, 'capacity' refers to a child being able to demonstrate sufficient understanding and intelligence to appreciate what is being proposed. This is sometimes referred to the child being 'Gillick competent'. Some texts may also refer to 'Fraser guidelines', so called after the Law Lord who ruled on the case. It should be stressed, however, that the Fraser guidelines apply only to girls and contraception, not the wider consent issues now associated with Gillick competency (Wheeler, 2006). It is important to consider what criteria are used for testing if a child is to be considered Gillick competent. According to Larcher (2005) the young person should be able to:

- Understand in simple terms, the nature, purpose and necessity for the proposed treatment
- Believe that the information applies to them
- Retain the information long enough to make a choice
- Make a choice free from pressure

Within the UK, *young people aged 16–17* can consent to treatment, but cannot necessarily refuse treatment that is intended to save their lives or prevent serious harm. This is crucially important in certain categories of disorder management such as eating disorders. The British Medical Association (BMA) guidelines of (2001) state that although the young person's right to consent to treatment is now firmly established, his or her rights to refuse treatment remains less certain. Because of this factor, a competent young person's refusal might be overturned in certain circumstances, for example in cases where the child's refusal means they are at risk of suffering 'grave and irreversible mental or physical harm' (Department of Health, 2001a). Where disputes cannot be resolved by negotiation and mediation, legal intervention may be required. Courts have overturned young people's refusal of psychiatric medication and, for example, blood transfusion in cases of leukaemia and heart–lung transplantation. The psychological effects of having a young person's consent decision over-ruled should be carefully considered. Forcing young people to have treatments they do not want may produce long-term psychological harm and lack of cooperation with future treatment. The question remains whether it is logically consistent that young people can seemingly consent to treatment, but their rights to refuse treatment are more limited (BMA, 2001).

Young *people aged under 16* may legally consent if they satisfy criteria of competence and voluntariness. In Scotland, the Age of Legal Capacity Act (1991) gives statutory power to mature minors under the age of sixteen to consent to treatment. The act effectively does through statute what the Gillick case has done through common law in England and Wales (Hope, 2003). It should be stressed, however, that competence is context-dependent and may therefore fluctuate. Pain, the environment of care, and psychosocial state may all reduce or adversely affect competence. Conversely, a child's past experience of illness may increase competence.

In law, it is the doctor's responsibility to assess competence, although other professionals with appropriate skills may be delegated to help (Larcher, 2005). The more complex the procedure, the more challenging it is for nurses involved with the care of certain children.

Coercion – whether subtle or overt – of young people to give consent is not uncommon. It is possible, for example, that failing to provide a child or young person with adequate time or facilities to receive and reflect on information will be perceived as coercive, even if it was unintentional. Additionally, young people may feel that their unquestioned acquiescence to the decisions of authority figures (such as health-care professionals and their parents) is required. Hence, pressurising children and young people to make decisions when they feel neither happy nor confident to do so may be coercive (Larcher, 2005).

Obtaining consent is a fundamental part of good practice, and any health-care professional who does not obtain valid consent may be liable to legal action by the patient and his or her family, in either a criminal offence of battery or a civil claim for negligence. Nurses may also find themselves having to account for their actions to their regulatory body, the NMC (Department of Health, 2001b).

Before any procedure in this book is performed, the practitioner must possess knowledge and understanding of the subject of consent, so that a valid and meaningful consent can be obtained before the procedure takes place. It is important to stress that consent is a process and not a one-off event. It is required whenever a nurse wishes to examine or treat a sick child, unless in an emergency.

Types of consent

Consent may be expressed explicitly or it can be implied. It can be given verbally, in writing, or implied by conduct, depending on the clinical situation, the treatment, and the degree of risk involved.

Implied consent

Implied consent is a universally accepted concept. It relates to behaviour of the patient, legal guardian or child that indicates to the health-care professional his or her agreement to the procedure. Implied consent is often obtained for simple acts of care, such as mobilising or personal hygiene. Aveyard (2002) advises caution when relying on implied consent prior to nursing procedures because of the difficulty in distinguishing between *consent* and *compliance*. If any doubt exists, it is prudent to obtain 'express' consent instead. Implied consent may be expressed verbally or non-verbally, whereby actions speak louder than words (such as a child holding out an arm to have his or her pulse taken).

Express consent

Express consent is an umbrella term that incorporates written and oral consent, and is used for procedures carrying a special risk. The law does not specify when consent should be written rather than oral (Kennedy and Grubb, 2000; Montgomery, 2003). Written consent is normally obtained using a consent form and it draws the child's, young person's or guardian's attention to the fact that he or she is consenting to a clinical procedure, and that it may carry risks or have major consequences. Dyer (1992) suggests that practitioners have a fixation about written consent, and describes this as a triumph of myth over reality – it is the reality of consent that matters, not its form. It is important to stress that written consent simply provides evidence of consent. If all the elements of consent have neither been undertaken nor satisfied, then a signature on a piece of hospital paper will not make the consent valid (Department of Health, 2001a,b). There is no legal, ethical or professional distinction to be drawn between the efficacy of written, oral and implied consent, except in evidential terms. The crucial factor in all cases is the validity of the consent (Kennedy and Grubb, 2000; Department of Health, 2001a; Dimond, 2003; Montgomery, 2003).

Validity of consent

Gillon (1986) defines valid consent as:

> *"...a voluntary and uncoerced decision made by a competent or autonomous person on the basis of adequate information and deliberation to accept rather than reject some proposed course of action that will affect them."*

For consent to be valid, certain conditions must apply. The consent must be given voluntarily without coercion by a mentally competent person who has been given adequate information (Kennedy and Grubb, 2000; Aveyard, 2001; Department of Health, 2001a; NMC, 2002; Montgomery, 2003).

Assent

Assent is when agreement is given by a child who is not competent to give legally binding consent under current legislation. Assent should always be obtained from children. It is a process in which the health-care professional is able to allow a child to indicate their willingness to participate, even when they are insufficiently mature to make a fully informed decision to consent (Callery *et al*, 2006). All children should be provided with information about procedures, and nurses must endeavour to seek the child's assent – any sustained dissent should be taken seriously (Harrison *et al,* 1997). Some hospitals may use a special assent form for younger children, written and couched in terms they will understand. Good practice suggests that a signed assent form, in addition to the consent form signed by the child's legal guardian, will help in the overall process of family-centred care.

Information

Information is a complex area and much debate exists over the amount of information that children and their families need. For consent to be legally valid, the child and legal guardian needs to understand in broad terms the nature and purpose of the procedure (Department of Health, 2001a). Although such measures would avoid a claim for battery, to avoid a claim for negligence and sufficiently fulfil the duty of care to the patient the information should be tailored to the patient's individual needs. In relation to procedures described in this book, the information given must demonstrate knowledge of the procedure, must be individualised, and must be given in an understandable format.

Kennedy (2001) recommends that information should be given in a variety of ways, that it should be given in stages, and that it should be reinforced over time. It should be tailored to the needs, circumstances and wishes of the individual. It should be based on current evidence, in a form that is comprehensible to the child and to his or her guardians. When performing nursing procedures, information should be given about what the procedure is, why it is necessary, the perceived benefits and risks, the available alternatives, and the consequences of not performing the procedure. Such information should be presented in a way that can be easily understood, and that avoids the use of jargon. The child and the legal guardians should be allowed time to ask questions and to have them answered honestly. The information-giving process should be ongoing, where possible, throughout the procedure, and these conversations should be documented to establish that valid consent and/or assent was obtained. Each family will require different amounts of information.

The *Children First* website is now referred to in the websites of many children's units. It is designed to help children and their families learn about illnesses, tests and treatments.

Voluntariness

Consent must be voluntary, free from force, deceit, duress, over-reaching or other ulterior forms of constraint. Such pressure can be evident from family members as well as health-care professionals. Children must know they can assent to care and ask questions (Alderson and Goodey, 1998).

Capacity

The NMC (2002) states you should *presume* that every patient and client is legally competent unless otherwise assessed by a suitably qualified practitioner. Capacity is generally characterised by understanding. If a Gillick-competent child refuses a procedure, it does not mean that he or she lacks capacity, it might just be that he or she has a different opinion and set of values. In this instance, the nurse must ensure that the child has received all the information needed to make a decision and that the refusal is documented.

Valid and invalid refusal

Children sometimes refuse treatment because their anxieties are focused on one aspect in particular, namely the short-term fear of pain (perhaps from an injection). When a child refuses treatment or a medical procedure, they may not be expressing a considered choice in favour of non treatment; indeed, the child might willingly accept the intervention if it were administered differently. With effective preparation, the use of local anaesthetic, sedation and analgesia, together with skilful use of distraction techniques and encouragement, the child can be enabled to cope with their anxiety and pain (Royal College of Nursing [RCN], 2003). Genuine refusal of treatment is, in contrast, based on awareness of the implications, and it is consistent over time, and compatible with the child's view of his or her best interests beyond the short term (BMA, 2001).

Care without consent

In emergencies where treatment is necessary to preserve life or where the capacity of the patient is permanent or likely to be longstanding, or *in the absence of a legal guardian*, it is lawful to carry out procedures that are in the best interest of the child (Kennedy and Grubb, 2000; Department of Health, 2001a; 2002; NMC, 2002; Cable *et al*, 2003; Dimond, 2003; Montgomery, 2003). Best interests are not confined to medical best interests but also include the patient's values and preferences when competent. These include their psychological health, well-being, quality of life, relationships with family and other carers, spiritual and religious welfare, and personal financial interests (Department of Health, 2001a).

Who should obtain consent?

Ideally, the individual performing the procedure should obtain consent. This is particularly appropriate for the procedures described in this book, where oral consent is likely to be sought at the point when the procedure will be carried out. At other times, it may not be possible for the person carrying out the procedure to obtain the consent. In such circumstances, the task may be delegated to nurses on behalf of a colleague. The NMC (2002) affirms that you may seek consent on behalf of colleagues if you have been specially trained in that area of practice. The Department of Health (Department of Health, 2002) acknowledges this practice as long as professionals are competent to do so, either because they are able to carry out the procedure or because they have received specialist training in advising patients about the procedure, and have been assessed and are aware of the limitations of their own knowledge and are subject to audit.

When should consent be sought?

The process of consent may take place at one time or over a series of meetings and discussions. The Department of Health (Department of Health, 2002) describes the former as single-stage consent and the latter as a process of two or more stages. The latter is particularly pertinent to elective surgery or procedures and treatments where there is an initial decision and when later discussions confirm that the child and family, after having had time to absorb the information and ensured understanding, still want to go ahead. Single-stage consent is the most likely process for obtaining consent for the procedures within this book, whereby the procedure is initiated immediately after the explanation and after ascertaining that the required competence and lack of coercion exist.

Withdrawal of consent during a procedure

A patient with capacity is entitled to withdraw consent at any time, including during the performance of a procedure. If this happens, it is good practice (if safe to do so) to stop the procedure and explore the child's concerns, but also provide an explanation of the consequences of stopping. Giving a sense of control back to the child can be valuable at this stage, as the child may be finding it difficult to cope with what seems an overwhelming situation. Allowing the child to have some element of choice regarding aspects of the procedure, such as the timing, location, or the way in which they are held, can help. *However*, if stopping the procedure is deemed to be life threatening, then the individual carrying out the procedure may carry on until the danger has passed.

This first section has explored the issues that nurses need to be aware of for obtaining consent prior to any nursing procedure. It has highlighted that consent is primarily concerned with protecting the patient's autonomy, placing them in the middle of the decision-making process. By adhering to these principles and supporting them with effective documentation, nurses can demonstrate their knowledge to their patient and can also enhance the quality of their patient's experience. This can include enhancing the patient's dignity, privacy and comfort – issues that are discussed next.

Risk and child-patient safety

Reason (1990) indicated that one in ten hospitalised patients suffers from an adverse event during a course of treatment. Children are especially vulnerable, and children's nurses must address the context in which they work and deliver care. In acute hospitals, accidents (especially falls), and errors of treatment and procedures, medication, clinical assessment (including diagnosis) and documentation constitute a large proportion of reported incidents.

Given the high incidence of procedures leading to an adverse incident, children's nurses need to be vigilant and to follow strict procedures and guidelines. Procedural guidelines must be evidence-based and updated regularly. Staff performing procedural skills must be trained to do so and their competency must be monitored through their personal development plans. Annual updating must be recorded.

An adverse incident can be defined as any health-care occurrence that has led to unintended or unexplained harm to a child. A 'near miss' is defined as an occurrence that may have led to a child being harmed, but either the mistake was aborted before harm occurred or no harm actually resulted by chance alone. Potential causes of harm for a child in a health-care setting include:

- Errors in delivery of medication
- Mismatch between the child and the treatment
- Equipment errors
- A health-care professional working beyond competency
- Failure to make or a delay in making an accurate diagnosis
- Sub-optimal handover
- Sub-optimal continuity of care
- Failure to ensure follow-up of investigations
- Lack of awareness of local procedures and policies

What can be done in your unit to protect children?

- Hold a governance forum where risk issues are discussed every month
- Ensure a local lead for risk management activities
- Identify specialty triggers
- Conduct regular reviews of adverse-event reporting
- Carry out full investigation (root-cause analysis) of all 'red' NPSA-graded (National Patient Safety Agency) incidents
- Provide evidence of lessons learned and practices changed (eg. checking of nasogastric tubes and cannula dressings)
- Link to an audit programme

Remember the mantra of the children's nurse:

"First do the child no harm"

Dignity and family-centred care in partnership

The concept of the maintenance of dignity is central to good nursing practice (Haddock, 1996; Walsh and Kowanko, 2002). Nurses are advised through the *Code of Professional Conduct* (NMC, 2002) that they are:

> *"...personally accountable for ensuring that they promote and protect the interests and dignity of patients and clients, irrespective of gender age, race, ability, sexuality, economic status, lifestyle, cultural and religious or political belief."*

In order to maintain child-patient dignity, it is necessary to treat the person inside the patient, not merely regard the child as an object or a disease in a body in a bed. Woogara (2001) links the concept of dignity to Article 8 of the Human Rights Act 1998, which highlights that individual patients should be treated as people, and that the quality of care is improved by respecting their wishes and dignity. Jacelon (2003) suggests that dignity is defined as an individual's self-worth, and is composed of individual and interpersonal attributes, and is something that is both bestowed by others in the immediate environment and exists independently of it.

However, when interviewing the parents of 300 hospitalised children, Rylance (1999) found that dignity, privacy and (importantly) confidentiality were poorly respected on children's wards, even though these children and their parents should have the same rights as adult patients. Reed *et al* (2003) highlighted the complex issue of promoting child dignity, comparing it with attitudes towards older adults – on the one hand reacting to an elderly individual who may no longer be the same person they once were, and on the other hand dealing with a child who is evolving into a person who is as yet unknown. Adults who care for children in health-care environments need to behave in a way that shows respect for the dignity of the person the child is yet to be – that is they must be an advocate through the temporal lifespan for both the present and the future individual.

The *Essence of Care* (Department of Health, 2001c) describes nine key areas of care that have been identified by patients as needing attention. Among these are privacy and dignity, which are now firmly re-established at the forefront of nursing. Privacy and dignity are also firmly embedded within the *National Service Framework for Children, Young People and Maternity Services* (Department of Health, 2003) and will be closely monitored through regular auditing of children's units by the Health Care Commission. Importantly, in children's units where there are no specific age-related divisions, close attention must be paid to privacy in the context of gender, ethnicity and developmental age. In addition to preserving each child's dignity the fundamental aspects of caring for sick children and young people are embedded within the concept of family-centred care in partnership. Smith *et al* (2006) reinforce family-centred care as one of the most significant concepts to have evolved from the realms of children's nursing over the last 50 years, whereby the child and family are perceived as an indivisible unit and the family occupies a central tenet in the sick child's life. Family-centred care has been defined by Smith *et al* (2002) as:

> *"...the professional support of the child and family through a process of involvement, participation and partnership underpinned by empowerment and negotiation."*

This has important ramifications for children's nurses who may not actually perform the skills themselves but may undertake them through a third party, in the guise of parents or guardians or the child-patients themselves. Hence the role of the children's nurse encompasses both skills tuition and delivery. When guardians and children are taught skills, they must follow a training schedule where competency is assessed and recorded within the patient record. Casey (1995), who is regarded as the architect of the concept of partnership in care with families, found in a hospital survey of 243 children that 85% of the children were receiving some or all of their nursing care from a member of their own family, usually their mother.

Walsh and Kowanko (2002) compared the perceptions of nurses and patients with regards to dignity. The emerging themes are identified in *Box 1.1*.

Box 1.1: Patients' and nurses' perceptions of dignity

Patients' perceptions of dignity	Nurses' perceptions of dignity
Not being exposed	Privacy of the body
Having enough time	Providing private space
Not being rushed	Consideration of emotions
Having time to decide	Giving time
Being seen as a person	Viewing the patient as a person
Not seeing their body as an object	Not treating the body as an object
Being acknowledged	Showing respect
Being treated with consideration	Giving control
Being treated with discretion	Affording advocacy

(From Walsh and Kowanko, 2002)

How to maintain dignity

All procedures in this book require that the dignity of the child is maintained as an essential component. This should be considered before, during and after the procedure.

Pre-procedure

The children's nurse should establish effective communication with the child and family by simple actions such as introducing him or herself and establishing how the child would like to be addressed. Although it is customary to use first names with children, never assume it is appropriate or acceptable to greet a parent or guardian on first-name terms. Failure to recognize and observe this courtesy can often threaten dignity. The nurse must ensure at the earliest moment possible that the child is informed about the planned procedure and that he or she is offered choices (see *Consent to treatment* below); Walsh and Kowanko (2002) established that patients felt that their dignity was maintained when they were given choice and control.

Not only should the child-patient be fully prepared before a procedure commences, but so should the environment. All necessary play and distraction equipment should be set up, all clinical equipment ready and checked, with a practitioner competent in its use and aware of any pertinent health and safety regulations, policies and procedures. Such measures enable the procedure to advance without interruption. Dignity is enhanced when the child-patient (and family) is made aware that he or she is the most important person at that moment in time.

During the procedure

Mains (1994) suggested that one of the characteristics of dignity is appreciation of individual standards, which are given little consideration unless a person becomes vulnerable or anticipates their loss. This is evident during nursing procedures, and emphasis should be given to maintaining personal standards. Patient dignity can be achieved by ensuring the patient's comfort (as discussed in more detail below), maintaining communication, giving reassurance, ensuring that the patient's body is not unnecessarily exposed or violated, and creating an environment that remains private throughout.

Post-procedure

Communication, once more, is of paramount importance in order to give consideration to the child's emotions and to provide time for him or her to ask questions or to express feelings. It is important to ensure that any clothing is replaced and that the child's appearance is acceptable to him or her. All interactions that take place need to be child- and family-focused – and not for the benefit of the nurse. Haddock (1996) suggests that the most powerful tool a nurse possesses to maintain and promote dignity is his or her own self, to work with feelings and to use them constructively to understand patients by treating them as valid, worthy and important at a time when they are most vulnerable.

Privacy

Privacy is inextricably linked to the concept of dignity. The profile and expectations of patients regarding non-violation of privacy by health-care professionals have been raised by the Caldicott Committee report (Department of Health, 1997), the professional guidelines of the NMC (NMC, 2002), the publication of *Essence of Care* (Department of Health, 2001c) and incorporation of the European Convention of Human Rights 1998 within UK law.

Woogara (2001) noted that respect for privacy is manifest in a multitude of ways – the right to enjoy and control personal space and property, the right to confidentiality, and the right to expect treatment with dignity. Rylance (1999) highlighted in particular the problems of maintaining privacy in the children's wards; he believes they stem primarily from problems of attitude, behaviour and thought. Breaches of privacy during nursing procedures can be avoided easily by thorough preparation of the environment.

One major area for concern within the realms of privacy is confidentiality. This can be compromised in a variety of situations, such as asking the child of family personal questions in front of other families during bedside handover and ward rounds (this is particularly pertinent for families with children in small rural communities and on offshore islands where issues of privacy and confidentiality are more acute). It must be remembered that while drawing curtains around a child's bed or cot can successfully protect their personal space, the curtains are not sufficient to prevent verbal confidential information from being overheard.

Documentation forms an essential component of nursing practice by demonstrating that competent care has been delivered. Part of the professionalism surrounding documentation is to ensure that data protection issues have been addressed regarding the storage of documents so that privacy is maintained.

In conjunction with the confidentiality of information, nurses must provide an environment that protects personal space and privacy. Woogara (2001) noted that violation of privacy occurred when curtains were not shut properly or when people walked through curtains while procedures were taking place, thereby leaving patients in a vulnerable state. This can be avoided by clipping curtains together or by using a 'Do not disturb' notice. An ideal environment is to be away from the ward area altogether. By adopting such an approach, the professional is not only respecting the family's privacy and dignity, but is also demonstrating an ability to maintain patient comfort.

Comfort

Comfort is an integral part of nursing care and has been cited as a desired goal from the time of Florence Nightingale. Achieving a state of comfort for a child-patient can be seen as a measure of quality care (Wurzbach, 1996; Malinowski and Leeseberg Stamler, 2002; Robinson, 2002; Siefert, 2002). The literature suggests that comforted patients heal faster, cope better, require less analgesia, have shorter stays, and are generally more satisfied with care (Walker, 2001; Kolcaba and Wilson, 2002). However, Tutton and Seers (2003) point out that the exact meaning of the term 'comfort' is unclear. Definitions have included comfort as an outcome of nursing, as a basic human need, and as a process for which no consensus of a definition exists (Malinowski and Leeseberg Stamler, 2002). What is apparent is that comfort is a broad, complex and individualized concept. Kolcaba (1992) provides a technical definition of comfort as:

> *"...the state of being strengthened by having needs for relief ease and transcendence met in four contexts of experience (physical, psychospiritual, sociocultural and environmental)."*

A patient attains relief by having his or her specific needs met, for example by alleviating severe discomfort such as pain or nausea. 'Ease' is enabling a state of calm or contentment, and transcendence is the state in which one rises above problems and pain when they cannot be eradicated or avoided. This is of relevance during procedures in which discomfort cannot be avoided (Kolcaba, 1992; Kolcaba and Wilson, 2002). The four contexts – physical, psychospiritual, sociocultural and environmental – are dynamic in nature, and individual (depending on the person and procedure).

- **Physical** comfort may include obvious needs such as pain relief (which should be considered and discussed before all procedures) as well as issues that patients are unaware of such as maintenance of homeostasis
- **Psychospiritual** comfort is not easily identifiable, but might include issues such as touch and communication
- **Sociocultural** factors include cultural sensitivity, reassurance and support. These needs can be met by employing good communication skills, by developing a therapeutic relationship with the child-patient, and by planning the procedure carefully, perhaps informing the child that you may have to perpetrate discomfort temporarily in order to achieve a higher degree of comfort
- **Environmental** issues include those that have already been discussed in relation to privacy and dignity to safeguard confidentiality and personal space. They also include providing comfortable furniture, diminishing odours, and maintaining a safe environment

A later definition by Siefert (2002) reflects these values and defines comfort as:

"...a state and/or process that is individually defined, multidimensional and dynamic; it may be temporary or permanent and requires that one's needs be satisfied in the physical, psychological, social, spiritual and/or environmental domains within a specific context."

For nurses to achieve a state of comfort in sick children there must be an understanding of the symptoms of discomfort (Robinson, 2002). Suggested symptoms of discomfort include:

- Fatigue
- Loss of appetite
- Being too hot or too cold
- Pain
- Bowel distress
- Loss of bodily control
- Vulnerability
- Fear
- Embarrassment
- Stress
- Depression

This list of symptoms underlines the fact that comfort is indeed a multidimensional concept. Consideration must be given to the child's comfort needs before, during and after the procedure, because his or her needs will change at each stage. The nurse should also ensure that the same rules of comfort apply to the family who is involved in the procedure with the child. Siefert (2002) adds that for patients to achieve a state of comfort they must feel that their personal safety and security is assured, feeling comfortable they are dependent on knowledgeable and competent caregivers who have access to appropriate facilities and technology to meet their needs.

Safeguarding

All children deserve the opportunity to reach their full potential based upon the five key outcomes from *Every Child Matters* (Department for Education and Skills [DES], 2003, 2004a,b), outcomes that are fundamental to the well-being of children and young people.

- Stay safe
- Be healthy
- Enjoy and achieve
- Make a positive contribution
- Achieve economic well-being

Every Child Matters outlines the principles for all professionals who have a responsibility for safeguarding children and young people. Consideration of these five outcomes is a significant issue for all children's nurses when carrying out clinical skills with children and young people. Additionally, within the UK there has been increasing awareness of children's rights. The United Nations Convention on the Rights of the Child was ratified by the UK in 1991; articles 3, 12 and 19 are particularly pertinent in affirming children's rights in relation to healthcare interventions (UNICEF, 1989). These articles relate to three areas:

- Ensuring the child's best interests are paramount in decisions concerning their welfare (article 3)
- Recognising the rights of the child to express their views (article 12)
- Protecting every child from abuse and mistreatment (article 19)

The Department of Health document (Department of Health, 2006) *Working Together to Safeguard Children* highlights how important it is that all healthcare professionals consider the potential of their actions to cause harm or even abuse to children.

It is essential when performing clinical skills that the potential to cause harm – both psychological and physical – is recognised.

"Abuse and neglect may occur when individuals or processes inflict or fail to intervene to prevent the infliction of harm to a child."

Department of Health, 2006

The *National Service Framework for Children, Young People and Maternity Services* (NSF, 2004) document also discusses the impact of physical, emotional or sexual abuse or neglect or domestic violence, parental mental ill health and substance misuse. It explains how all or any of these problems can have a significant effect on all aspects of a child health, development and well-being. Any of these problems can last into and throughout adulthood, so children's nurses are in a unique position to work collaboratively with agencies that support children and their families. The joint document of the Department of Health, Home Office and Department for Education and Employment *Working Together to Safeguard Children* (2006) states that by doing so, children's nurses can help to:

- Protect the child from maltreatment
- Prevent impairment of the child's health or development
- Ensure that the child grows up in circumstances that are consistent with the provision of safe and effective care

Safeguarding children is the process of protecting children from abuse or neglect, and preventing impairment of their health or development. Children's nurses have a duty to safeguard and promote the welfare of children within their care. This duty cannot be carried out without effective joint working between professionals and agencies, working collaboratively with those professionals who have a particular professional expertise. The children's nurse may on occasions be required to liaise with a range of professionals including those working in education, children's social care, the voluntary sector and the youth justice services. To facilitate safeguarding of children while carrying out clinical procedures, the children's nurse should:

- Work collaboratively
- Respect diversity
- Promote equality
- Provide child-centred care
- Apply the processes of safeguarding and encourage participation of children and their families

Safeguarding of children during procedures will be assured if children's nurses:

- Understand the risk factors and recognise a child in need or one who needs support
- Assess the child's needs and the parenting capacity of the parents before undertaking a procedure
- Adopt a child-centred approach that ensures the needs of the child are respected and that his or her views are taken into consideration
- Decrease the child's anxiety before carrying out procedures
- Master stressful situations
- Encourage active involvement of the parents
- Provide significant pain control for invasive medical procedures
- Help the child to cope with subsequent procedures
- Consider and respect the issues of restraint within an ethos of caring and respect for the child's rights – restraint, holding or containing a child without his or her permission should be a last resort, never a first-line intervention (RCN, 2003)
- Carry out the clinical skill while ensuring that the child is not at risk of abuse (is the procedure really necessary or is there an alternative?)
- Obtain consent from a child who is old enough and able to understand
- Ensure that the procedure is carried out ethically in order to minimise the child's pain and suffering
- Are adept and skilled in carrying out the procedures

Overarching principles of safeguarding children

The most important things to remember as a children's nurse are summarised as follows:

- Be familiar with your organisation's policies and procedures for safeguarding and promoting the welfare of children within the area your practice
- Know the signs and symptoms and indicators of potential abuse or neglect in children and young people, and be alert and observe for indicators of abuse (this may include parental conditions that have an impact upon the child or young person)
- Ensure any concerns are referred to social services or police (after discussion with a senior colleague or designated nurse)
- Document all concerns and issues relating to the procedure
- Do not promise confidentiality
- If a child makes a disclosure to you, do not question them but convey that you believe them

Concerns may arise during a procedure because of one or more of the following factors:

- A discrepancy in a child's story regarding the cause of an injury
- Repeated attendances of the child at accident and emergency
- The pattern of injuries (old and healing)

- The ability of the parents or carers to respond to the child's needs
- Certain behavioural indicators

The context of the concern is vital to ensuring that children and young people are safe. It is as important as gaining and sharing information with other agencies and professionals. When carrying out clinical skills, the children's safety is paramount, and the nurse needs to consider all aspects in order to ensure that children and young people are able to fulfil and reach their potential.

Remember that you are not alone and there are other professionals to help and support you within your organisation. Working to ensure that children and young people are protected requires sound professional judgement. All children's nurses should have access to advice and support from their peers, managers and named and designated professionals. Supervision is key to promoting good standards of practice and it ensures that practice is based upon the procedures of your local Safeguarding Children Board.

Conclusions

This chapter has identified some of the key issues that must be considered before commencing any procedure in this book. It has also identified the importance of following health and safety, infection control, and local and national policies and procedures to ensure a safe environment is maintained. In addition, it has emphasised the importance of backing up every action with accurate documentation to demonstrate that the duty of care has been fulfilled, to enable continuity of care, and to demonstrate the nurse's professionalism. Importantly, this chapter has outlined the areas of practice that you must consider and abide by before you undertake any procedures with children and their families. Only by doing so will you ensure that children and their families receive quality care from a competent professional nurse.

References

Alderson P, Goodey C (1998) Theories of consent. *BMJ* **317:** 1313–15

Aveyard H (2001) The requirements for informed consent prior to nursing care procedures. *J Adv Nurs* **37:** 243–49

Aveyard H (2002) Implied consent prior to nursing care procedures. *J Adv Nurs* **39:** 201–07

Beauchamp TL, Childress JF (2001) *Principles of Biomedical Ethics, 5th edn.* Oxford University Press, Oxford

Beckett C (2007) *Child Protection: An Introduction,* 2nd edn. Sage Publications, London

British Medical Association (2001) *Consent, Rights and Choices in Health Care for Children and Young People.* BMJ Books, London

Cable S, Lumsdaine I, Semple M (2003) Informed consent. *Nurs Stand* **18**(12): 47–53

Callery P, Neill S, Feasey S (2006) The evidence base for children's nursing practice. In: Glasper EA, Richardson J, eds. *A Textbook of Children's and Young People's Nursing.* Churchhill Livingstone, Edinburgh

Casey A (1995) Partnership nursing: influences on involvement of informal carers. *J Adv Nurs* **22**(6): 1058–62

Corby B (2005) *Child Abuse: Towards a Knowledge Base*, 3rd edn. Open University Press, Maidenhead.

Department for Education and Skills (2004a) *Every Child Matters: Change for Children.* DES, London

Department for Education and Skills (2004b) *Every Child Matters: Next Steps.* DES, London

Department of Health (1997) *The Caldicott Committee: Report on the Review of Patient Identifiable Information.* DH, London

Department of Health (2000) *The NHS Plan.* DH, London

Department of Health (2001a) *The Royal Liverpool Children's Inquiry: Summary and Recommendations.* The Stationery Office, London

Department of Health (2001b) *Reference Guide to Informed Consent for Examination or Treatment.* DH, London

Department of Health (2001c) *Essence of Care.* DH, London

Department of Health (2002) *Model Policy for Consent to Examination or Treatment.* DH, London

Department of Health (2003b) *National Service Framework for Children, Young People and Maternity Services. Standard for Hospital Service.* DH, London

Department of Health, Home Office, Department for Education and Employment (2006) *Working Together to Safeguard Children.* The Stationery Office London

Dimond B (2003) *Legal Aspects of Consent.* Quay Books, Salisbury

Dyer C (1992) *Doctor Patients and the Law.* Blackwell Science, London

Gillon R (1986) *Philosophical Medical Ethics.* Wiley, Chichester

Haddock J (1996) Towards further clarification of the concept 'dignity'. *J Adv Nurs* **24:** 924–31

Harrison C, Kenny NP, Sidareous M, Rowell M (1997) Bioethics for clinicians 9: Involving children in medical decisions. *Can Med Assoc J* **156**(6): 825–28

Hope T, Savulescu J, Hendrick J (2003) *Medical Ethics and Law. The Core Curriculum.* Churchill Livingstone, Edinburgh

Jacelon CS (2003) The dignity of elders in an acute care hospital. *Qual Health Res* **13**(4): 543–56

Kennedy I (2001) *Bristol Royal Infirmary Inquiry. Learning from Bristol: the Report of the Public Inquiry into Children's Heart Surgery at the Bristol Royal Infirmary 1984–1995.* The Stationery Office, London

Kennedy I, Grubb A (2000) *Medical Law*, 3rd edn. Butterworths, London

Kolcaba K (1992) Holistic comfort: operationalising the construct as a nurse sensitive outcome. *Adv Nurs Sci* **15**(1): 1–10

Kolcaba K, Wilson L (2002) Comfort care: a framework for perianesthesia nursing. *J Perianesth Nurs* **17**(2): 102–14

Larcher V (2005) Consent, competence and confidentiality. *BMJ* **330:** 353–56

Mains ED (1994) Concept clarification in professional practice: dignity. *J Adv Nurs* **19:** 947–53

Malinowski A, Leeseberg Stamler L (2002) Comfort: exploration of the concept in nursing. *J Adv Nurs* **39:** 599–609

McHale I, Fox M, Murphy J (1997) *Health Care Law Text and Materials.* Sweet and Maxwell, London

Montgomery J (2003) *Health Care Law,* 2nd edn. Oxford University Press, Oxford

Nursing and Midwifery Council (2002) *Code of Professional Conduct.* NMC, London

Reason J (1990) *Human Error*. Cambridge University Press, Cambridge

Reed P, Smith P, Fletcher M, Bradding A (2003) Promoting the dignity of the child in hospital. Nurs Ethics **10**(1): 67–76

Robinson S (2002) Warmed blankets: an intervention to promote comfort for elderly hospitalized patients. *Geriatric Nurs* **23:** 321–23

Royal College of Nursing (2003) *Restraining, Holding Still and Containing Children and Young People*. RCN, London

Rylance G (1999) Privacy, dignity and confidentiality: interview study with structured questionnaire. *BMJ* **318**: 301

Siefert ML (2002) Concept analysis of comfort. *Nurs Forum* **37**(4): 16–23

Smith L, Coleman V, Bradshaw M (2006) Family-centred care. In: Glasper EA, Richardson J, eds. *A Textbook of Children's and Young People's Nursing*. Churchill Livingstone, Edinburgh

Smith L, Colman V, Bradshaw M (eds) (2002) *Family-Centred Care: Concept, Theory and Practice*. Palgrave, Basingstoke

The Royal Australasian College of Physicians Paediatrics and Child Health Division (2005) *Guideline Statement: Management of Procedure related Pain in Children and Adolescents*. Royal Australasian College of Physicians, Sydney

Tutton E, Seers K (2003) An exploration of the concept of comfort. *J Clin Nurs* **12:** 689–96

Walker AC (2001) Safety and comfort work of nurses glimpsed through patient narratives. *Int J Nurs Pract* **8:** 42–48

Walsh K, Kowanko I (2002) Nurses' and patients' perceptions of dignity. *Int J Nurs Pract* **8:** 143–45

Wheeler R (2006) Gillick of Fraser? A plea for consistency over competence in children. *BMJ* **332:** 807 (editorial) was cited with author BMJ

Woogara I (2001) Human rights and patients' privacy in UK hospitals. *Nurs Ethics* **8**(3): 231 46

Wurzbach ME (1996) Comfort and nurses' moral choices. *J Adv Nurs* **24:** 260–64

Further reading

Department of Health (1999) *Making a Difference*. DH, London

Department of Health, Home Office, Department for Education and Skills, Department for Culture, Media and Sport, Office of the Deputy Prime Minister, Lord Chancellor (2003) *What to Do if You're Worried A Child is Being Abused*. DH, London

Morse I (2000) On comfort and comforting. *Am J Nurs* **100**(9): 34–38

Useful websites

Children First
www.childrenfirst.nhs.uk/kids

National Service Framework for Children
www.dh.gov.uk

National Society for the Prevention of Cruelty to Children (NSPCC)
www.nspcc.org.uk

Chapter 2

Fundamental aspects of safe, clean care of the infant

Joanna Millar

Infants rely on their carers to fulfil and meet all of their needs. Their basic needs include feeding, hygiene, comfort, safety and development. Whenever you are caring for an infant you should always remember to communicate with them, by talking and singing to them, smiling at them and touching them.

Handling an infant

There are numerous ways to hold and cuddle an infant. Although it may seem scary to begin with it will get easier the more you do it. Infants, especially neonates (newborn to 28 days of age) need to be held gently, but firmly. Their head and neck should be supported at all times and consideration should be made as to the infant's developmental age because this will affect their head control and their ability to wriggle.

Picking-up an infant

- Slide one hand under the infant's shoulders and neck, using your fingers to support their head
- Reach over the infant, and slide your other hand between their legs and under their bottom
- You can now pick the infant up

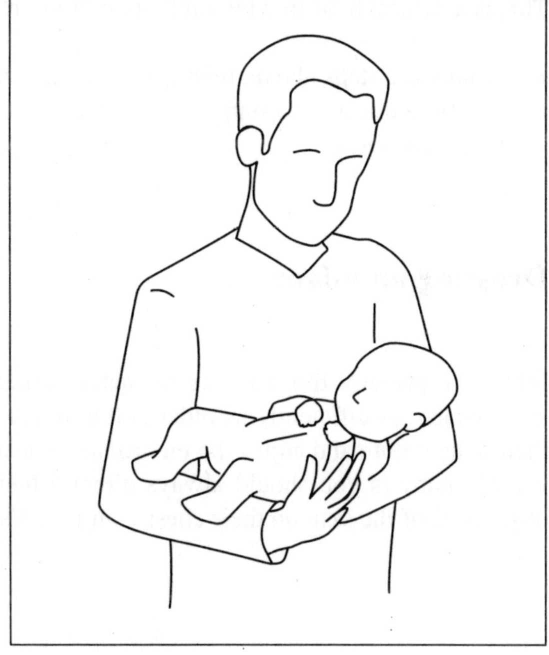

Figure 2.1: Cradling an infant in the arms

Cradling an infant

This is a simple, supportive way to cradle an infant (*Figure 2.1*):

- Once you have picked the infant up as described above, carefully slide your hand along their bottom up their back, transferring support of their head to the arm they are lying along, so that the infant lies on his or her back along your inner forearm
- Cradle infant in both arms, ensuring that infant's head is head being supported in the nook of your arm (especially important during the neonatal period)

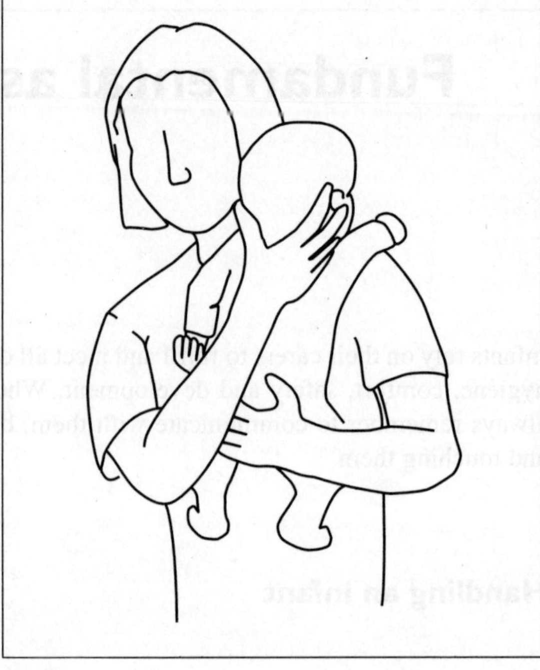

Figure 2.2: Holding an infant on the shoulder

Holding the infant in the shoulder hold

This is a natural hold in which infants will often fall asleep (*Figure 2.2*).

- Follow the steps above, then gently lift the infant onto your shoulder
- Use the same arm to support under the infant's bottom and use your spare hand to support the infant's head

Dressing an infant

Infants (especially those in the neonatal period) cannot regulate their own temperature and environment as efficiently as older children and adults. Therefore it is crucial that you monitor their temperature and adjust the environment accordingly (Lee and Hilton, 2004). To check how warm a baby is you should always directly feel, with the back of your hand, for warmth (or otherwise) of the skin on their chest – an infant's hands and feet are often cool.

Pre-procedure

Equipment required

- Clean vest
- Babygrow
- Socks
- Mittens (if required)

Specific preparation

- First collect everything you will need
- Wash your hands
- Examine the clothes to see if there are poppers, buttons or zips
- Consider whether each garment needs to go over the baby's head, or does up at the front, back or bottom

During the procedure

- Gather the infant's vest up around the neckline and then place it on top of the infant's head. Smoothly pull the vest from the crown over the face and head
- Pick up one of the infant's arms and gently push their hand into the sleeve. With your other hand lightly pull their arm through from the cuff end of the garment sleeves. Repeat with the other arm
- Hold the infant's ankles and lift their bottom up with your non-dominant hand. Using your dominant hand, pull the vest down their back
- Secure the poppers together
- Lay out the babygrow on the changing surface, lift the infant, lay them down on top of it
- Using the same techniques as above, put the infant's arms and legs through the babygrow
- If the babygrow does not have enclosed feet, place socks on the infant's feet
- Finally, working from the top down, do up all the poppers and place the infant somewhere safe
- Wash your hands

Infant hygiene

Changing a nappy

Infant nappies may need changing up to ten times a day, and many babies do not like having their nappies changed and may cry or even scream. Young children are not usually toilet trained until they are 3 years old and they will wear nappies until this time (Royal College of Nursing [RCN], 2006). An infant's skin, particularly in the neonatal period, is very delicate and is in almost constant contact with moisture, bacteria and ammonia (Darmstadt and Dingles, 2000); therefore their skin is at risk of breaking down (McManus, 2001).

Do not use talcum powder as there is risk of aspiration (Department of Health [DH], 2006). If a parent specifically requests talcum powder to be used, then sprinkle it onto your hand and rub it onto the infant's skin while shielding their face from any dust. Use it sparingly.

Pre-procedure

Equipment required

- Gloves
- Apron
- Waste bag
- Clean nappy
- Changing mat
- Cotton-wool and warm water (if under 28 days) or wipes (if over 28 days)

Specific preparation

- First collect together all the things you will need
- It is important to follow standard precautions when changing an infant's nappy as you will obviously come into contact with bodily fluids. You should always wear an apron and gloves, and wash your hands before and afterwards (Department of Health, 2003)

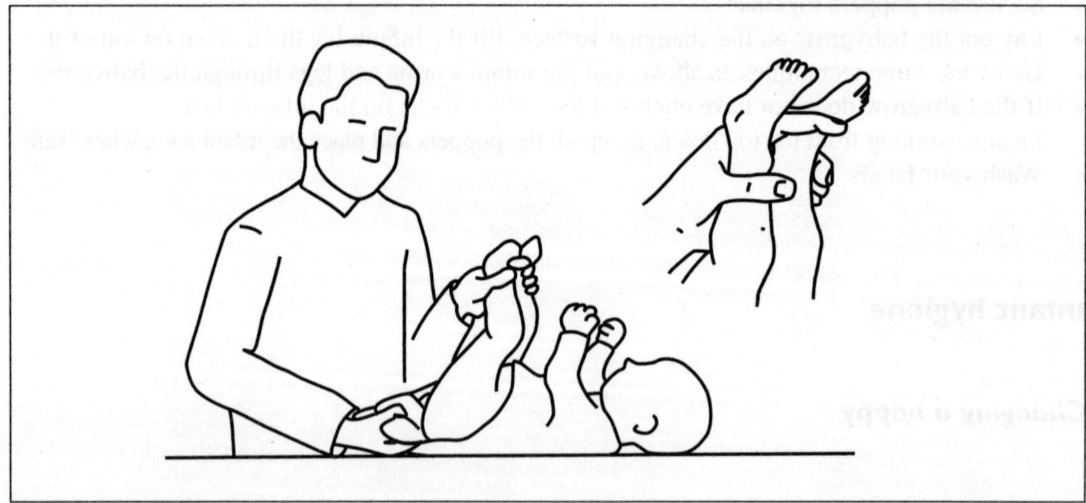

Figure 2.3: Lifting an infant's legs during a nappy change

- *NEVER leave an infant unattended when being changed in a raised cot or changing mat* (Harold *et al*, 2003)

During the procedure

- Lift the infant onto a changing mat at waist level (Smith, 2005), laying them supine (on their back), positioning the head gently to one side. Undress the infant from the waist down
- Remove the infant's nappy by undoing the adhesive tabs and re-fastening them back onto themselves to prevent them from sticking to the infant's delicate skin
- Securely hold the infant's ankles with your non-dominant hand and then lift them up (*Figure 2.3*). Beware that infants often urinate on removal of their nappy – especially boys
- Use your dominant hand to slide the front of the nappy underneath the infant's bottom. If the infant has opened their bowels wipe away most of the mess towards their back, using the inside of the nappy, and then fold it over so that the mess is inside the nappy. The infant is now laying on the folded nappy
- Use warm water and cotton-wool to gently cleanse the infant's skin.
  - In boys, never pull the foreskin back – this is an unnecessary and damaging practice (Department of Health, 2006)
  - In girls, cleanse from the front to the back in one swipe and discard the piece of cotton-wool or wipe to prevent vaginal and urethral contamination (Chon *et al*, 2001). Repeat as needed
- Carefully blot (never rub) the infant dry, paying special attention to any creases (McManus, 2001)
- Lift the infant's legs, as before, and slide a clean nappy under their bottom. Always make sure that the penis is tucked downwards so that urine will flow into the nappy and not out the top (Lund, 1999). Make sure that the nappy is fastened securely, but not so tightly that is pinches the skin (McManus, 2001)
- Re-dress the infant and place them somewhere safe
- Discard the dirty nappy and cotton-wool in the clinical waste bin (Department of Health, 2003), throw away the water and wash out the bowl with hot water and detergent. Dry them and store them in a dry place
- Remove gloves and apron and dispose of in a clinical waste bin (Department of Health, 2003)
- Wash your hands

Post-procedure

- Maintain appropriate records (Nursing and Midwifery Council [NMC], 2004)

Topping and tailing

Infants do not need a bath everyday (Department of Health, 2006) and can just have a 'top and tail'. Again, it is important to follow standard precautions as you may come into contact with bodily fluids (Department of Health, 2003). Gloves and aprons should always be worn. Avoid 'top and tailing' an infant immediately after a feed as this can induce vomiting (Lee and Thompson, 2007). Topping and tailing gives you a good opportunity to observe how the infant handles and behaves (Department of Health, 2004).

Pre-procedure

Equipment required

- Gloves
- Apron
- Changing mat
- Cotton-wool/sponge
- Warm water
- Clean nappy
- Baby soap
- Bowl
- Face-cloth
- Two warm towels
- Clean clothes

Specific patient preparation

- First collect everything you will need
- Bathing of infants (especially neonates) can induce hypothermia (Rudolf and Levene, 2006) so steps should be taken to reduce this possibility. Shut all windows and doors and make sure you have everything you need to hand
- Check the temperature of the water; it should be between 32°C and 35°C, which feels neither hot nor cold when you test it with the back of your hand or elbow (Young, 2004)

During the procedure

- Lay the infant on the changing mat and remove clothes
- Wrap them in one of the warm towels to prevent them from becoming cold
- Use a damp face-cloth to wash the infant's face, neck and head with water (White and Denyer, 2006)

- Use the other warm towel to dry them
- Remove the infant's nappy and use wet cotton-wool or wet wipes to cleanse the nappy area
- Put on a clean nappy and clothes
- Place the infant somewhere safe
- Discard the dirty nappy and cotton-wool or wet wipes into the clinical waste bin (Department of Health, 2003)
- Throw away the water and place the towels into the correct linen bin
- Wash out the bowl and sponge with hot water and detergent, dry it and store in a dry place
- Discard your gloves and apron
- Wash your hands (Department of Health, 2003)

Post-procedure

- Maintain appropriate records (NMC, 2004)

Bathing an infant

Bathing can be an enjoyable way to interact and play with an infant. However, some infants enjoy baths more than others and this should be taken into consideration. In some clinical situations, infants may not benefit from being given a bath, which can be discussed with a senior member of staff. Newborns and infants aged under 1 month of age (neonates) should be washed in plain water only; avoid soap or bubble-bath (Department of Health, 2006). Remember that neonates should not be bathed until their cord has fallen off, and topping and tailing will adequately meet their hygiene needs until then (Department of Health, 2006). Standard precautions should be followed, namely hand washing, disposable gloves and aprons because of the potential leakage and contamination with body fluids.

Never leave an infant alone in a bath

Pre-procedure

Equipment required

- Clean nappy
- Clean clothes
- Two warm towels
- Sponge
- Jug
- Cotton-wool
- Baby bath, baby soap and shampoo (if over 28 days of age)

Specific preparation

- First collect together everything you will need
- Close any windows and doors to reduce the chance of baby getting cold
- Fill the bath up by a few centimetres with cold water first, as this will prevent scalding. Then top up the bath with hot water. The water should be 5–8 cm deep to prevent accidental drowning (Lee and Thompson, 2007)
- Always test the temperature of the water with the back of your hand or elbow. It should be neither hot nor cold to your touch (Young, 2004)
- Wash your hands

During the procedure

- Undress the infant and remove their nappy
- Swaddle the infant in one of the warm towels to help maintain comfort and body temperature, leaving only their face exposed
- First cleanse the infant's face using a cloth and plain water (soap should not be used on an infant's face as their skin is particularly sensitive) (Cowan and Frost, 2006)
- To wash the infant's hair, keep them swaddled in the towel and expose their head. Hold securely along your non-dominant forearm, with the head supported in your hand. The infant will be lying at a slightly downwards angle. Using your dominant hand, gently splash water from the bath onto the head. Apply a small amount of baby shampoo and gently massage. Use a jug or your cupped hand to rinse the soap off with water from the bath. Once the soap is completely rinsed off, immediately dry the infant's head with the second towel to prevent heat loss
- Add baby soap to the bath as directed by manufacturer, remembering that excessive use of baby soap can dry out an infant's sensitive skin (Cowan and Frost, 2006)
- Remove the towel swaddling from the infant. Without letting go of the infant, move the hand supporting the head round their back and shoulders, and hold on to the distant arm. The head should naturally rest and be supported in your forearm. Place your other hand between the infant's legs and under the buttocks
- Slowly and smoothly lift the infant in this cradle-hold and lower down gently into the bath. Slide your hand out from their bottom. Most of the infant's body and head will be out of the water
- Still supporting the infant's head, neck and upper torso, use your free hand to cup bath water over the infant to wash and keep them warm (*Figure 2.4*). Pay particular attention to the creases around the neck, under the arms, the tops of the thighs and the genital area (Samaniego, 2003)
- Have fun! Talk and play with the infant
- Young infants, especially neonates, can become cold quite quickly so they should not stay in the bath too long (Department of Health, 2006). Lift the infant out of the bath and onto the dry towel using the cradle-hold in reverse. Take extra care because the infant will be slippery (Lee and Thompson, 2007)

- Wrap the infant up in the towel to keep them warm
- Keeping the infant covered as much as possible, use the second towel to dry thc body, beginning with the torso, taking care to dry in between any creases around the neck, under the arms and in the genital area to prevent soreness
- When the infant is totally dry, put on a clean nappy and clothes
- Place the infant somewhere safe
- Throw the dirty nappy into the clinical waste bin and put the towels into the linen bin
- Wash and dry out the bath using hot water and detergent
- Remove your gloves and apron and dispose of as appropriate (Department of Health, 2003)
- Wash your hands (Department of Health 2003)

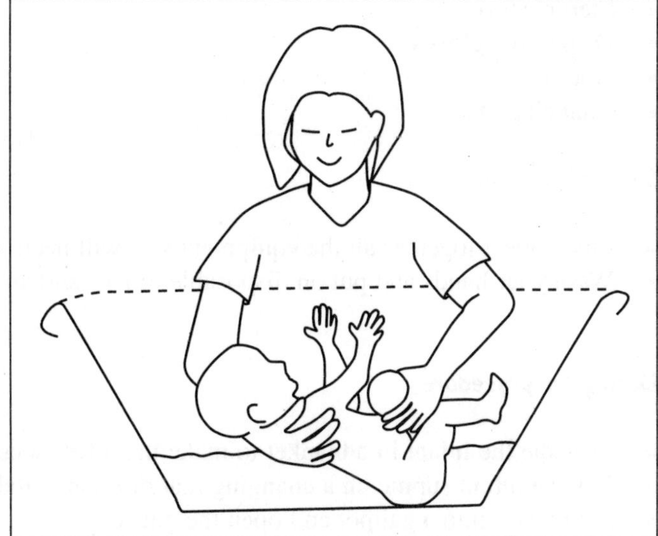

Figure 2.4: Washing an infant in a bath

Post-procedure

- Maintain appropriate records (NMC, 2004)

Caring for the eyes

Eye care should only be performed when it is clinically indicated, for example if infant has 'sticky' eyes. In the first few weeks of life infants cannot secrete tears, which serve as a barrier against infection (Lissauer and Fanaroff, 2006). Eye care may need to be performed three or four times a day until the eyes are clear.

Pre-procedure

Equipment required

- Cooled boiled water/sterile water
- Sterile container

- Sterile gauze
- Disposable gloves
- Apron
- Changing mat

Specific preparation

- First collect together all the equipment you will need
- Wash your hands and put on disposable gloves and an apron (Department of Health, 2003)

During the procedure

- Swaddle the infant in a blanket to make them feel secure and stop them wriggling
- Lay the infant supine on a changing mat or other suitable surface
- Pour water into a galipot and open the gauze
- Dip the gauze into the water and squeeze out any excess
- Gently wipe from the inner eye outwards in one single action and discard, repeating until clean
- Check that the infant is safe and comfortable
- Discard the water, galipot, gauze, apron and gloves as clinical waste (Department of Health, 2003)
- Wash your hands (Department of Health, 2003)

Post-procedure

- Maintain appropriate records (NMC, 2004)

Caring for the umbilical cord

It is important to keep the umbilical cord stump clean as it is a direct portal for infection (Boxwell, 2001). However, the stump should only be cleaned if clinically indicated by the presence of debris (World Health Organization [WHO], 1998; Zupan *et al*, 2004). The umbilical stump normally falls off between 5 and 15 days after birth (Zupan *et al*, 2004). It is normal for there to be a few spots of blood on the stump, but if the area looks red and inflamed this should be reported to a doctor. The WHO (1998) recommend keeping the stump dry and only covering loosely with clothes or a nappy. Dressings should not be applied to the cord stump.

Pre-procedure

Equipment required

- Disposable gloves and apron
- Sterile container
- Sterile water
- Sterile gauze swab

Specific preparation

- First collect together everything you will need
- Close all windows and doors to ensure the infant does not get too cold (Boxwell, 2001)
- Wash your hands and put on gloves and apron

During the procedure

- Place the infant on a flat surface that is waist height
- Undress the infant from the feet up to the waist (it may be helpful to undo the nappy to expose the cord stump, but leave the nappy covering the infant in case they urinate)
- Examine the stump for signs of debris and infection, and only clean the stump if debris is present
- Dip the gauze into the sterile water and gently wipe around the stump (Zupan *et al*, 2004), then discard after one swipe and repeat with a new piece of gauze
- Gently dry the cord area, but do not rub (the cord will naturally fall off and should not be pulled or picked at)
- Leave the cord exposed for as long as possible and be careful when putting the nappy back on not to knock the stump
- Dress the infant and place them somewhere safe
- Discard the plastic container, gauze, gloves and apron in a clinical waste bin (Department of Health, 2003)
- Wash your hands

Post-procedure

- Maintain appropriate records (NMC, 2004)
- Report any concerns to medical staff

Feeding an infant

It is accepted that breast-feeding is the best form of infant nutrition (WHO, 2003; Department of Health, 2005). Babies should ideally be breast-fed exclusively for the first 6 months and then have solids introduced. UNICEF recommends that health workers should actively support breastfeeding. However, if the mother prefers not to or is unable to breast-feed then healthcare practitioners should support their decision.

Sterilising feeding equipment

All equipment used for feeding must be sterilised to reduce the risk of the infant developing gastroenteritis (vomiting and/or diarrhoea) (Department of Health, 2005).

Cold-water sterilising

- Always follow manufacturer's instructions
- Wash your hands
- Make sure all equipment is clean, washing it with hot soapy water if needed
- Make sure the sterilising solution is changed every 24 hours
- Completely submerged all equipment under the solution and leave for at least 30 minutes

Steam sterilising

- Always follow manufacturer's instructions
- Wash your hands
- Make sure all equipment is clean, washing it with hot soapy water if needed
- Once the equipment has been steamed it should be used immediately (if stored in the steamer and used later, it must be re-sterilised)

Making up formula feed

Numerous powdered formula feeds are available for infants (Renfrew *et al*, 2003), and use of them is a parental choice which must be respected and adhered to.

> *NB: Incorrectly reconstituted formula feeds can have serious consequences for babies* (Renfrew *et al*, 2003).

Pre-procedure

Equipment required

- Kettle with freshly cooled boiled water
- Sterilised feeding bottle(s)
- Infant formula
- Measuring scoop

Specific preparation

- Collect together everything you will need
- Wash your hands and put on a disposable apron

During the procedure

- Clean down surfaces using hot water and soap and dry
- Follow the manufacturer's or dieticians' guidelines on how to make up the feed (powder to water ratio)
- Remove a bottle from the steriliser, handling it as little as possible
- Add the directed amount of water to the bottle
- Loosely fill a scoop with formula feed powder and add to the water
- Remove the teat and ring from the steriliser by either using sterilised prongs or holding onto the edge only. Screw them onto the bottle
- Remove the lid from steriliser and push onto the bottle
- Shake the bottle well to mix up the formula feed
- Safely store the bottle (see below)
- Wash your hands

Storing formula feed and breast milk

It is always best to make up a feed just before it is needed, but this is not always practical. Formula and breast milk can be stored in sterile bottles in a fridge for up to 24 hours (the fridge must be below 5°C) and breast milk (not formula) can be stored in a sterile bottle in the freezer for up to 3 months. It can be defrosted at room temperature, or in the fridge or in a jug of warm water. Only remove the feed from the fridge just before it is needed, and warm it up by placing in a jug of warm water. Do not leave it in the water for more than 15 minutes. Always shake the bottle to ensure it is warmed through evenly.

Bottle-feeding a baby

Feeding an infant can be a very enjoyable experience. Newborn infants can feed up to every 3 hours and as they get older they may start to feed in larger amounts less often. Try to keep the environment calm and quiet during feeding time.

> *Do NOT heat bottles in the microwave as they do not heat evenly and there may be 'hot spots' of milk that could burn the baby. Always use a jug of hot water and shake the bottle before use* (Maclean, 1991 [cited in Stehlin, 1991]).

Pre-procedure

Equipment required

- Apron
- Bottle of formula or breast milk
- Jug of hot water
- Bib or cloth
- Comfortable chair

Specific preparation

- First collect together everything you need
- Wash your hands and put on a disposable apron

During the procedure

- Put the feed bottle in the jug of water to warm up
- After a few minutes shake the bottle and check the temperature of the milk by tipping a few drops of milk onto the inside of your wrist (Department of Health, 2005). Be careful not to let the teat actually touch your wrist. The milk should feel warm (not hot or cold). Just in case they have a preference, ask the parents whether their baby prefers milk at room temperature or warmed up
- Nurse the infant in your lap with the head and neck supported by forearm, and lying slightly upright at about an angle of about 45 degrees
- Gently introduce the teat to the infant's lips, who should naturally open his or her mouth. If not, try dropping a few drips of milk onto the infant's lips (if the infant has not fully woken for their feed, but it is time to feed them, consider changing their nappy first; if you do so, this remember to wash your hands and change your gloves before you recommence feeding)

- Once the infant's mouth is open, tip the bottle up until the teat is full of milk and insert it into the mouth (*Figure 2.5*). If the teat is not full of milk air may be swallowed (Department of Health, 2005)
- When the infant is about half way through their feed, remove the bottle and place it somewhere safe with the lid on and 'wind' the infant. Most infants need help to bring up wind. There are numerous methods, as described below
- Once the infant has burped, start to feed them again
- When the infant has finished the bottle, try winding them once more. Afterwards, perhaps after a nappy change, you can gently lay them down or put them in a slightly upright position in an appropriate infant chair

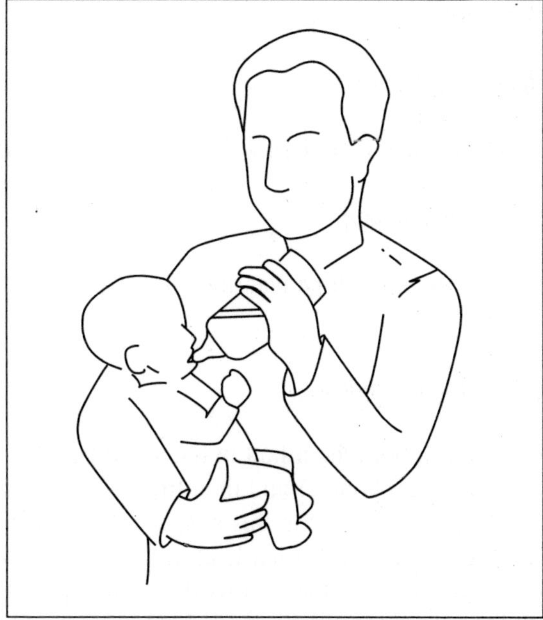

Figure 2.5: Feeding an infant with a bottle

Post-procedure

- Wash out the bottle and teat with hot soapy water
- Place the bottle, teat and lid into the steriliser
- Remove your apron and dispose of in a non-clinical waste bin (Department of Health, 2003)
- Wash your hands
- Maintain appropriate records (NMC, 2004)

Winding an infant

Infants often need winding, not just during feeding and after feeding. It is normal for babies to bring up a small mouthful of milk during winding, which is known as 'posseting'. All babies are individuals and like to be 'winded' in different ways; some can be winded very easily and others take longer.

Pre-procedure

Equipment needed

- Have ready a cloth or soft bib in case the infant 'possets'

Specific preparation

- You should still be wearing an apron from feeding or handling the infant

During the procedure

- You can hold the infant in the shoulder hold, as described previously. First place a cloth over your shoulder and then lift the infant up, resting on your chest and over your shoulder. Once the infant is in this position, leave one hand on their bottom and use your spare hand to gently rub his or her back in a circular motion or pat it gently
- If this position does not work, sit the infant on your lap, facing to one side. Use one hand to support the infant's back, and the fingers of your other hand along the jaw-line to support the infant's head (do not to put your fingers across the neck as this may block the airway). Now lean the infant forward. Use the hand that was supporting their back to gently rub or pat the back (*Figure 2.6*)
- If this position does not work, lay the infant across your knees in a prone position. Gently turn his or her head to one side and let the arms fall naturally. Gently pat or rub the back

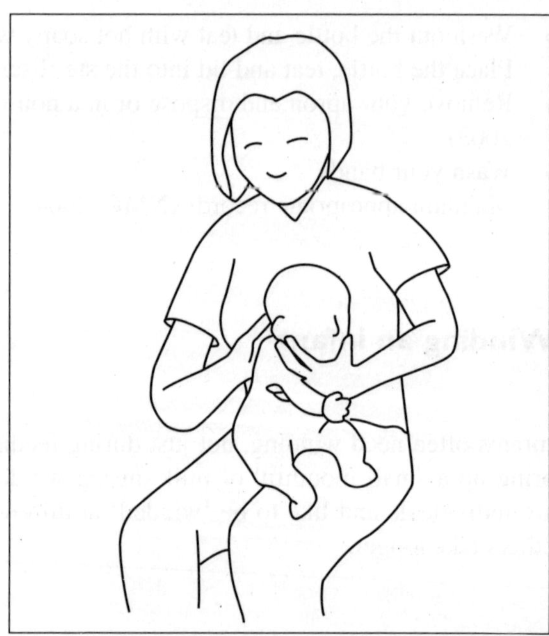

Figure 2.6: Winding an infant in an upright position

Settling an infant

Infants cry for many reasons, when they are upset, hungry, need winding or a change of nappy, or are in pain or discomfort. Sometimes it is very hard to tell why an infant is crying but there are certain things you can do.

- First, simply pick up the infant and try to comfort him or her
- Does the infant like hearing your voice? Talk gently, sing, hum or put on the television or some music in the background

- Is the infant happier lying down in your arms or being in a more upright position? If upright, try winding
- Does the infant need a nappy change? Check the nappy and change it if necessary
- Is the infant hungry? When was the last feed? Try offering a bottle
- Is the room too hot or cold? Does the infant feel warm enough? Put on another layer of clothes or remove a layer or a blanket

If the baby is still crying and you have run out of options, try gently rocking him or her in your arms, or put them in a pram and go for a walk. Look carefully at the infant. Are they crying continuously? Are they drawing their legs up as if in pain? Is there an obvious reason for their discomfort (teething, post-operative pain or a sore bottom)? Do they stop crying when you do a certain thing?

There may not be a reason for an infant to be unsettled. Perhaps the infant was woken up and wants to go back to sleep. If you are sure that he or she is not hungry, cold, hot, dirty or in pain, try putting them down in their cot (see *Putting an infant down to sleep* below). Turn the lights down (if appropriate) and leave them to settle for a few minutes. If they do not settle, try giving them another cuddle.

Getting an infant to sleep

Infants should have as much routine as possible (Department of Health, 2006) to help them get into a sleep–wake pattern. Newborn infants can sleep between 10 and 20 hours a day. Infants do not sleep for much more than 3 or 4 hours at a time, and most do not sleep through the night until they are at least 4 months old (many take much longer). An example of a suitable routine is described in *Box 2.1*.

Box 2.1: Example of infant's routine

Wake at 07:00	Feed, change nappy, top and tail, change clothes, put down for nap
Wake at 09:00	Feed, change nappy, play, put down for nap
Wake at 12:00	Feed, change nappy, put down for nap
Wake at 15:00	Feed, change nappy, playtime,
Wake at 18:00	Bathe (if needed) or top and tail, feed, dress for bedtime, put down in cot at 19:00
Wake at 22:00	Feed, change nappy
Wake at 01:00	Feed, change nappy
Wake at 04:00	Feed, change nappy

Putting an infant down for bed

Make sure the room is neither hot nor cold. It should be around 18°C (Department of Health, 2007). Babies should sleep in the same room as their parents, in their own cot or basket until they are 6 months old (National Institute of Child Health and Human Development [NICHD], 2003; Department of Health, 2007); this is not always possible, but it is best for the baby. The cot or basket should have a firm surface with a fitted sheet on it. Turn down the lights and/or draw the curtain to create a calm environment.

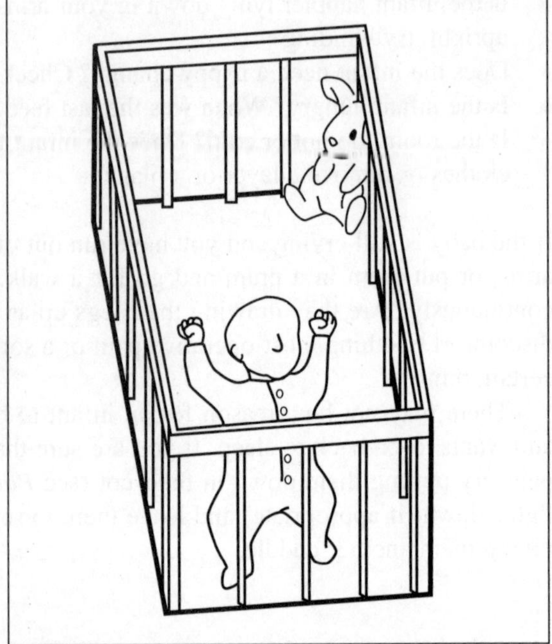

Figure 2.7: Laying an infant down towards the bottom end of a cot

During the procedure

- Lay the infant down supine (on their back) with their feet near the foot of the cot or basket (*Figure 2.7*).This position is thought to reduce the risks of sudden infant death syndrome (SIDS) (NICHD, 2003; Department of Health, 2007). Depending on their developmental ability, an infant may naturally roll over, but the risk of SIDS has passed by that stage (NICHD, 2003)
- Place a sheet or one layer of blanket over the infant. It is important to avoid over-heating (NICHD, 2003; Department of Health, 2007)
- If the infant does not settle, try singing or talking to them. Some will settle quickly and others will take a while; try not to pick an infant up instantly if they do not settle

When an infant wakes for a feed during the night, avoid playing with them. This will help them to learn the difference between night-time and day-time.

> *Never allow a neonate (under 28 days of age) to sleep for more than 6 hours without waking.*

To prevent infants from developing 'head flattening' let them spend some time on their stomach during the day, for a few minutes or more, if tolerated, when awake and under your supervision (Department of Health, 2007).

References

Boxwell G (2001) *Neonatal Intensive Care Nursing*. Routledge, London

Chon DH, Frank CL, Shortliffe LM (2001) Pediatric urinary tract infections. *Pediatr Clin N Am* **48:** 1441–59

Cowan ME, Frost MR (2006) A comparison between detergent baby bath additive and baby soap on the skin flora of neonates. *J Hosp Infect* **7:** 91–95

Darmstadt GL, Dinuos JG (2000) Neonatal skin care. *Pediatr Clin N Am* **47**(4): 375–82

Department of Health (2003) *Winning Ways: Working Together to Reduce Healthcare Associated Infection in England*. Department of Health, London

Department of Health (2004) *National Service Framework for Children, Young People and Maternity Services*. Department of Health, London

Department of Health (2005) *Bottle Feeding*. Department of Health, London

Department of Health (2006) *Birth to Five*. Department of Health, London

Department of Health (2007) *Reduce the Risk of Cot Death*. Department of Health, London

Harold SK, Tamura T, Colton K (2003) Reported level of supervision of young children while in the bathtub. *Ambulat Pediatr* **3**(2): 106–08

Lee LK, Thompson KM (2007) Parental survey of belief and practices about bathing and water safety and their children: guidance for drowning prevention. *Accid Analysis Prevent* **39:** 58–62

Lees S, Hilton A (2004) Maintaining body temperature. In: Hilton P (ed) *Fundamental Nursing Skills*. Whurr Publishers, London

Lissauer T, Fanaroff A (2006) *Neonatology at a Glance*. Blackwell Publishing, Oxford

Lund C (1999) Prevention and management of infant skin breakdown. *Nurs Clin N Am* **34:** 907–20

McManus J (2001) Skin breakdown: risk factors, prevention and treatment. *Newborn Infant Nurs Rev* **1**(1): 35–42

National Institute of Child Health and Human Development (2003) *Safe sleep for your baby: Ten ways to reduce the risk of sudden infant death syndrome (SIDS)*. Government Printing Office, Washington DC

Nursing and Midwifery Council (2004) *Code of Professional Conduct*. NMC, London

Renfrew MJ, Ansell P, Macleod KL (2003) Formula feed preparation: Helping to reduce the risks; a systematic review. *Arch Dis Child* **88**(10): 855

Royal College of Nursing (2006) *Paediatric Assessment of Toilet Training Readiness and Issuing of Products*. RCN, London

Rudolf M, Levene M (2006) *Paediatrics and Child Health*, 2nd edn. Blackwell Publishing, Oxford

Samaniego IA (2003) A sore spot on pediatrics: Risk factor in pressure ulcers. *Pediatr Nurs* **29**(4): 278–82

Smith J (ed) (2005) *The Guide to the Handling of People*, 5th edn. National Back Pain Association, Teddington

Stehlin D (1991) *Feeding Baby: Nature and Nurture*. US Food and Drug Agency, USA

White R, Denyer J (2006) *Paediatric Skin and Wound Care*. Wounds UK, Aberdeen

World Health Organization (1998) *Care of the Umbilical Cord: A Review of the Evidence*. World Health Organisation, Geneva

World Health Organisation (2003) *Global stratergy for infant and young child feeding*. World Health Organisation, Geneva

Young AE (2004) The management of severe burns in children. *Curr Paediatr* **14:** 202–07

Zupan J, Garner P, Omar AAA (2004) Topical umbilical cord care at birth. *Cochrane Database Syst Rev* **3:** CD001057

Chapter 3

Fundamental aspects of basic life support

Jan Heath

Basic life support

Basic life support (BLS) is also known as cardiopulmonary resuscitation (CPR). It was first described in the Old Testament as the prophet Elisha revived a seemingly lifeless child using mouth-to-mouth breathing. However, slow progress was made with these skills until the middle of the twentieth century, but from 2000 there has been exponential growth and advances in the formalisation of these skills (Byrne and Phillips, 2003). Basic life support is best defined as a series of simple but important skills. If more people knew how to perform these skills there would be less death from life-threatening events. This chapter outlines the key steps involved in basic life support and includes the management of casualties found collapsed, applying the ABC principles throughout:

- A is for *airway*
- B is for *breathing*
- C is for *circulation*

Before proceeding, it is important to acknowledge the age ranges to be covered. The Resuscitation Council (UK) (2005) aimed to produce guidelines that are as simple as possible. Many people who have no experience in resuscitating children worry about causing harm, whereas doing nothing to a collapsed child is obviously harmful. Therefore, the guidelines released in 2005 attempt to provide advice for lay people in which children and adults are treated as similarly as reasonably practicable. Because 'doing *something'* – as opposed to 'doing *nothing'* – certainly improves the chance of survival, the lay person is advised to adopt the same ratio of 30 compressions to 2 ventilations for the infant or child *and* the adult. However, for those rescuers with a 'duty to respond' the ratio should be:

- 15 compressions to 2 ventilations for the child BUT
- 30 compressions to 2 ventilations for the adult (or young person beyond puberty)

These guidelines should be practiced and they can be rehearsed using appropriate training manikins under the supervision of an experienced life support trainer to help you feel comfortable in delivering psychomotor skills (Resuscitation Council, 2004).

The terms 'children' and 'child' in this chapter refer to individuals from aged from birth to puberty. There are parts of the guidelines where the management of the infant differs to that of the child. The age groups are defined in Box 3.1.

Box 3.1: Classification of age groups

Infant	Birth to 1 year
Child	1 year to puberty
Young person	Puberty to adulthood

Key points of the Resuscitation Council (UK) 2005 guidelines

Mouth-to-mouth rescue breathing

- Occasionally rescuers undertaking CPR have caught infections (European Resuscitation Council, 2005)
- There have been a few isolated incidents of tuberculosis (TB) and severe acute respiratory distress syndrome (SARS)
- There have been no reports of HIV virus (AIDS)

It may be preferable to do mouth-to-mouth rescue breathing using a basic airway device such as a face-shield if you have been trained to do so. There are a number of these devices on the market, but you should use one that is readily accessible and easy to store or carry around.

Mouth-to-nose rescue breathing

- This is as effective as mouth-to-mouth and should be used if it is difficult to open the casualty's mouth
- It is a good method for casualties in water where achieving a good seal for mouth-to-mouth is difficult

Mouth-to-tracheostomy ventilation

- This is for casualties who have a tracheostomy tube or tracheal stoma (depending on the underlying reason for the tracheostomy)

Bag-valve–mask ventilation

- Training is vital to support the use of a bag-mask device
- A major advantage is that they allow supplementary oxygen to be delivered

Compression-only CPR

- On occasions you may be unable or unwilling to give mouth-to-mouth but you can give chest compressions only at a rate of 100 per minute
- There is evidence to suggest this may be as effective as rescue breathing, particularly immediately after a cardiac arrest
- In any situation, it is certainly better than nothing at all

Basic life support for young people beyond puberty

Safety

- Check for danger
- Is the situation safe for the casualty, yourself and any bystanders?

Response

- Check the casualty for responsiveness
- Gently shake the shoulders and ask loudly 'Are you alright?'
- **If responding:**
  - Leave in the position you found them providing there is no risk of harm
  - Assess the situation and get appropriate help
  - Observe the patient for any change in condition
- **If *not* responding:**
  - If you are alone, shout for help
  - If you are not alone, ask someone to stay as you may need assistance once you have fully assessed the casualty
  - Turn the casualty onto their back and begin the ABC assessment

Airway

- Open the airway by a chin lift (put your fingers under the chin, place one hand on the forehead and tilt the head back)

Breathing

- With the airway open look listen and feel for and signs of normal breathing and signs of life such as swallowing, gasping, movement
- Look at the casualty's chest for any movement
- Listen at the casualty's mouth for sounds of breathing
- Feel for any expired air on your cheek
- **If breathing normally:**
  - Turn the casualty into the recovery position and get help
- **If *not* breathing normally:**
  - This is a seriously ill person and resuscitation must be started
  - Begin chest compressions as described under *Circulation*

Circulation

- Kneel by the side of the casualty's chest
- Place the heel of one hand on the centre of the casualty's chest in line with the armpits
- Place the heel of the other hand on top of the first hand.
- Interlock your fingers to avoid applying pressure over the casualty's ribs
- Position yourself so that your shoulders are over the casualty's sternum
- Press down on the breast bone to a depth of 4–5 cm
- After each compression release the pressure and repeat at a rate of 100 compressions per minute
- After 30 compressions go back to the airway
- Open the airway again
- Close the casualty's nose by pinching the soft part of the nose using your thumb and index finger
- Continue with chin lift allow the casualty's mouth-to-open
- Place your lips around the casualty's mouth and with a good seal blow steadily into their mouth watching their chest rise
- Take your lips away and allow the air to come out and watch the chest wall fall
- Take another breath and repeat to give a total of 2 effective breaths
- Go back to the landmarks (in line with the armpits) on the chest and repeat the 30 chest compressions

Basic life support must *continue until:*

- Help arrives to take over, *or*
- The casualty starts to breathe normally, *or*
- You are physically too exhausted to continue

A summary of basic life support in young people is given in *Box 3.2.*

Performing basic life support is very tiring, so where possible share the workload with another rescuer who can do the breathing or compressions to work with you, or get another rescuer to take over from you (Resuscitation Council, 2001). If there is more than one rescuer, it is good practice to perform about 2 minutes of basic life support then swap over with another rescuer to prevent tiredness. The change over should be done with minimum delay.

Box 3.2: Summary of basic life support for young people beyond puberty

Danger	Check for danger
Response	Check for response
Shout	Shout for help
Airway	Open the airway
Breathing	Check for normal breathing
CPR	*Ratio* – 30 : 2 (30 compressions to 2 breaths)
	Rate – 100 compressions over 1 minute
	Depth – 4–5 cm

The Resuscitation Council's procedure for adult basic life support is reproduced in *Figure 3.1.*

Basic life support for children

Resuscitation of children and infants is different from that of adults and older teenagers. Adults are more likely to collapse due to a cardiac event, but children generally have a primary respiratory event, which – if not recognised or dealt with – will rapidly deteriorate to a cardiac event (Jevon, 2004). Dealing with seriously ill children is difficult and can be very frightening. Thankfully there are relatively small numbers of resuscitation events involving children emergencies, which means that few people have the opportunity to manage these events. It is helpful therefore to use recognised guidelines and follow a systematic approach in the management of such emergencies.

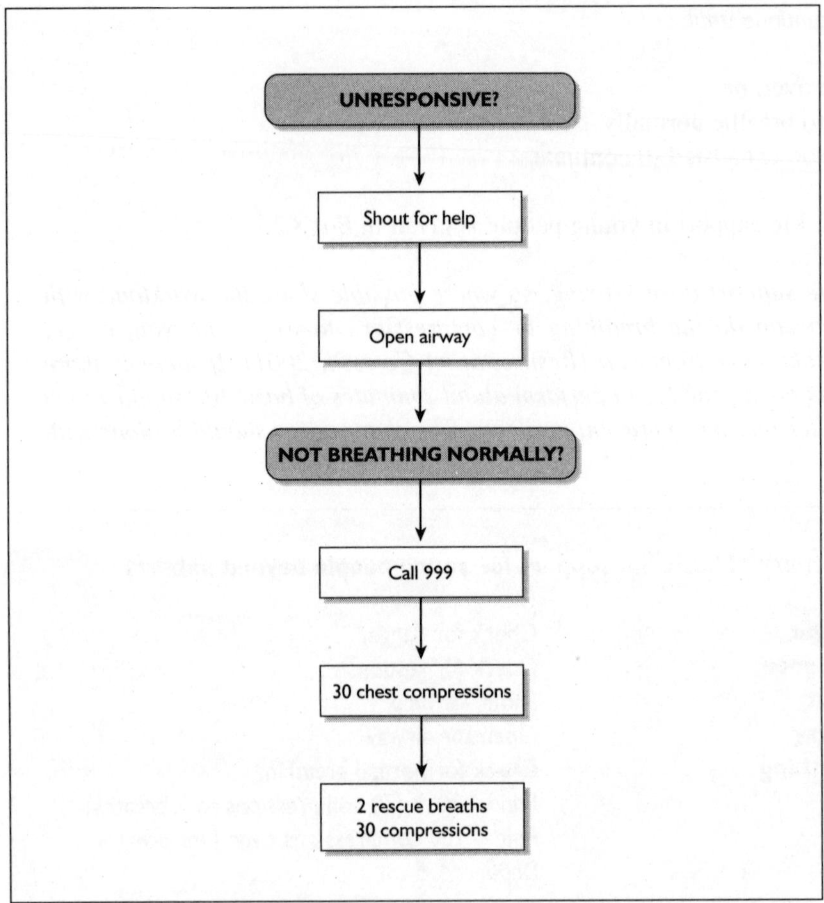

Figure 3.1: Adult basic life support (reproduced with kind permission of the Resuscitation Council, UK)

Different age groups are at different risks and hence need appropriate intervention. Resuscitation is not always appropriate, and for some children with life-limiting conditions it may be argued that any attempt to resuscitate that child would not be beneficial. Furthermore, the outcome from a paediatric cardiac arrest is extremely poor, so early intervention in a child who appears very unwell is vital. Resuscitation of a child is emotive for families and staff caring for that child, both in and out of hospital. It is important that after a paediatric resuscitation, particularly an unsuccessful attempt, that a debriefing session should be held. This should be led by an experienced facilitator (European Resuscitation Council, 2005).

Causes of paediatric emergencies

Causes include:

- Trauma
- Drowning
- Congenital abnormalities
- Respiratory disease
- Infections

See *Box 3.3* for interventions to prevent paediatric deaths.

Box 3.3: Interventions aimed at prevention of paediatric death

Prevention of accidents
Road safety
Playground safety
Fire safety
Reducing the effects of an accident
Wearing a cycle helmet
Wearing protective clothing to handle fireworks
Education in the management of injury
First-aid training for babysitters and childcare givers
Courses in basic life support

Safety

- Check for danger
- Ensure you are safe before approaching the casualty
- Make sure you are safe from hazards from (eg. fire, water, electricity). In hospital, consider any hazards such as needlestick injury. Treat all body fluids as potential dangers and put on gloves to minimise risk of infection.
- When approaching the child, look for any clues that may suggest why this child may have collapsed, which may dictate the way the emergency is managed (eg. empty bottles of hazardous substances, any suspicion of trauma)

Response

- Ask the child loudly to open his or her eyes or call his or her name if known
- Gently stimulate the child and ask loudly 'Are you alright?'
- Do not shake the child if you suspect a cervical spine injury
- **If responding:**
  - Leave the child in the position you find them in (unless in danger) and get assistance
- **If *not* responding:**
  - Ask someone to get an ambulance or call the cardiac arrest team (if in hospital)
  - If you are alone, shout for someone to help you (do not leave the child to go for help or to use a phone)
  - If no-one comes to help provide 1 minute of BLS before going for help yourself

Danger

- Ensure the safety of the rescuer and child
- If there is no danger leave the child in the position you find them in and get assistance (only leave the child alone if you cannot raise help)

Airway

- Only ever put a finger into a child's mouth if you can see or suspect there is something in their mouth which you are confident you can remove with a with a pincer grip
- Open the airway (the aim is to move the tongue away from the posterior pharyngeal wall)
- **In the infant:**
  - Place the infant's head in the neutral position. Put your fingertips on the bony part of the jaw and lift the chin upwards while resting your other hand on the infants' forehead
- **In the child:**
  - The head and neck need to be tilted more than in infants
  - If there is still difficulty in opening the airway, attempt the jaw thrust manoeuvre: place two fingers behind each side of the child's jaw bone and push the jaw forward
  - This manoeuvre is much more difficult in small children without full dentition (to get an idea of the correct position, push your lower jaw forwards so that your bottom teeth are in front of your upper teeth)
- Only when this step is complete should you attend to *Breathing*

Breathing

Take *no more* than 10 seconds to assess the child's breathing:

- **Look:** Is the chest moving?
- **Listen:** Can you hear any breath sounds from the child's mouth or nose?
- **Feel:** Can you feel expired air from the casualty on your cheek?

If there is no breathing or only occasional ineffective gasps, deliver rescue breaths, which may prevent cases of respiratory arrest proceeding to cardiopulmonary arrest.

- **In the infant** (*Figure 3.2*):
  - Cover the mouth and nose where possible to create a seal to deliver expired-air rescue breaths
  - Make sure the head is in the neutral position and apply chin lift
  - Breathe whilst maintaining a neutral airway position
  - Attempt 5 initial rescue breaths, each lasting 1 to 1.5 seconds
  - Watch for chest movement
  - Any gag or cough response to your actions will contribute to your assessment of the casualty
- **In the child** (*Figure 3.3*):
  - Occlude the nose by pinching the nostrils and perform mouth-to-mouth, blowing steadily into the casualty's mouth
  - Make sure the head is in the neutral position and apply chin lift
  - Breathe whilst maintaining a neutral airway position

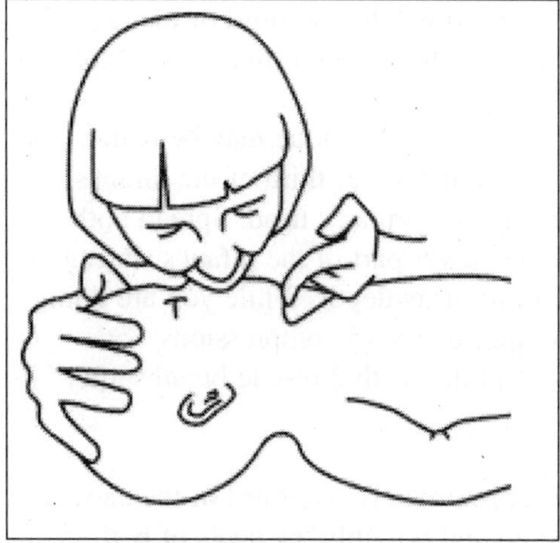

Figure 3.2: Delivery of rescue breaths to an infant with mouth over the infant's mouth and nose

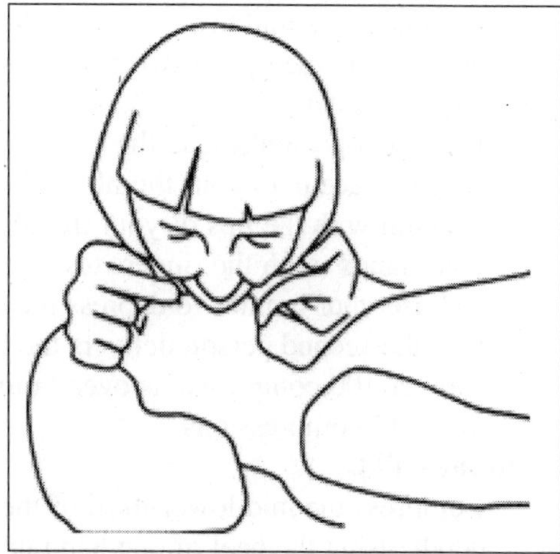

Figure 3.3: Delivery of rescue breaths to a child. With nose pinched and mouth sealed over the child's mouth. Breathe whilst maintaining a neutral airway position

  - Attempt 5 initial rescue breaths, each lasting 1 to 1.5 seconds
  - Watch for chest movement
  - Any gag or cough response to your actions will contribute to your assessment of the casualty
- If there is no chest movement, adjust the position of the infant or child's head and repeat
- If (despite repositioning) you are still unable to move the chest, consider a foreign-body airway obstruction (see below)
- When you have delivered 5 initial rescue breaths, attend to *Circulation*

Circulation

Take *no more* than 10 seconds to assess for signs of life:

- Is there any movement, coughing or normal breathing (not gasps)?
- Is there a pulse? (you should be trained to do this and experienced, because it can be difficult)
- **In the infant:**
  - Feel for a brachial pulse, inside the inner aspect of the upper arm
- **In the child:**
  - Feel for the carotid pulse in the neck
  - If there is a pulse, continue with rescue breaths
  - If breathing but unconscious, put the child in the recovery position
- If there is no pulse or only a slow pulse (less than 60 beats per minute), or you are not sure, or there are no signs of circulation, proceed to manage circulation
- **In the infant:**
  - Compress the mid lower-third of the sternum by approximately one-third of the chest's depth using the tips of two fingers on the lower third of the sternum (this is good for the single rescuer)
  - For a two-person rescue the chest compression (encircling) technique may be better. You should place both your thumbs flat and side by side on the lower third of the infant's sternum with the tips of your thumbs pointing towards the infant's head. Spread both your hands (with the fingers together) to encircle the lower part of the infant's rib cage and use your thumbs to depress the chest by one-third of its depth. While you are doing this, the second person delivers the breaths – 2 to after every 15 compressions
  - Deliver 100 compressions over 1 minute, but interrupt this with 2 rescue breaths after every 15 compressions
- **In the child:**
  - Compress the mid lower-third of the sternum by approximately one-third of the chest's depth, using the heel of one hand in smaller children and possibly the heels of both hands in larger children (whichever enables you to compress the chest by one-third)
  - Deliver 100 compressions over 1 minute, but interrupt this with 2 rescue breaths after every 15 compressions

A summary of basic life support for children is provided in *Box 3.4*, and the Resuscitation Council's recommended procedure is reproduced in *Figure 3.4*.

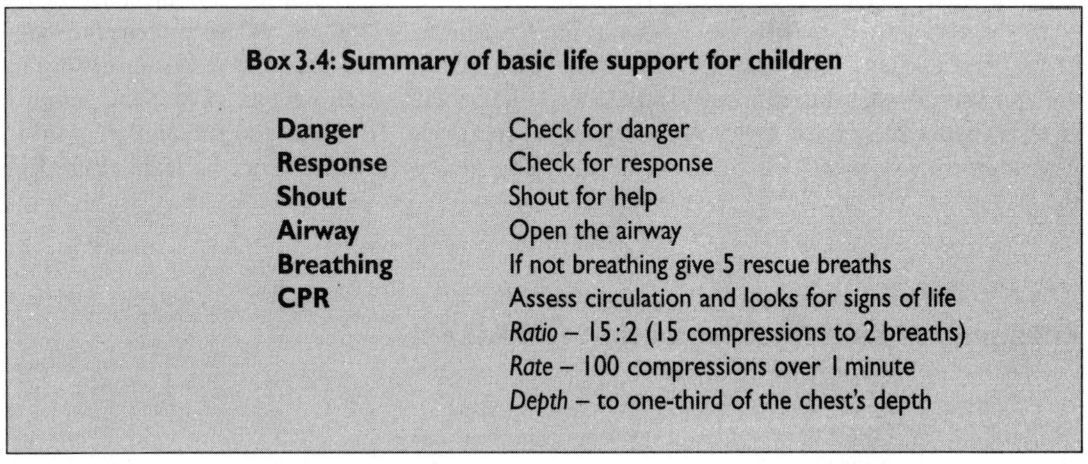

Box 3.4: Summary of basic life support for children

Danger	Check for danger
Response	Check for response
Shout	Shout for help
Airway	Open the airway
Breathing	If not breathing give 5 rescue breaths
CPR	Assess circulation and looks for signs of life
	Ratio – 15:2 (15 compressions to 2 breaths)
	Rate – 100 compressions over 1 minute
	Depth – to one-third of the chest's depth

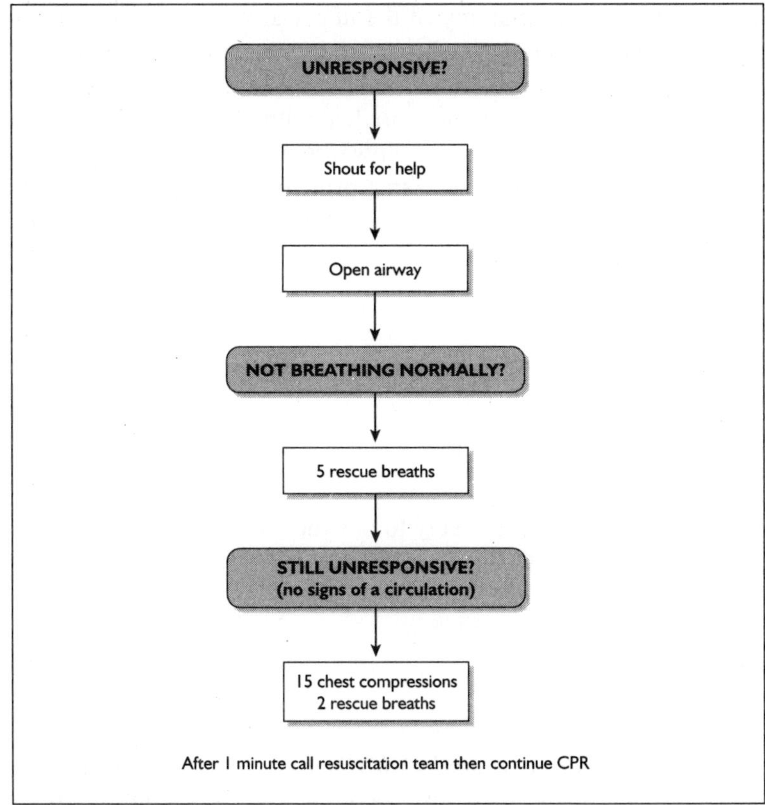

Figure 3.4: Paediatric basic life support (reproduced with kind permission of the Resuscitation Council, UK)

Parents of the child or infant

When a child is being resuscitated, provision should be made to consider the presence of his or her relatives. An experienced member of staff must stay with them and keep them informed of progress and any interventions. This person can also prevent the relatives from disturbing the staff during this difficult time. It has been shown that when parents have been presence at resuscitation they have fewer difficulties after the event. However, the person delegated to look after the relatives should *not* be the most inexperienced member of the team (European Resuscitation Council, 2005).

Foreign body airway obstruction (FBAO)

Choking in children is a frightening yet common occurrence (D'Amore and Campbell Hewson, 2002). Children often put things in their mouths –sweets, pieces of toys, beads and pieces of food – whilst playing. Remember the anatomy of the upper airway. Items which are in the nostril can therefore be inhaled. The upper airway is shaped like a cone and thus inhaled objects can become lodged in the larynx, which can cause the child to asphyxiate. Simple yet effective methods can deal with such problems. The actions to deal with an airway obstruction aim to force air out of the lungs by a sudden inwards and upwards movement which in turn should push the obstruction out of the airway. This is the same principle as a powerful cough. The choking casualty is usually unable to cough for themselves. If he or she is coughing, then encourage them to keep doing so.

Signs and symptoms of FBAO

- The incident occurred without warning
- The child is otherwise well
- The child was seen eating or playing with objects likely to obstruct airways.
- The child is suddenly silent or unable to breathe

FBAO procedure in children

The smaller size of infants makes them easier to deal with when choking (Dickson and Anders, 2004), but remember that abdominal thrusts are too dangerous to use in infants below the age of 1 year.

In infants:

- Support the infant on your knee (if possible)
- Turn the infant face down, supporting the chin with the fingers of your left hand and the chest resting on your palm or forearm
- With the infant face down, head lower than the chest, apply up to 5 firm back blows with flat of hand between the shoulder blades or until the foreign body is cleared
- Re-assess the child after every five interventions
- If the foreign body is expelled, assess the infant's condition, and seek emergency assistance if it still gives cause for concern
- If these back blows do not solve the problem, turn the infant into a supine position (face up) and place him or her on a firm surface (eg. your thigh). Make sure the head is still lower than their chest, and apply chest thrusts in the same manner as chest compressions in CPR, but deliver them more slowly and more forcefully, at a rate of 1 thrust every 2 seconds

In children:

- Try to place smaller children across your lap and then give up to 5 firm back blows between the shoulder blades as described above
- If this position is not possible, support the child in a forwards leaning position and deliver back blows between the shoulder blades
- Re-assess the child
- If the foreign body is still not cleared, apply abdominal thrusts:
  - Stand behind the child and place a clenched fist midway between the umbilicus and xiphisternum
  - Cover your fist with your second hand and pull upwards and inwards
  - Repeat up to five times and re-assess the child
- If the foreign body is expelled, assess the child's condition, and seek emergency assistance if it still gives cause for concern
- Do not attempt blind finger sweeps because they may push the object further down and cause injury

The Resuscitation Council's recommended procedure for dealing with a foreign body airway obstruction (FBAO) is reproduced in *Figure 3.5*.

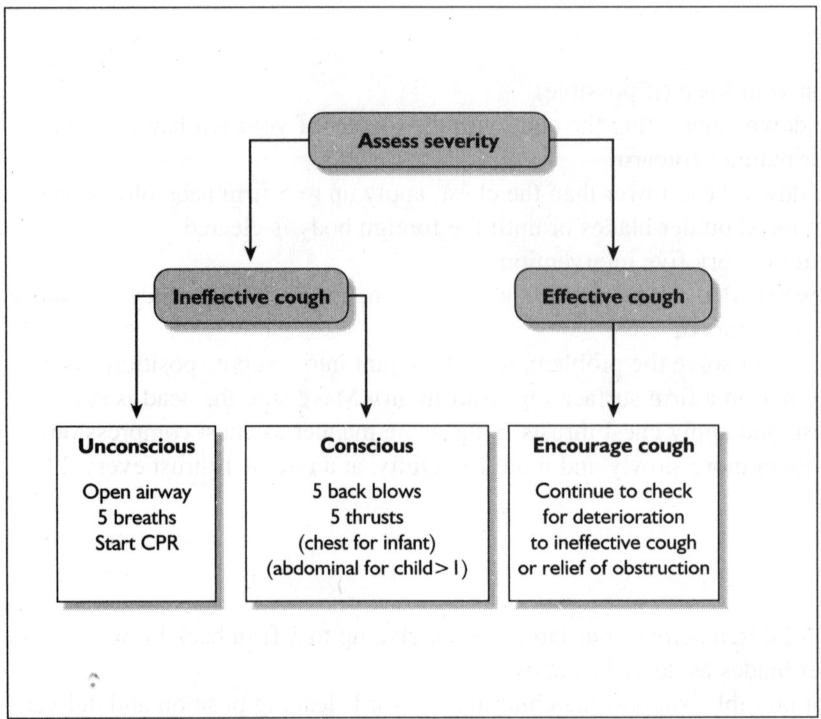

Figure 3.5: Paediatric foreign body airway obstruction (FBAO) treatment (reproduced with permission of the Resuscitation Council, UK)

An example of applying FBAO treatment to an infant

While you are having a picnic with one of your friends, you notice her 10-month-old daughter is having difficulty breathing while eating from a bowl of grapes. What do you do?

You pick up the baby to see if she is making any noise or moving air in or out. She is not, so you sit down, placing her head down on your lap, and deliver five back blows. If the grape were expelled at this point you could stop and re-assess the baby's condition, but it is not, so you turn the baby over, with the back of her head in your hand to support the airway, and deliver five chest thrusts in the centre of her chest. After the third chest thrust, a partially chewed grape is expelled. You sit the baby up and she has a good cry, which fills her lungs with air (and you can all enjoy the rest of the picnic).

Anaphylaxis

Anaphylaxis is rare but life-threatening reaction to an allergen. There is not a definitive definition for anaphylaxis but it should be considered when more than two systems are affected – skin, respiratory, circulatory, neurological, or gastroenterological.

Other features which are usually present include:

- Erythema
- Generalised pruritis
- Urticaria
- Angioedema
- Wheezing
- Rhinitis
- Conjunctivitis
- Itching of the palate or external auditory meatus
- Nausea, vomiting, abdominal pain
- Palpitations
- A sense of 'impending doom'

What happens during anaphylaxis?

An anaphylactic reaction occurs following exposure to an allergen to which a person has been sensitised. People who have asthma and allergies are at high risk of anaphylaxis (Resuscitation Council, 2005). Repeated exposure results in specific immunoglobulin (Ig)E antibodies recognising the allergen and creating a reaction to it. This encourages mast cells to release inflammatory mediators, which cause an anaphylactic reaction. It is the rapid release of large quantities of mediators, causing leakage of capillaries and mucosal oedema, and cardiovascular and respiratory shock.

Anaphylaxis may be due to a whole host of things, most commonly:

- Foods (sea-food, peanuts, sesame and dairy products)
- Drugs (aspirin and antibiotics)
- Latex
- Stinging insects (bees and wasps)

When dealing with someone who presents with difficulty with breathing, a severe rash or circulatory problems following exposure to an element that may cause anaphylaxis, urgent action is required.

How to treat anaphylaxis

Act immediately!

- Remove the item causing the event if possible (eg. stop any antibiotics, or scrape away any insect parts at the site of a sting – without squeezing!)
- Place the casualty in a position in which they can breathe more easily, if possible
- If the casualty feels very faint or looks very pale, lie him or her down
- Give 100% oxygen if possible (an experienced anaesthetist is mandatory if in hospital)
- Give medication according to the guidelines of the Resuscitation Council UK (2005)
- **In young people:**
  - Epinephrine (adrenaline) 0.5 mL 1 : 1000 solution (500 μg) intramuscularly – if there is no improvement after 5 minutes repeat the dose
  - Chlorphenamine 4 mg orally or 10–20 mg by slow intravenous injection
  - Fluids given intravenously are usually necessary
  - Salbutamol 5 mg by nebuliser (can be used to relieve bronchospasm)
- **In children:**
  - Give epinephrine (adrenaline) to all children with signs of circulatory failure, airway swelling or difficulty with respirations
  - Repeat after 5 minutes if there is no improvement
  - Doses must be given intramuscularly
- Age-adjusted doses for epinephrine (adrenaline) are shown in *Table 3.1*
- After giving epinephrine, it may be appropriate to give an antihistamine (chlorphenamine)
- If the patient does not respond to the epinephrine it is advisable to give intravenous fluids (20 mL/kg 0.9% saline)
- For severe reactions, or patients with asthma, hydrocortisone may follow

Antihistamines, fluids and hydrocortisone should be given only after epinephrine (adrenaline), which is a life-saving drug in anaphylaxis, that is carried by large numbers of the population who should be capable of administering the drug themselves if they find themselves unwittingly exposed to a substance that they are allergic to.

Table 3.1: Age-adjusted doses of epinephrine (adrenaline) for treatment of anaphylaxis in children

Age	Dose (1 : 1000)	EpiPen equivalent
Under 6 months	50 µg (0.05 mL)	–
6 months to 6 years	120 µg (0.12 mL)	150 µg
6–12 years	250 µg (0.25 mL)	300 µg
Over 12 years	500 µg (0.5 mL)	300 µg

The in-hospital resuscitation team

Each organisation will have its own action plan to attend to individuals who collapse. There should be a team which responds to cardiac arrest. The composition of the team will vary within different organisations but it should have a minimum of two doctors trained to deal with such emergencies. Collectively, the team should have the skills to deal with:

- Airway interventions
- Routes for drug administration
- Monitoring and defibrillation
- Knowledge of drugs and fluids
- Post-resuscitation management
- Team-leader skills

Ideally there should be a separate paediatric team with appropriately trained individuals (Resuscitation Council, 2004). Members of paediatric cardiac arrest teams should attend one of the national paediatric resuscitation courses, among which are the European Paediatric Life Support Course, the Advanced Paediatric Life Support Course, and the Newborn Life Support Course. Details of all of these courses and the National Audit of Paediatric Resuscitation study can be found on the Resuscitation Council (UK) website www.resus.org.

Conclusions

Resuscitation is a stressful subject – and the degree of stress is inversely proportional to the size of the casualty (the smaller the child, the scarier the situation!). Simple guidelines are available and they should be adhered to as appropriate for the age of the casualty. Survival from cardiac arrest is poor but early intervention can reduce mortality. Good training and preparation optimises the delivery of these skills and hopefully leads to the reward of a successful outcome.

Choking in the unconscious child is not covered in this chapter, but more can be found on this subject in the about it in The Resuscitation Council (UK) website at www.resus.org.

References

Byrne E, Phillips B (2003) The physiology behind resuscitation guidelines. *Curr Paediatr* **13:** 1–5

D'Amore A, Campbell Hewson G (2002) The management of acute upper airway obstruction in children. *Curr Paediatr* **12:** 17–21

Dickson EM, Anders NRK (2004) Infant resuscitation. *Curr Anaesth Crit Care* **15:** 53–60

European Resuscitation Council (2005) European Resuscitation Council Guidelines for Resuscitation 2005. *Resuscitation* **67**(Suppl 1): S1–S190

Jevon P (2004) *Paediatric Advanced Life Support: A Practical Guide*. Butterworth Heinemann, London

Resuscitation Council (UK) (2001) *Guidance for Safer Handling During Resuscitation in Hospitals*. Resuscitation Council, London

Resuscitation Council (UK) (2004) *Cardiopulmonary Resuscitation: Standards for Clinical Practice and Training*. Resuscitation Council, London

Resuscitation Council (UK) (2005) *Resuscitation Guidelines 2005*. Resuscitation Council, London

Useful websites

EpiCentre Lifeline (Epipen)
www.epipen.co.uk

Advanced Life Support Group
www.alsg.org.uk

Resuscitation Council (UK)
www.resus.org

Chapter 4

Fundamental aspects of moving and handling

Maureen Harrison

When thinking about manual handling, one of the first thoughts that may come to mind is assisting frail and disabled adults, and how there is so little correlation between those procedures and handling children. Why do children's nurses and other caregivers (lay and professional) involved with children need to know about manual handling, and why is such a topic included in a book about skills that may be more relevant or useful to a children's health-care provider?

Regardless of whether you work with children or adults, or clients with learning disabilities or mental health difficulties, anyone working within the caring industry will be involved in manual handling to a varying extent.

Surveys have demonstrated (Jones *et al*, 1997; Jones *et al*, 2001; Health and Safety Executive [HSE], 2007) that employees in health and social work have statistically significantly higher rates of musculoskeletal disorders connected to manual handling tasks within their jobs than most other industries (with the exception of the construction industry!). On a daily basis, manual handling is almost unavoidable. Common examples are lifting a baby from its cot, putting a toddler in its highchair, helping a child climb out of the bath, and holding a child steady during a procedure.

Unlike many of the skills discussed in this book, manual handling is probably the only one that is governed by statutory legislation. The Health and Safety at Work Act 1974 (HSE, 1974) makes:

> *"...provision for the health, safety and welfare for persons at work and for protecting others against risks to health or safety in connection with the activities of persons at work..."*

There are sections in this Act that apply to both employers and employees. Additionally, the Management of Health and Safety at Work Regulations 1999 gives employers a legal obligation to provide safety in the work place, thereby protecting the health and safety of their workforce. Employers must ensure that any risk is managed 'so far as is reasonably practicable' (HSE, 1999, section 8.2a).

As well as the general risk assessment requirements set out in the Management Regulations, the need to 'risk assess' was also addressed in the Manual Handling Operations Regulations (MHOR) of 1992. The MHOR were enforced from January 1993 and these regulations specifically govern the moving and handling of people in the workplace, and as identified, would include caring industries such as nursing.

These regulations were implemented to meet the challenge of the number of reported musculoskeletal injuries from manual handling activities. By the time the MHOR were enforced, employers had already accepted the need to control risks regarding manual handling (Lancaster *et al*, 2001). But the number of accidents being reported did not change significantly. The survey conducted by Lancaster and colleagues found that the attitudes and behaviour of management and employees were variable regarding compliance with the law. The culture of an organisation of workers is very important, especially in situations where employees accept that handling is part of their job but do not seek to reduce risks or draw the risk to the attention of others.

In a survey of manual handling practices amongst student nurses, Swain *et al* (2003) found that students did not use the recommended techniques that they had been taught in school in clinical practice. The most frequent explanation given was the influence of other nurses who were undertaking *poor practice*. The authors identified the susceptibilities of socialisation into poor ward practice and the individual student's need to be accepted as a member of the team. This again highlights the huge influence of workplace culture.

There is a considerable danger for an employee working with children who takes the view that handling children is just a 'normal' daily activity, and just an accepted part of the job. This view is possibly perpetuated by many parents, who accept or view the tasks related to handling children as 'normal'. As a consequence little consideration is given to the assessment, planning and performance of these tasks. Sanders and Morse (2005) acknowledge that there are very few studies that examine the ergonomic risks involved in caring for children, who obviously are dynamic and change with time and across the age continuum. When children are at their youngest (and lightest) they are very dependant; as they grow in size and weight their independence increases. They also go through various stages of assisting and resisting the performance of daily routines such as bathing and dressing (Wilson, 1998). The behaviour seen in the home situation, and the manner in which their parents handle them, is reflected in the inpatient environment. Hence the values and beliefs regarding child handling are transferred to children's nurses and become part of the work culture.

Wilson (1998) and Sanders and Morse (2005) have identified the risks to parents from poor handling in terms of musculoskeletal injury. Both studies identify lower back pain as the most common evidence of injury.

It is almost impossible to avoid handling children in the workplace, and employers have a duty to avoid as far as reasonably practical any manual handling activities which carry the risk of injury to their employees (MHOR 1992, Section 4, 1a) and where it is not reasonably practical to avoid manual handling tasks, an example being the handling of young children, employers must carry out a suitable risk assessment on all those manual handling tasks (MHOR 1992, Section 4,b,i). Examples of tasks are holding a child, the load, away from the trunk, stooping, and handling loads where there is a risk of sudden movement (Section 4, (b),(i), (Columns 1 and 2).

Employees must adhere to safe handling principles and activities, including risk assessment, using the appropriate handling techniques correctly (MHOR 1992, Section 5) informing employers if they identify any potential hazards, and being very careful to ensure that that none of their activities put themselves or others at risk (HSE, 1974, section 7; HSE, 2004.

In addition to the above acts of Parliament, clause 8 of the Nursing and Midwifery Council's code of conduct (NMC, 2004) charges all registered practitioners to 'act to identify and minimise the risk to patients and clients' and to 'work with other members of the team to promote healthcare environments that are conducive to safe, therapeutic and ethical practice'.

In order to practice within the boundaries of 'reasonable care' five simple steps (HSE, 1999) should be used when assessing risk. They are targeted predominately at employers, but it is good practice for employees to take responsibility for their immediate work environment).

The five steps of risk assessment

Step 1: Look for hazards

A hazard is something with the potential to cause harm. Examples are equipment (beds, cots), monitoring devices; methods of working (lifting children, holding children), and working environment (lighting, obstructions such as toys and spillages). Hazards are not only physical, but also include workplaces that are psychologically stressful and mentally tiring.

Step 2: Decide who might be harmed and how

The risks will never be the same for all individuals in an environment. The risks to a nurse will be different to those of a patient. Is the nurse physically fit and adequately trained? At what stage of development are the children who are being cared for, and what is their level of physical ability? A parent caring for her child might be pregnant – there are specific regulations for pregnant and nursing mothers. Risks must be considered for others people in the area too, friends and family, other members of the health-care team, cleaners, clerks, and anyone else who visits the environment. In addition to promoting safety in the workplace, all employees have a duty to promote the health of others. All nurses have responsibility to ensure that parents are advised of safe handling techniques, especially if any intervention requires that parents change the way they handle their child.

Step 3: Evaluate the risk and decide whether existing precautions are adequate or whether more should be done

What is the likelihood of harm arising? Would the potential of that harm include risk of injury to oneself or others? How severe could that injury be (worst-case scenario)? How many people would be involved in that risk? What has been already done to prevent risk? What more could be done? If unsure, has more expert advice been sought?

Step 4: Record your findings

All employers of five or more employees should keep a written record of their risk assessment and the employees must know about the findings. 'Significant findings' should be kept on record. In the ward environment there is not a specific duty for an employee to keep a record of potential hazards, but is best practice for this to happen. If a patient is involved and there are concerns for the patient's safety, undertake a risk assessment and place it in the patient's notes. Be aware of local trust policies regarding 'risk assessment' and 'clinical incident reporting'. The record may be accessed by safety representatives. Record what action was taken, if any.

Step 5: Review your assessment and revise it if necessary

Is the situation now safe? Do any further measures need undertaking? There is no excuse in the law for ignorance or failing to undertake the risk assessment procedure described above, thereby avoiding hazardous techniques when handling children. The MHOR of 1992 identifies that a risk assessment should be carried out prior to any manual handling task. The main areas to focus on are given by the acronym TILE – **T**ask, **I**ndividual capability, **L**oad and working **E**nvironment (Lancaster *et al*, 2001). During manual handling training, employees may be taught to remember this TILE (or LITE) checklist. It is illustrated in detail in *Box4.1*. Employees and (in this context) children's health practitioners need to adopt the TILE tool as part of their everyday working activities and encourage and educate others, including parents, to do so too. It is *not* just a checklist to be completed mindlessly and then filed away and forgotten (Johnson, 2005).

Box 4.1: The TILE assessment (adapted from Neathey et *al*, 2006)
PART 1: TASK (the activity)

Does the task involve holding next to the trunk? In a study of manual handling activities performed by mothers, Wilson (1998) found that on average a mother performed 96 lifts over a 24-hour period for 6-month-old babies, and 82 lifts for 2.5-year-old toddlers. Lifting activities reduced considerably after the age of 2.5 years. Children's nurses have similar manual handling activities, although it is very unlikely that they would need to lift children as often as the mothers in the study. Additionally, improvements in equipment in ward areas mean that some of the mothers' handling activities (such as lifting a baby for the purpose of changing its nappy) are not necessary. Whenever possible, children should be encouraged to move themselves, but younger and less mobile children need assistance. Ideally a child should be held firmly between the caregiver's shoulder and hip. Babies tend to be held at chest level; older children tend to be held with their trunk against the caregiver's trunk. The main risk is not the holding of the child, but the lifting and lowering of the child in to and out of the holding position. The Health and Safety Executive (HSE, 2000) produced guidelines for lifting and lowering weights both close to and away from the body, the guide weights being reduced when lifted or lowered away from the trunk; among the many examples are lifting a child from the floor to a highchair, from a cot to a changing mat, and from a bath to the floor. The weights for lifting and lowering assume that the weight can be grasped with both hands.

Guideline weights for lifting and lowering activities close to the body for men and women

Shoulder height	Women 7 kg	Men 10 kg
Elbow height	Women 13 kg	Men 20 kg
Hip height	Women 16 kg	Men 25 kg
Knee height	Women 13 kg	Men 20 kg
Floor level	Women 7 kg	Men 10 kg

The Health and Safety Executive guidelines (HSE, 2000) are for infrequent operations and refer predominantly to inanimate loads, but the principles can also be applied to children. Wilson (1998) measured the loading levels and disc pressures on the L5 and S1 spinal joints for different postures when mothers were handling 6-month-old, 2.5-year-old and 4.5-year-old children. The highest pressures were recorded for the older and heavier children. The pressures were particularly high when lifting a child from the floor into the carrying pose, and lowering the child from the carrying pose to the floor. Most of these lifts were undertaken close to the body, but Wilson (1998) noticed that differing techniques were used, some of which caused higher pressures.

Does the task involve holding away from the trunk? Such as when holding a child's leg while a colleague applies skin traction, or lifting or holding a child who is wearing a plaster cast, whereby the child's weight cannot be aligned close to the holder's body. Lifting a child in and out of a highchair can be problematic if the design of the chair makes it difficult to keep the child close to the body during the lift.

Guideline weights for lifting or lowering children or weights away from the body

Shoulder height	Women 3 kg	Men 5 kg
Elbow height	Women 7 kg	Men 10 kg
Hip height	Women 10 kg	Men 15 kg
Knee height	Women 7 kg	Men 10 kg
Floor level	Women 3 kg	Men 5 kg

Does the task involve twisting? Such as putting a baby in a car seat, sitting on a child's bed and attending to Intravenous equipment, and holding a child who is undergoing procedures.
Does the task involve stooping? Such as picking up a baby or toddler from the floor, helping a child out of a bath, or taking a child out of a buggy.
Does the task involve excessive pushing or pulling of loads? Such as moving equipment (cots, beds, heavy trolleys) around the ward environment.
Does the task involve excessive carrying distances? Such as carrying a child from one area to another.
Does the task involve risk of sudden movement of loads? Such as holding a child who is very distressed and unpredictable in their movements.

contd....

PART 2: INDIVIDUAL CAPABILITY (of the handler)

Are all staff capable of the same manual handling procedures? Many manual handling procedures, for example making beds and using hoists, involve two handlers – whenever possible, these individuals should be 'matched' (for example, be of similar heights).
Is the handler pregnant or is there a known health problem? For either of these situations, reasonable adjustments need to be made and individualised risks identified.
Has the handler been trained in safe techniques? No employee should be involved in any handling procedures without training (HSE, 1974).
Does clothing affect the task? Handlers should wear suitable clothing that will allow a full range of movement, including footwear that provides a stable base.
Is the handler physically fit? Wilson (2002) identified several risk factors for musculoskeletal disorders caused by work. These included lack of exercise, obesity, prolonged sitting, poor posture with prolonged, repetitive or awkward movements (as when feeding children).

PART 3: LOAD (the child)

How much help does the child need? The child may need help to stand, crawl, or walk, or may have a physical disabilities. If the child needs specialist equipment such as hoists, is the nurse trained in the use of that equipment?
What is the child's age and stage of development? This might give a rough guide on the weight of the child and their potential attainment of milestones. It is important to interpret 'safe' weights into age groups of children.

Average weights of children according to age

Age	Weight
Birth–1 month	3 kg
4–6 months	7 kg
6–10 months	9 kg
11–13 months	10 kg
22–25 months	13 kg
3 years	15–16 kg
5.5 years	20 kg

Before lifting a child, make a quick risk assessment. Many children are 10 kg or more before they can walk unaided. If a baby of 10 kg is lifted from the floor to the waist, this is a risky procedure for a woman (see HSE guideline weights above), and only if the baby can be held close to the body is it safe for men. If the lift involves any twisting or stooping, such as getting a child out of a car, or lifting the child from a playpen, the baby's weight will exceed the 'safe' guidelines for both men and women. If the child is very unpredictable, again the lowest guideline weight should be considered.

What are the child's or the parents' expectations and wishes? Parents regularly lift their children (Griffin and Price, 2000) and even with the build-up of their musculature and strength as the child increases in weight, they are prone to manual handling injuries (Finkelstein, 1995). Many manual handling injuries build up over a period of time and are a result of many factors rather than being caused in a single incident (Robins and Buckle, 2002) and even though the expectation of the parent and the child is to 'lift', nurses must be aware of the risks.
Is the child able to weight bear? Babies learn to stand and support themselves while holding on to stable objects – long before they can walk independently. Caregivers should use this developmental milestone as it is far safer to lift a child from standing rather than from a lying down position, because the child's weight can be spread over the handler's trunk.
What about the child's predictability and behaviour? Children of all ages can never be entirely predictable; this must be built into the risk assessment. Toddlers who are distressed and who start kicking while being held will result in more challenging handling.
What about physical abilities/operations or interventions? Does the child have cerebral palsy or muscle weakness? If so, a risk assessment involving specialists such as physiotherapists and occupational therapists may be needed. Children with normal mobility post-operatively can revert to a 'helpless' mode and it is easy for parents and carers to take over and physically help them, rather than encourage independence.

PART 4: ENVIRONMENT

Are there any space constraints on posture? Working in a high-dependency or intensive-care environment poses potential risks regarding posture because of the number of machines and associated wires needed to care for a child. Other problems are caused by the extra furniture, such as put-you-up beds for parents, which can reduce the space available to monitor a child.
What about the heating, lighting, ventilation, and floor surface? Employers have the responsibility for maintenance of these things, but it is how employees use the environment which will determine safety.
Is there any equipment that can help? Are employees aware of equipment that can be used in a variety of settings? In the case of a post-operative child who is unwilling to move, the handler should consider using slide sheets to reduce the friction caused by bed linen, and to ease movement. If hoists are used, has the equipment been checked and does it comply with equipment regulations?

The HSE (2003) states that there is no completely *safe* manual handling operation. However, working outside the above guidelines increases the risk of injury. But even before lifting is considered, awareness of scientifically based principles for conventional, two-handed, symmetrical lifting (Graveling *et al*, 2003) is vital. This type of lifting is very common with workers with children and parents. The recommendations of Graveling *et al*, (2003) are used in the following discussion. Further information and guidance can be gained from Smith (2005).

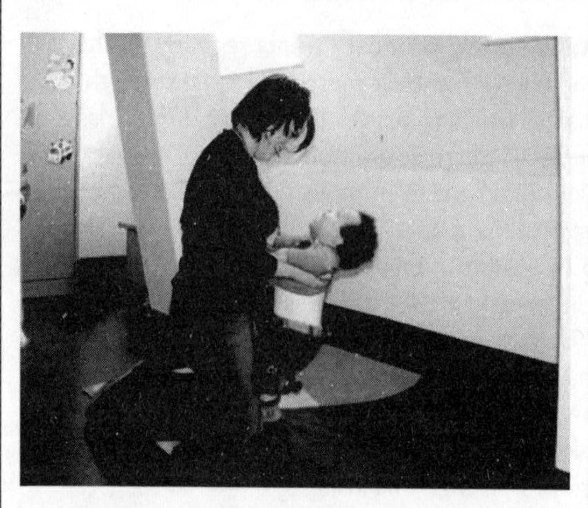

Figure 4.1: Lifting children can be dangerous because of their unpredictability. In this instance, the handler was on a stable base, with a straight back and a good grip on the child (weight approximately 12 kg). As the handler was about to lift, the child threw his head back to laugh, at which point the 'load' became unsafe because it was away from her body and any further twisting or pulling movements were unpredictable

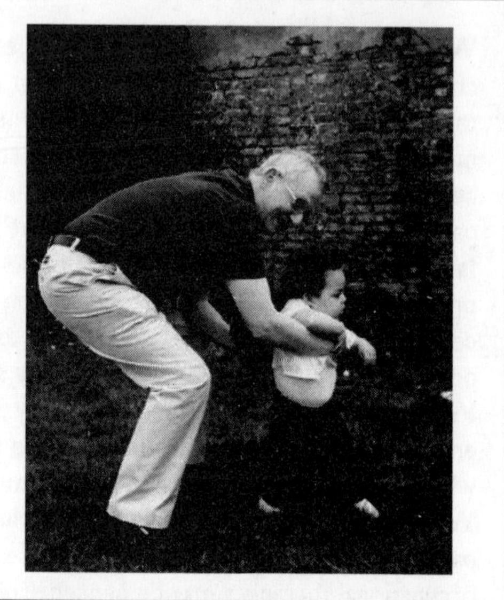

Figure 4.2: This is another very common handling situation. The handler has a stable base, a slightly bent back and flexed knees, and a potentially good grip on the child. The lift will be from knee height and with the child's weight away from the body – the recommended weight for men is 10 kg which is less than the HSE (2004a) guideline weight. However, this handler does not lift the child frequently and so the risk of injury is minimal

Figures 4.1 and *4.2* illustrate some typical scenarios of adults and children at play, and clearly demonstrate the problems that might arise when handling younger children, particularly because of the unpredictability of their movements.

Two-handed symmetrical lifting in the context of lifting a child

Reasons for the procedure

- To lift a child from one surface to another
- To undertake a procedure that involves some lifting such as stabilising limbs

Complications

- The unpredictability of the child

Pre-procedure

Equipment required

- A healthy and reasonably fit handler

Think TILE (task-individual-load-environment)

- Think before you lift; is the task necessary? Plan the task
- Consider the weight of the child – the heavier the child, the greater the risk
- Where is the child being lifted from and where will he or she be placed? Can the child help with the lift in any way?
- Is the environment safe? Is there enough room for manoeuvre? Are there any slippages or obstructions such as toys on the floor?

During the procedure

- Before the lift, keep the child's trunk as close to your waist as possible. For infants who are able to stand, encourage them to stand in line with the your body
- Adopt a stable position with feet set apart and one foot slightly forward. This maintains the balance. If the child is heavier than expected, your feet may have to be adjusted during the lift in order to keep stable
- Ensure that you have a secure hold of the child. This is particularly important if the child is wriggling. Hug the child close to your body and encourage him or her to hold onto you
- At the start of the lift, slight bending of your back, slight flexing of hips and knees is preferable to fully flexing your back (called 'stooping') or full flexion of the hips and knees (squatting). This means that it is always better to break down the lifting movement. If you were to lift a child from the floor to the waist, it would involve either considerable stooping or squatting. It is better to lift the child from the floor onto a small chair (at knee level), while half-kneeling, then, while still holding the child, stand up. The lift would then be completed using the correct principles, but the height of the lift would be reduced (the child having been lifted from knee to waist height)
- Do not flex your back any further as you lift. This might happen if you had not anticipated the weight of the child properly. It also happens if the legs are straightened before starting to raise the load and the hands have remained where they were placed at the start of the lift
- When lifting, keep your shoulders level and facing in the same direction as your hips. When your back is bent, avoid twisting your trunk or leaning sideways – it is better to turn, using your feet – after the lift is complete

- Keep your head up when handling a child. It is safer to look ahead than to look at the child – even though the latter can be very tempting!
- During the process of the lift, move smoothly, and try not to jerk. If a child does not feel safe during a lift, they will move to grasp at the handler and their movements can increase the risk of injury
- If there is ever any doubt about your ability to manage a child, owing to the child's size or weight or other factors that might influence the lift, do not lift. Seek advice from the experts such as back-care advisers or physiotherapists
- If you have lifted the child and feel that you have not got a good grip, or good control of the child, it is better to put the child down and start the lift again, rather than trying to adjust your hold while carrying the child

Post-procedure

- Think carefully about where you are going to put the child if you know that he or she will need to be lifted again in a short while
- If the procedure was difficult, you must record the reasons why, risk assess the situation and try other strategies in the future; the next time you may need to consider handling aids
- If a child needs lifting frequently during the day, you must undertake a personalised risk assessment on all handling procedures required during the day. Part of this assessment would identify the level of independence that the child has – remember, if the child can move himself, you must not do it for him

Tools for specific tasks

For examples of individualised tools that can be used to perform various tasks see Johnson (2005). These tools are based on the principles of TILE. The tasks include everyday activities such as helping a child to:

- Turn themselves in bed
- Reposition themselves in bed
- Get up off the bed
- Stand from a sitting position
- Get on and off the toilet
- Transfer from a bed to a chair

Conclusions

This chapter has introduced you to the importance of knowing and being compliant with the law in respect to manual handling. Never fall into the trap (whether through misconception or culture) of believing that handling children is just a 'normal' and 'routine' part of your workload and that all moves are 'acceptable' – think before you act.

Risk assessment is statutory for employers and employees. The focus is on:

- The Task
- The Individual
- The Load
- The Environment

And finally, although the safest method of lifting a child has been described here, before it is done 'think before you lift'.

References

Dimond B (2002) Risk assessment and management to ensure health and safety at work. *Brit J Nurs* **11**(21): 1372–74

Finkelstein MM (1995) Back pain and parenthood. *Occup Environ Med* **52**: 51–53

Graveling RA, Melrose AS, Hanson MA (2003) *The Principles of Good Manual Handling: Achieving a Consensus*. HSE Books, Norwich

Griffin SD, Price VJ (2000) Living with lifting: mothers' perceptions of lifting and back strain in childcare. *Occup Ther Int* **7**(1): 1–20

Health and Safety Executive (1974) *Health and Safety at Work Act 1974*. HMSO/HSE, London. www.hse.gov.uk/legislation/hswa.pdf/

Health and Safety Executive (1992) *Manual Handling, Operations Regulations 1992*. HMSO/HSE, London. www.opsi.gov.uk/si/si1992/Uksi_19922793_en_1.htm/

Health and Safety Executive (1999) *Management of Health and Safety at Work Regulations*. HMSO/HSE, London. www.opsi.gov.uk/si/si1999/19993242.htm/

Health and Safety Executive (2000) *Getting to Grips with Manual Handling: A Short Guide for Employers*. HSE Books, Sudbury

Health and Safety Executive (2003) *The Principles of Good Manual Handling. Achieving a Consensus*. HSE Books, Sudbury

Health and Safety Executive (2004) Manual Handling Operations Regulations 1992 (as amended). Guidance on Regulations L23, 3rd edn. HSE Books, Sudbury

Health and Safety Executive (2004a) *Getting to Grips with Manual Handling: A Short Guide*. HSE Books, Sudbury

Health and Safety Executive (2007) *Musculoskeletal Disorders Risk Assessment*. www.hse.gov.uk/msd/risk.htm/

Johnson C (2005) Manual handling risk assessment – theory and practice. In: Smith J , ed. *The Guide to the Handling of People*, 5th edn. National Back Pain Association, Teddington

Jones JR, Huxtable CS, Hodgson JT (2001) *Self Reported Work-Related Illness in 1998/99: Results from EUROSTAT Ill-Health Module in the 1999 Labour Force Survey Summer Quarter*. Health and Safety Executive, London

Jones R, Hodgson T, Osman R (1997) *HSE: Self-Reported Working Conditions in 1995 a Household Survey*. HMSO, Norwich

Lancaster R, Jacobson Maher C, Alder A (2001) *Second Evaluation of the Manual Handling Operations Regulations (1992) and Guidance*. Health and Safety Executive, London

Manual Handling Operations Regulations (1992) *Statutory Instruments 1992, no. 2793, Health and Safety*. Health and Safety Executive, London

Neathey F, Sinclair A, Rick J, Ballard J, Hunt W, Denvir A (2006) *An Evaluation of the Five Steps to Risk Assessment*. C Books, Norwich

Nursing and Midwifery Council (2004) *Code of Professional Conduct*. NMC, London

Robins V, Buckle P (2002) *Health and Safety Executive: Work, inequality and musculoskeletal health. Research Report 421*. HSE Books, Sudbury

Sanders MJ, Morse T (2005) The ergonomics of caring for children and exploratory study. *Am J Occup Ther* **59**(3): 285–95

Smith J (ed.) (2005) *The Guide to The Handling of People*, 5th edn. National Back Pain Association, Teddington

Swain J, Pufahl E, Williamson GR (2003) Do they practise what we teach? A survey of manual handling practice amongst student nurses. *J Clin Nurs* **12**(2): 297–306

Wilson A (2002) *Effective Management of Musculoskeletal Injury: A Clinical Ergonomics Approach to Prevention, Treatment and rehabilitation*. Churchill Livingstone, Edinburgh

Wilson K (1998) The manual handling of children: a 24-hour exposure. *Safety Sci Monit* **2**(2): 1–14.

Useful websites

Health and Safety Executive
www.hse.gov.uk

Office of Public Sector Information
www.opsi.gov.uk

Chapter 5

Fundamental aspects of play in hospital

Katy Weaver and Joanna Groves

Why is play important?

Play is essential for all aspects of a child's 'normal' growth and development, enabling the child to advance emotionally, socially, physically and intellectually. Another very important reason for play is simply because it is enjoyable and fun for children, yet it has many functions. Play enables children to learn because while they are playing they are absorbing new information and processing it in such a way that it then becomes part of their knowledge base, and this, in turn, enables them to change or adapt their views and opinions. McMahon (2003) describes play thus:

> *"Play is not a mindless filling of time or a rest from work. It is a spontaneous and active process in which thinking, feeling and doing can flourish since they are separated from the fear of failure or disastrous consequences."*

Play is important for children and adults alike. However, with play there are no limits or restrictions and children are free to be as creative, imaginative and adventurous as they choose to be. And because there is no right or wrong about playing there is no risk of undesirable consequences – unlike in the everyday world. According to Lansdown (1996):

> *"The food and drink of mental growth, play, is an essential requirement for a child's well-being and development."*

Play in hospital

Whatever the child's previous experiences of hospital are, a visit to hospital can be not only a challenge, but also potentially frightening and very traumatic, whether as an inpatient or an outpatient. As emphasised above, play is vital for any child, including those in hospital. However, in a hospital environment, and for children who are unwell, play is intended to fulfil different functions, and is often used to fulfil a purpose.

The functions of play in hospital

- To link to home
- To aid feelings of normality
- To provide an outlet for feelings and frustrations
- To reduce stress and anxiety
- To help the child to regain confidence and self-esteem
- To teach in an enjoyable way (eg. About procedures)
- To encourage involvement of families and siblings
- To facilitate communication for all children, whatever their age, stage of development, language, or ability
- To minimise regression
- To provide fun!

In addition, play is believed to help speed up recovery of children in hospital.

The role of the hospital play specialist

Hospital play specialists (HPS) are trained professionals who work within the paediatric team. They have completed the BTEC qualification in Professional Diploma in Specialised Play for Sick Children and Young People. The role of the hospital play specialist can vary significantly depending on the setting in which he or she is based.

However, the fundamental role of the hospital play specialist remains the same, as listed here.

The role of the hospital play specialist

- Organise activities
- Make the environment child-friendly
- Support patients and families (including siblings) using therapeutic play techniques during their stay in hospital
- Act as the child's advocate
- Use various techniques to help children to master and cope with anxieties
- Use play to prepare children for hospital procedures
- Contribute to clinical judgements through play-based observations
- Be an active member of the multidisciplinary team and to aid and/or support other professionals
- Work closely with the child psychology department
- Teach the value of play to other members of staff and volunteers
- Use play to promote development and prevent regression for children and young adults while in hospital (particularly important for long-stay patients and those in isolation)
- Develop and execute individual play programmes
- Facilitate obtaining informed consent

Young children often find it difficult to play spontaneously, particularly in a hospital environment, and when play does occur it isn't always as productive as it would be if it was guided by a professional (Lansdown, 1996). Taylor *et al* (1999) state:

> *"In the absence of familiar persons, objects and routines and with the real or perceived threat of injections, medications and procedures, many children while hospitalised cannot spontaneously play."*

Additionally when a child is sick he or she may need specific help, possibly even physical help when movement is restricted, in order to facilitate play. This according to Walker (2006):

> *"While all paediatric staff can use play in their care of the child, the play specialist holds the responsibility for ensuring the essential functions of play are built into the fabric of the child's journey through the hospital experience."*

Types of play

Messy play

This can take many forms and is a positive outlet for feelings and frustrations, allowing the child to gain confidence and cope with difficult situations. Messy play can be wonderful for initiating discussions with the child as an activity such as drawing or painting can often highlight any feelings – positive or negative – that the child may be experiencing. Furthermore, the child has created something personal to them, which they can keep. Some good examples of messy play are:

- Painting with syringes
- Sticking and cutting
- Cornflour 'gloop' (mix cornflour (or custard powder) and water together, and add paint or glitter)
- Playing with play dough or salt dough (see *Box 5.1*)
- Printing with paints

Box 5.1: Simple dough recipes

Play-dough
1 cup flour
½ cup salt
2 teaspoons cream of tartar
1 cup water
2 tablespoons oil
Food colouring (if desired)
Heat the oil in a saucepan. Add the other ingredients to the oil and cook, stirring throughout, for 3 minutes over a medium heat (or until consistency is like PlayDough). Carefully tip the dough out of pan – it will be hot!

Salt dough
1 cup flour
½ cup salt
2 tablespoons cream of tartar
1 tablespoon oil
1 cup boiling water
Food colouring (if desired)
Mix and knead all the ingredients together. This dough does not require cooking, and it is not quite so sticky and does not dry out so quickly.

***NB:** When using either type of dough be aware of the potential for cross infection. For health and safety reasons you should make separate dough for each patient or divide it up before play, and always discard it after use. However, if the same patient would like to continue playing with the dough later it can be stored in the fridge to stop it from drying quickly.*

Imaginative play and role play

Examples of imaginative play are dressing up in healthcare staff costumes, playing with dolls and dolls houses, hospital toy sets and figurines, train sets and puppets. Story telling also comes into this category.

Construction play

This includes any activity that involves building something. There are a variety of construction toys available including building blocks, shapes that click together or connect together, and stacking toys.

Physical play and physical activities

Many games and activities can be linked to the physiotherapy treatment. Hence it is valuable for healthcare professionals to first discuss the child's needs with the physiotherapist where appropriate. Suitable games are throwing and catching a ball, kicking a ball, and making and throwing paper aeroplanes. Also use toys like balloons, sit-in cars, and dance mats.

Sensory play

This type of play can be especially beneficial to children with special needs or sensory impairments. This type of play might make use of musical instruments, fibre optic lights, bubble tubes, tactile toys, soap bubbles, ceiling mobiles, music CDs, story CDs and water play.

Interactive toys and games

These can often be useful as distraction toys because they actively involve children and take their focus away from their surroundings. Some ideas include board games, puzzles, computer games, cause-and-effect toys, and activity centres.

Therapeutic play techniques

> *"All staff concerned with children contributes to creating an environment which encourages children to play and supports parents. Play Specialists, unlike other staff, have as their major responsibility the social and emotional welfare of the child and family."*

These comments about the role of play specialists were made by the Play in Hospital Liaison Committee (Hogg, 1990). While the hospital play specialist will have gained a relevant qualification to develop his or her essential knowledge and skills required for the role, as professionals within a healthcare setting all should all be aware of the techniques available and the way in which they can be applied within their role.

Firstly, when approaching or interacting with any child remember to consider the aspects summarised in *Box 5.2* at all times.

Box 5.2: How to interact effectively with a child

Language	Use appropriate language to the child's age and understanding while taking into account the language and words used by their parents or carers. Consistency enables healthcare professionals to build up a rapport (for example, a child may refer to a scar by using the word 'zip')
Approach	A child will usually respond better if they are approached at eye level
Body language	Don't forget body language and using your hands to stress a point – they are essential to all forms of communication. Adults are aware of and respond to these communication cues, and this is no different with children
Tone of voice	Remember that tone of voice is often as important as what is being said
Special needs	The child or family may have specific needs, such as hearing or visual impairments. Children with special needs and those for whom English is a second language still benefit from explanations and attempts to communicate, whatever their level of understanding. Parents may benefit too. However, in such cases professionals need to be particularly aware of the language and tone of voice used to maximise the effectiveness
Communication	In hospital situations it is easy to overlook issues about general communication with children, although most of it is common sense

There are many ways in which professionals can use play to make hospital experiences for sick children and their families more positive. The following information might help professionals put this into practice.

Preparation of the child

The aims of preparation are to help the child to understand his or her illness and treatment, and to provide an opportunity to correct any misconceptions the child or family may have. It is important to allow the child to express the whole range of feelings they may be experiencing through play activities. It can be very difficult to do this in a strange and unfamiliar environment. Preparatory play, therefore, aims to increase and improve the child's ability to cope in the hospital setting. The process of preparation can return to the child the feeling of control, by facilitating discussion of all options and allowing the child to participate and make his or her own choices. Examples of such choices are letting the child choose whether to have their medication as a liquid or tablets, or whether to have a local anaesthetic cream or cold spray for a blood test.

Preparation also gives staff the opportunity to build a rapport with the child and encourages trust which is crucial and of great benefit throughout the child's time in hospital. When there is little time available to prepare children it is vital that use is made of any information obtained from the parents or carers, who generally know the child better than anyone else. Such information can help in the selection of more appropriate techniques. A well-prepared child is less likely to suffer long-term psychological effects, which in turn will make any subsequent visits to hospital more positive. According to the National Association of Hospital Play Staff (NAHPS, 1987):

> *"Over the years, several controlled studies have been completed and they show that well-prepared children suffer less emotional trauma post-procedurally than children who have had no preparation."*

Using play to prepare a child is an effective way of gaining informed consent for the child and their parents or carers and siblings. This is of paramount importance before any procedure or treatment is carried out. The Department of Health (2003) describes the type of information that is required:

> *"Children, young people and parents need valid, relevant, accurate, up-to-date, easily accessible and well presented information, that is appropriate to their level of understanding, before they can decide whether to consent to, or refuse, treatment."*

Preparation can take many forms and it provides one form of support for a child going through the three stages of a planned admission. The three main stages are:

- The pre-admission period
- The admission
- The specific preparatory intervention

Such preparation ensures that the child is well supported and informed throughout the experience as much as possible. Play preparation has many benefits but principally it may also contribute to a speedy recovery, and therefore can minimise the length of stay.

Encouraging children to attend a pre-admission group whenever this service is available is vital because it is a good opportunity for children and parents or carers to ask questions, to voice their concerns, to meet some of the staff, to visit relevant sites (theatres, recovery rooms) and to experiment with some of the equipment. Importantly it lays firm foundations for any subsequent preparatory techniques used.

Methods that might be selected in order to prepare a child for a procedure can be simple, such as spending a little time with the child and explaining the procedure in a suitably detailed yet age-appropriate manner, or showing the child the real tools and equipment used for the forthcoming procedure. Additionally this allows the child to meet the staff who will be involved, and this empowers the child by clarifying the choices open to them, enabling them to take part in deciding how things are done. Other useful techniques are looking at photograph books that show children who are experiencing the same procedure or situation, or reading story books about relevant life experiences, or role play with real equipment and dolls.

There are some important things to remember when preparing a child. Always try to implement the principles described in *Box 5.3*.

Box 5.3: Principles to follow when preparing a child

Be honest

Use appropriate and child-friendly language

Use the correct terms for equipment to avoid confusion

Stay calm and relaxed to instil confidence and reassure the child and family

Spend time with siblings whenever possible

Be aware that the child may not necessarily be fearful of the procedure itself but may be worried about the implications (with an intimate invasive procedure the child may be very embarrassed)

Consider timing when undertaking preparation. For some young children doing this too early can exacerbate fears because they have a limited concept and understanding of time and so struggle to manage their fears in relation to this; but if done too late, when a child is already distressed, it may not be successful because stress impairs the ability to absorb information. Always be vigilant and look for non-verbal clues that the child is no longer paying attention

Needle play

This carefully supervised play can be beneficial for children who have fears or phobias of needles; it can help to allay their fears considerably. The technique can be used for fear of other types of medical equipment. It is important to remember that young children are animistic and confer life on inanimate objects. This is not surprising as many popular children's television programmes feature machines that suddenly burst into life, a process known as personification. Many adults recall childhood fears of being swept into the vacuum cleaner or being sucked down the plug hole of the bath!

Some examples of needle play include the use of venesection dolls. These are specially designed to enable the child to 'take blood'. Calico dolls can be personalised and used in a similar way. This form of play can also be linked to desensitisation techniques.

The four stages of needle play are shown in *Box 5.4*. For more information, see the National Association of Hospital Play Staff guideline on needle play (NAHPS, 2002)

Box 5.4: Four stages of needle play

Assessment	Discuss the benefits of needle play with parent or carers and the child. Allow the child and his or her parents or carers to decide whether they feel this would be beneficial, or appropriate. Explain that it often leads to a better understanding of the procedure and provides an opportunity for feelings to be discussed
Preparation	Warn the child about possible dangers of handling needles outside the needle play session. Demonstrate the procedure using appropriate equipment and visual aids. You need to ensure that you are well prepared for this and have all the correct information. Allow time for questions
Procedure	Follow the child through the procedure offering support and distraction therapy if this is what the child wants
Post-procedure	Give feedback to the child and praise their achievements, however minor. Discuss if further needle play sessions might be beneficial. It is important to recognise your limitations and involve other professionals if necessary (perhaps the psychologist)

Post-procedural play

This can take practically any form because one of its sole purposes after a procedure is to allow the child to evaluate the experience and make sense of what happened. It gives them the opportunity to discuss the parts of the procedure that went well and the parts that didn't. It is important for revealing areas that could be improved should another intervention be required. Additionally, post-procedural play allows praising, rewarding and reinforcement of all the positive elements (Iles, 2007). Taking the time to do this can also enable staff to create a positive end to the experience, whether or not it was successful.

Desensitisation

Desensitisation can be a lengthy process in which the child is subjected to controlled exposure of an object or situation that they are afraid of. For example, it might begin by introducing a child to a butterfly needle in its wrapper, at the opposite side of the room, and may eventually progress to the child having the confidence to handle the butterfly needle directly. Obviously, this technique involves detailed planning and constant monitoring and must always be carried out under professional supervision. The technique is not always successful or appropriate, and so careful consideration is needed.

Distraction therapy

The primary aim of distraction is to take the child's focus and attention away from the procedure itself. A wide variety of techniques and tools are used to do this. When distraction is successful it can help to form a temporary barrier between the child's fearful mind and the physical experience of the procedure. This, in turn, can reduce any anxieties or perceptions of pain and take the child's thoughts away from the emotional turmoil they may be feeling inside.

Other aspects of preparation of the child

Positioning

Positioning depends hugely on the procedure and the specific circumstances, but there are always alternative positions, however small the differences may seem. For example, moving the pillow slightly may mean the child is more comfortable, or moving the couch a little may allow one or both carers to be close and visible to the child.

Choice of techniques

All techniques must be age-appropriate and stage-appropriate.

Timing

Timing applies both to the distraction and to the medical staff. Good timing is essential, and it is important to ensure that staff members are aware of the situation and the plans which have been formulated. All the necessary equipment should be ready and all staff well prepared for the procedure. Be ready as soon as the child says he or she is ready. It is also important to remember that children often get bored or lose interest quickly, so it is necessary to assess the situation constantly and adapt the distraction methods accordingly. If distraction is commenced too early, the child's focus may have been lost before the procedure has even begun.

Positive reinforcement

All efforts of the child should be praised, no matter how small they may seem and whatever the outcome. Make sure you use comments like: 'Thank you for listening' and 'Well done for trying so hard'.

The people involved

Consider what the child wants. Which people would be most supportive for the child? How many people are needed?

Useful play activities and toys for different ages

Remember that some children like to watch the procedure and take a more active role, even though this may not be a good idea. Whilst professionals can advise and help children to make a decision that will suit them best, the final decision is theirs. In a situation like this, whatever the outcome or the child's response, it is often useful to approach things in a relaxed manner, offering lots of praise and reassurance. Explaining exactly what is happening in simple terms can help to reduce fear, and asking questions or finding a little light-hearted humour can help to relax children. Always involve the child in things, even if only a little.

When distracting children, even if the techniques don't appear to be successful, the professional should still endeavour to continue. Changing the method or even just changing the approach a little may help. Either way, it's not impossible to calm a child who appears to be distressed, so do keep trying! Where possible, give parents or carers and other staff the confidence to distract the child if needed. Nominate just one person to be the distracter because too many distracters can have an undesirable effect. Empowering children with their own coping skills can ultimately help them to achieve independence and enable them to have more positive experiences in the future.

Below are some specific ideas for dealing with children across all age ranges.

Babies and toddlers

Multisensory toys, such as noisy musical toys, visually stimulating toys (mobiles and toys that light up or move), talking toys, bright 'touch and feel' books, and soap bubbles are really good for this age group.

Young children

Make use of the child's interests or hobbies. These can provide easy sources of distraction for children who become very engrossed talking about something they really enjoy or that they have done. Interactive toys are often successful too because of the level of involvement required. Examples are pop-up toys, activity books, talking computers, hand-held computer games, soap bubbles, story books, interactive puzzle and picture books. Children in this age group usually have a vivid imagination that can be a useful tool and can prompt some interesting and distracting discussions. Use the distraction boxes made by Starlight Children's Foundation whenever possible, particularly in emergency care situations. Such boxes contain all the play equipment needed for a distraction episode.

Older children

For this age group successful distraction can be found with interactive books of optical Illusions and picture puzzles, for example. There are many suitable games and activities, from card games, counting games, to telling jokes, and old favourites like 'I spy'. Exploring the child's interests and hobbies will also initiate discussions. Even if you know little about their interests, most children will be happy to educate you and will probably find your attempts to discuss them amusing!

Teenagers and young people

Hand-held computer games are very good for this age group, as are videos, DVDs, music, and their own developed or practised coping techniques. In many instances a general chat about school or hobbies can make all the difference.

Children with special needs

For children with learning disabilities it is useful to elicit as much information from the parents or carers about their specific needs before considering any procedure. For example, if a child is visually impaired, try to be more vocal and also more aware of the tone of your voice. It is important for the nurse to know if the child can understand what is being communicated, even if the child finds it difficult to communicate or respond. Consider all five of the sense (sight, hearing, smell, touch, and taste). It is always a good idea to ask the child or their parents or carers about the kind of toys or activities they enjoy.

Guided imagery

Whitaker (2003) gives the following definition:

> *"Guided imagery is a therapeutic technique that allows two people to communicate based on a reality that one of them has chosen to construe through a process of imaging."*

The choice of imagery is always the child's and the adult should guide while being guided by the child's own imagery. To practice this technique some training is recommended, but it can be used by play specialists, medical/nursing professionals and parent or carers alike. The technique can be effective and successful with any child as long as that child is capable of using their imagination. Imagery can be used with children in hospital as a coping technique, as well as a form of pain management. However, it should be used to compliment other traditional methods of pain control, not replace them.

Before attempting guided imagery, and after training, professionals should spend time with the child to build a rapport and learn a little more about them. They can begin with some basic relaxation (see below). However, as with any technique, this will not work or be appropriate for everybody. Each individual case will need to be reviewed in advance. It may not be suitable for children who have learning disabilities.

Relaxation therapy

A good way to begin relaxation therapy is with progressive muscle relaxation whereby regions of the body are relaxed in sequence, working from the toes, through the body, to the head and neck. Children sometimes find this quite difficult so it may help to encourage them to contract the chosen muscle initially. This focuses their attention on how it feels and enables them to then do the opposite, to relax the muscle. When the relaxation time is over, bring the child out of it slowly. Ask them to count backwards from 5, and to slowly open their eyes when they reach 1, for example.

Therapeutic uses of relaxation therapy and guided imagery

- To help control pain
- To control nausea and vomiting
- Stress management

As with guided imagery, relaxation can only be used as an adjuvant to control pain and not as a replacement.

How can you help the child in hospital?

- Involve a hospital play specialist as soon as possible
- Start preparing the child at the earliest opportunity – it's everybody's job
- Use age-appropriate language with the child
- Be consistent with words the child and family may already use
- Always be honest and encourage parents or carers to do the same
- Don't make promises you cannot keep (eg. 'You won't have to have a blood test' 'It won't hurt')
- Give praise and positive reinforcement
- Work as part of a team (teamwork is essential)
- Communicate effective and appropriately
- Be guided by the child
- Don't distract the child from the distracter (too much input will overwhelm and confuse him or her)
- Take time to play and interact with the child whenever time allows, to help build rapport and trust
- Remember that parents are usually the experts
- Remain relaxed and calm – the child may be easily affected by other people, which can affect his or her mood and responses

Conclusions

Through the use of preparation, distraction and post-procedural play, the child can be encouraged to gain and practice their own coping skills. Irrespective of the play intervention selected, it cannot be overemphasised how important it is to assess the child's individual needs and abilities as much as possible before attempting any preparation techniques. However, hospital environments are unpredictable, and when there is so much to consider not all attempts will be successful (and there is often an element of luck involved). The better informed the professional, the greater the degree of success. Measuring success in these play situations is not always straightforward, however. While evaluations of a play experience may be negative, there may actually have been a marked improvement compared to previous experiences. For some children, shouting can be an effective coping technique, so don't be discouraged.

References

Department of Health (2003) National Service Framework for Children. Standard for Hospital Service. Department of Health, London

Hogg C (1990) *Play in Hospital Quality Management for Children.* Play-in-Hospital Liaison Committee, London

Iles P (2007) Preparation and post-procedural play. In: Glasper EA, McEwing G, Richardson J, eds. *Oxford Handbook of Children's and Young People's Nursing.* Oxford University Press, Oxford

Lansdown R (1996) *Children in Hospital.* Oxford University Press, New York

Mcmahon L (2003) *The Handbook of Play Therapy.* Routledge, London

National Association of Hospital Play Staff (1987) *Let's Play: Play Preparation for Surgery and Unpleasant Procedures.* NAHPS, Middlesex

National Association of Hospital Play Staff (2002) *Guidelines for Professional Practice No. 6: Needle Play.* NAHPS, Middlesex

Taylor J, Müller D, Wattley L, Harris P (1999) *Nursing Children – Psychology Research and Practice,* 3rd edn. Stanley Thornes, Cheltenham

Walker J (2006) *Play For Health: Delivering and Auditing Quality in Hospital Play Services.* National Association of Hospital Play Specialists, London

Whitaker BH (2003) Distraction, relaxation and imagery as adjuvants to managing acute pain. Western Hospital Department of Emergency Medicine, Continuing Medical Education Seminar, October 2003

Useful websites

National Association of Hospital Play Staff
www.nahps.org.uk/

Starlight Children's Foundation (for seriously and terminally ill children)
www.starlight.org.uk/

Distraction Therapy and Guided Imagery Course (Great Ormond Street Hospital Trust)
www.ich.ucl.ac.uk/education/short_courses/courses/distract/

Chapter 6

Fundamental aspects of nursing assessment and monitoring

Jane Shelswell and Catherine Bentley

This chapter covers a range of assessments to make an overall assessment of a child's condition, which, in isolation, may have little meaning. These are:

- Temperature
- Pulse and heart rate
- Oxygen saturation
- Respiration
- Blood pressure
- Blood glucose

Temperature

Body temperature is a physiological variable that is usually precisely controlled by the body. Just as adequate oxygen is essential to cellular metabolism, appropriate temperature is critical to the function of the enzymatic systems regulating cellular functions (Tortora, 2005). Normal body temperature represents the optimal thermal condition needed to support the internal functions. Thermoregulatory responses balance heat production and heat loss in order to maintain normal body temperature.

Temperature measurement is a useful observation in children and helps us to identify thermal imbalance. Normal body temperatures in children are shown in *Box 6.1*. Most commonly, temperature is measured to identify the presence of infection and to monitor the effectiveness of treatment. Many parents are anxious about the presence of a high temperature but it can, of course, be beneficial to the patient by increasing metabolic rate, destroying micro-organisms and speeding up removal of them from the body (Harrison, 2007). The height of the fever does not necessarily relate to the seriousness of an infection, nor does it necessarily identify a bacterial infection (Rudolf and Levene, 2006). It must be remembered, however, that both hypothermia and hyperthermia have profound effects on the cardiovascular, pulmonary, neurological and haematological systems of the child who is presenting with serious illness (Smith *et al*, 2005). Recording a temperature may reveal a trend, but it is also important to observe the child for other signs associated with a raised temperature – a raised heart rate and altered conscious level, for example (Monaghan, 2005). Remember that body temperature varies throughout the day and is often higher in the afternoon and evening (Rudolf and Levene, 2006).

Box 6.1: Normal paediatric body temperatures (Brown, 2007)

Infant ≤6 months	36.8–37.2°C
Infant 7 months–1 year	37.5–37.7°C
Child 2–5 years	37.0–37.2°C
Child >6 years	36.6–36.8°C

Core temperature

The aim of measuring a child's temperature is to determine their 'deep core' temperature. This core temperature is relatively constant despite possibly wide fluctuations in the environmental conditions. Even when the skin and superficial tissues are influenced by the environment, the 'core' remains more constant (Childs *et al*, 1999). The most reliable measurement of body core temperature is obtained through a pulmonary artery catheter, the so-called gold standard. However, this is much too invasive for use in general care. The other methods used in this chapter – oral, axilla and tympanic – vary by 0.4–0.6°C (on average) from the core temperature (National Institute for Clinical Excellence [NICE], 2006). For the purposes of this chapter these are considered to be 'core' sites.

Signs and symptoms of pyrexia (Harrison, 2007)

- Tachycardia
- Tachypnoea
- Discomfort
- Pallor – due to vasoconstriction
- Mild cyanosis
- Mottled limbs and poor circulation
- Irritability
- Lethargy
- Clammy skin
- Reduced oral intake

Common sites for core temperature measurement

- Tympanic membrane
- Oral cavity (in children over 5 years of age who are fully conscious)
- Axilla

The rectal site is not commonly used in general practice because of the risk of perforation. Indeed, it is rarely performed in intensive care. When used in intensive care it is continuously monitored using a specially designed probe made of a soft, pliable material.

Types of thermometers

The three most commonly used methods are digital probes, tympanic thermometers and thermometer strips (Taylor, 2006). Tympanic thermometers are widely used within the hospital setting although there is much controversy regarding the accuracy of tympanic thermometry (Craig *et al*, 2003). It is reported that children prefer tympanic membrane thermometry to the digital under-arm device (Pickersgill *et al*, 2003). Although it is deemed that the axilla site is both accessible and safe in young children (NICE, 2006), taking and recording a temperature of a wriggly, ticklish or shy young child can be challenging.

For a child under 5 years use:

- Electronic digital thermometer in the axilla
- Single-use thermometer in the axilla
- Tympanic membrane thermometer (in the ear)

Temperature measurement

Reasons for the procedure

- To identify hypothermia or hypothermia
- To monitor the effectiveness of antibiotic treatment for hypothermia or hyperthermia (Smith *et al*, 2005)

Pre-procedure

Equipment required

- A watch or easily visible clock
- Appropriate thermometer
- Observation chart

Specific patient preparation

- Ensure the environment is child friendly, providing toys and a quiet area, and ensuring privacy and dignity is maintained
- Explain all the procedures and care in an age/developmentally appropriate manner to both the child and family. Encourage parental participation to promote child cooperation and understanding (National Patient Safety Agency [NPSA], 2004)
- Obtain consent prior to the procedure. The child, or their carer, may give consent so long as they are informed of the implications, potential side-effects and alternatives. If they are competent, seek informed consent directly from the child (British Medical Association [BMA], 2001; Department of Health, 2001)
- Offer reassurance where appropriate (parents are often anxious about pyrexia, so provide reassurance)
- Consider the age of the child when choosing the most appropriate thermometer (NICE, 2006)

During the procedure

Electronic digital thermometer (oral measurement)

- Follow the manufacturer's guidelines at all times
- Ensure the patient has not had anything to eat or drink for 20 minutes
- Check that the lens is clean and if required apply a disposable lens cover
- Place the probe into the child's mouth and place under the tongue, explaining to the child the importance of keeping his or her mouth closed
- Activate the thermometer and leave it *in situ* until a reading is displayed
- Dispose of the cover or clean the thermometer following local guidelines

Electronic digital thermometer (axilla measurement)

- Follow the manufacturer's guidelines at all times
- Ensure that the area under the child's arm is clean and dry
- Place the thermometer under the child's arm, ensuring that the surface of the skin is touching the end of the thermometer
- Where possible, explain the importance of keeping still to the child
- Activate the thermometer and leave *in situ* until a reading is displayed

Single use thermometer (oral or axilla measurement)

- Follow the manufacturer's guidelines at all times
- Place the device in the child's mouth or axilla
- Leave *in situ* for the time specified in the manufacturer's guidelines
- Remove and read the temperature
- Dispose of the single use thermometer following local guidelines

Tympanic membrane thermometer (aural measurement)

- Follow the manufacturer's guidelines at all times (Rush and Wetherall, 2003)
- Ensure the thermometer is charged and calibrated
- Apply a disposable lens cover, making sure the lens is clean
- Place the probe into the external auditory meatus. Make sure that infants and young children are held firmly but gently by a parent to avoid any head movement. For older children, explain the importance of keeping still
- Activate the thermometer and leave *in situ* until a reading is displayed
- Dispose of the cover appropriately

Post-procedure

- Record as appropriate (Nursing and Midwifery Council [NMC], 2004)
- Report any abnormalities to medical staff immediately (refer to the normal parameters as shown in *Box 6.1*)
- Administer antipyretics as prescribed (but consider treating the cause rather than the temperature in isolation). Also, only give antipyretics if the child appears uncomfortable or has symptoms requiring antipyretics (Taylor, 2006)

Pulse and heart rate

Pulse rate measurements are used in conjunction with other observations, such as blood pressure, temperature and respiration rate, to assess the overall condition of the child. In isolation, the pulse may have little meaning but may alert the nurse to carry out a full set of observations (Aylott, 2006b). Each ventricular contraction ejects a volume of blood into the aorta, producing an increase in the blood pressure which causes an expansion of the artery. During ventricular diastole, the elastic recoil of the aorta moves the blood into the next portion of the artery, which stretches and then recoils. This alternating expansion and recoil spreads along the whole arterial system, producing a pulse wave. Each pulse wave corresponds to a heart beat (Tortora and Derrickson, 2007). The sinoatrial node is the pacemaker, initiating each wave of contraction, giving the heart its characteristic rhythms or arrhythmias (uncoordinated contractions) (Marieb, 2004).

Pulse points

Pulse waves can be felt at a site chosen appropriately for the age of the child. It is best to palpate where an artery is nearer to the surface and in an area that can be compressed against underlying bone (see *Figure 6.1*). Assessing pulses in central and peripheral sites may also be necessary because some forms of cardiac disease can cause a variance. Also, comparative palpation of both peripheral and central pulses can give an indication of perfusion. Absent peripheral pulses and weak central pulses are serious signs of advanced shock and comparison with blood pressure readings would show hypotension (Advanced Paediatric Life Support Group [APLSG], 2005). It is sometimes difficult to assess a child who may not be still or is not happy to have this procedure carried out.

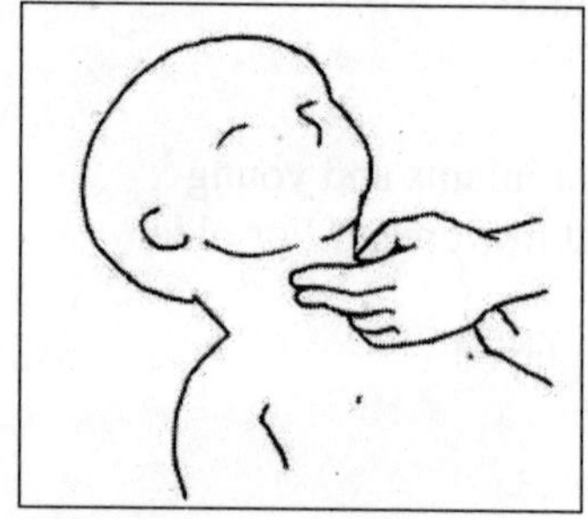

Figure 6.1: a) on the neck – carotid

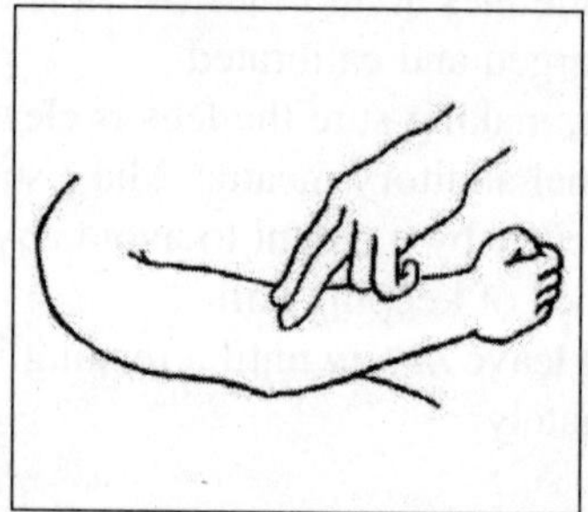

Figure 6.1: b) inside the elbow – brachial

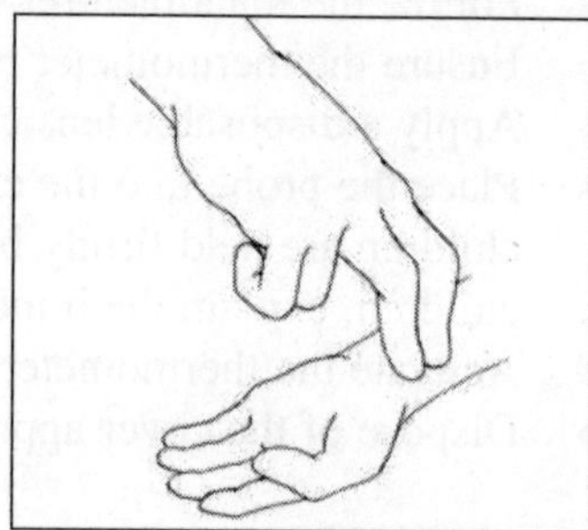

Figure 6.1: c) inside the wrist – radial

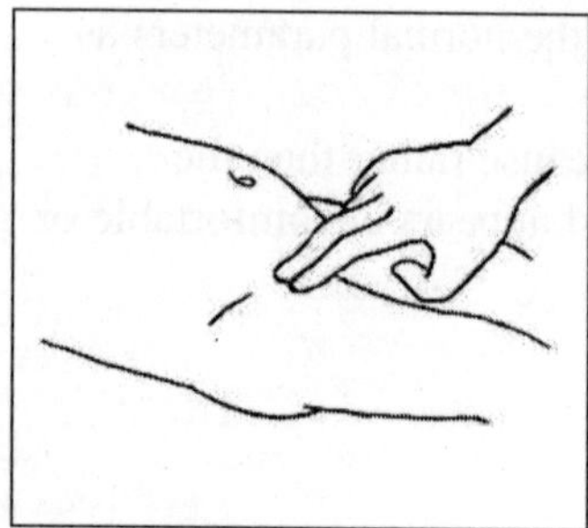

Figure 6.1: d) on the thigh – femoral

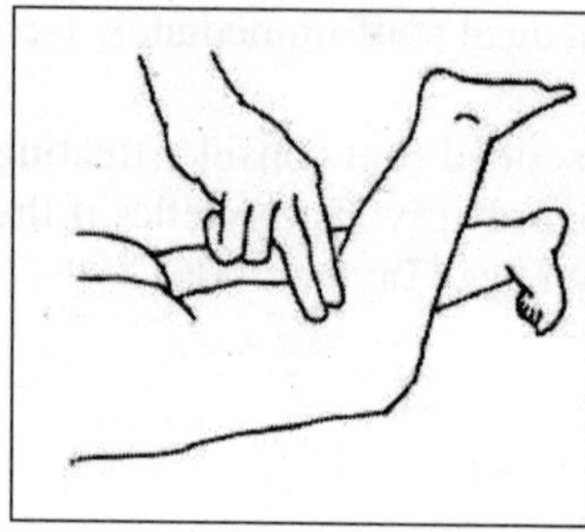

Figure 6.1: e) behind the knee – popliteal

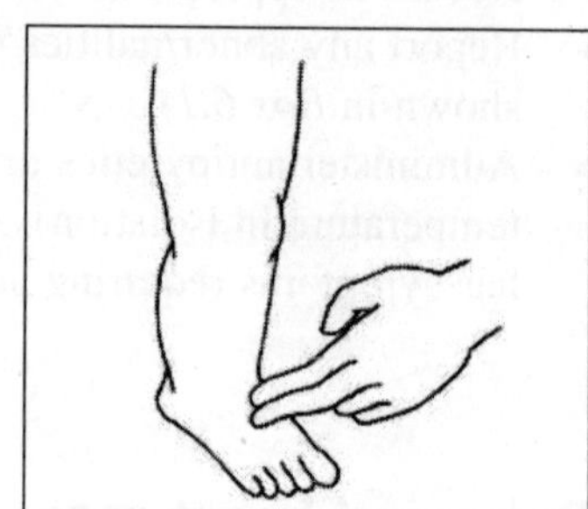

Figure 6.1: f) on the foot – dorsalis pedis

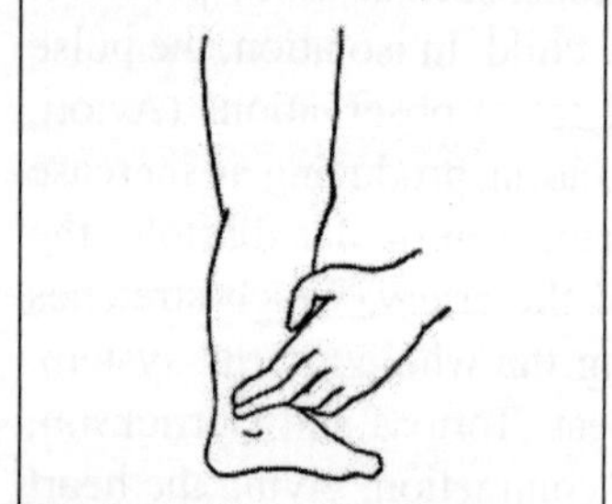

Figure 6.1: g) on the ankle – posterior tibial

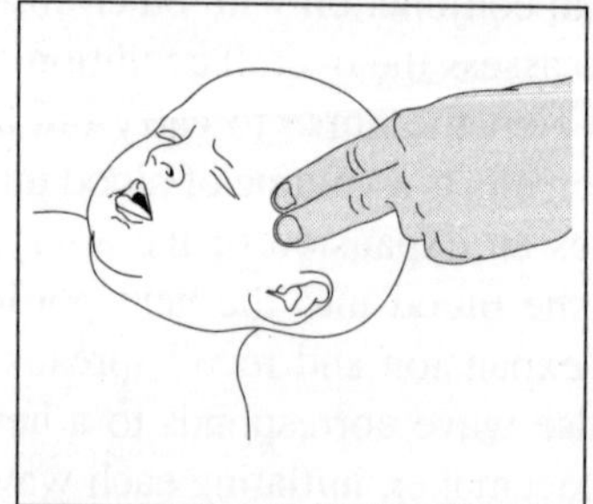

Figure 6.1: h) on the temple – temporal

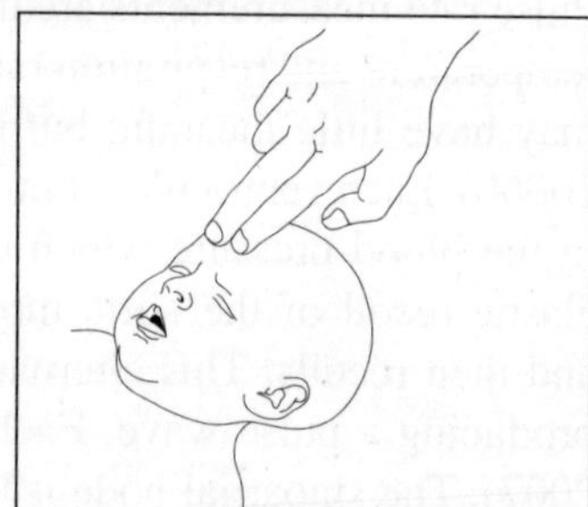

Figure 6.1: i) on the forehead – facial

Arterial pulse sites

- Carotid artery (*Figure 6.1a*)
- Brachial artery (*Figure 6.1b*)
- Radial artery (*Figure 6.1c*)
- Femoral artery (*Figure 6.1d*)
- Popliteal artery (*Figure 6.1e*)
- Dorsalis pedis artery (*Figure 6.1f*)
- Posterior tibial artery (*Figure 6.1g*)
- Temporal artery (*Figure 6.1h*)
- Facial artery (*Figure 6.1i*)

Heart rate

A child's normal heart rate can vary with age (*Box 6.2*), medical status, for example shocked state, head injury, conscious level, fever or pain. It is advisable to be aware of such variations when undertaking observations in children (European Resuscitation Council [ERC], 2004). Heart rate can increase under certain conditions; dehydration and fluid balance may affect the circulating volume within the body. The heart rate increases to ensure the body receives the same amount of oxygenated blood to the tissues – a compensatory mechanism (Aylott, 2006a).

An increase in temperature also affects the heart rate as the metabolic rate is increased and the demand of oxygen by the tissues is increased accordingly. Activity increases heart rate also because of the increased demand for oxygen (Neill and Knowles, 2004). It should be noted that the heart rate is normally higher in babies and young children because of their higher metabolic rates.

In some children there is an increase in heart rate on inspiration, and a decrease on expiration (Neill and Knowles, 2004). On inspiration, more blood is pooled in the lungs, causing a decrease the return to the left side or the heart, which in turn affects the stroke volume (Marieb, 2004).

Box 6.2: Normal paediatric heart rates (APLSG, 2005)

Infant <1 year	110–160 beats per minute
Infant 1–2 years	100–150 beats per minute
Child 2–5 years	95–140 beats per minute
Child 5–12 years	80–120 beats per minute
Child >12 years	60–100 beats per minute

The apex beat

You may still find it useful to auscultate the heart in neonates or children with a stethoscope over the apex of the heart. How to find the location of the apex is described below and this location is shown graphically in *Figure 6.2*.

Locating the apex beat (Aylott, 2007b)

- **Locate the suprasternal notch:** Feel for the hollow U-shaped depression just above the child's sternum and between the clavicles
- **Locate the sternum (breastbone):** This has three parts – the manubrium, the body and the xiphoid process
- **Locate the manubriosternal angle:** Walk your fingers down the manubrium a few centimetres until you feel this as a distinct bony ridge; it is continuous with the 2nd rib and a useful place to start counting ribs
- **Locate the 2nd rib:** Palpate lightly to the second rib on the left side and slide down to the second intercostal space
- **Locate the 4th intercostal space:** Count down the intercostal spaces till you reach the 4th one, under the 4th rib

Note that each intercostal space is always numbered by the rib above it.

Pulse measurement

Reasons for the procedure

- To ascertain a baseline rate at time of initial assessment
- To identify any initial arrhythmia indicating the need for ECG monitoring
- To assess the quality and characteristic of pulse
- To monitor the effects of drug treatment for a possible underlying arrhythmia (eg. digoxin)

Pre-procedure

Equipment required

- Stethoscope cleaned with alcohol-impregnated swab (Hudson, 2003)
- Watch with a second hand
- Observation chart to record findings

Specific patient preparation

- Ensure the environment is child friendly, provide toys and a quiet area and ensure privacy and dignity is maintained
- Explain all procedures and care in an age/developmentally appropriate way to both the child and family. Encourage parental participation to promote child cooperation and understanding (NPSA, 2004)
- Obtain consent prior to the procedure. The child, or their carer, may give consent so long as they are informed of the implications, potential side-effects and alternatives. If they are competent, seek informed consent directly from the child (British Medical Association, 2001; Department of Health, 2001)
- Before approaching the child, consider his or her age when selecting most appropriate method to use (Lockwood *et al*, 2004)

During the procedure

- Be aware of the normal parameters for different age group and any underlying problems beforehand that may affect the heart rate (eg. pyrexia, dehydration)

Neonates and infants

- Wash your hands to ensure there is reduced risk of infection (Department of Health, 2003)
- Ensure the baby is secure and comfortable before undertaking the procedure because crying will increase the heart rate significantly and affect the reliability of the clinical judgement made
- Ensure the stethoscope has been cleaned using appropriate preparation
- Locate the apex beat (*Figure 6.2*) and listen over the apex of the heart for 60 seconds (Lockwood *et al*, 2004)

Children less than 5 years of age

- Wash your hands to ensure there is reduced risk of infection (Department of Health, 2003)
- Try to use the medial aspect of the brachial artery of the antecubital fossa or the femoral artery in a sick child. The carotid artery is difficult to palpate in this age group due to their short stature and fatty tissue in this area (and a very unwell child may protest)
- Press gently on the artery of choice for 60 seconds
- Don't confuse your own thumb and finger pulses with the underlying pulse. Avoid using these two fingers or be able to differentiate between your own pulses and the child's (Lockwood *et al*, 2004)

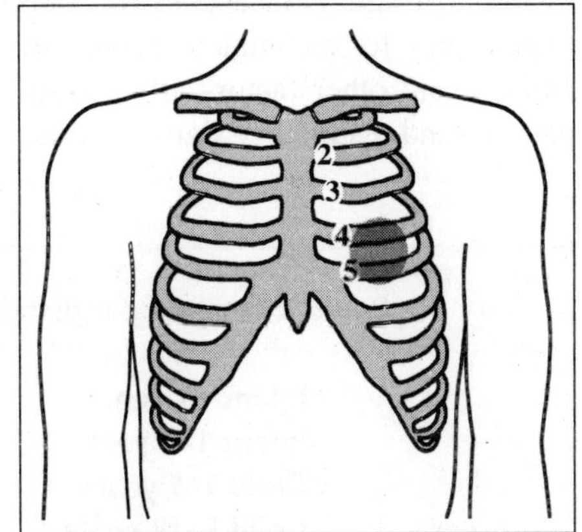

Figure 6.2: Location of the apex beat between the 4th and 5th ribs

- In children aged under 2 years, you may still find it more accurate to use a stethoscope over the apex of the heart for 60 seconds (*Figure 6.2*), especially when the child is tachycardic (Hwu *et al*, 2000). Although using a stethoscope to auscultate the heart rate, a pulse check is still required to determine pulse volume and strength

Children of 5 years of age and over

- Wash your hands to ensure there is reduced risk of infection (Department of Health, 2003)
- Ensure you explain the forthcoming procedure to reduce the child's anxiety
- Use your fingertips to feel for the appropriate artery (the radial artery is usually more accessible)
- Press gently for 60 seconds and record
- If recording for 30 seconds double the count (record over 60 seconds if there is discrepancy in the rate, rhythm or quality of the pulse; Lockwood *et al*, 2004)
- Although using a stethoscope to auscultate the heart rate, a pulse check is still required to determine pulse volume and strength

Post-procedure

- Record findings on the observation chart (NMC, 2004)
- Report any significant changes (>10% difference from the expected norm) to a medical practitioner for further review if necessary

Respirations

Respiratory rate is measured by counting each cycle of respiration – one inspiration plus one expiration – for a complete minute (Barber *et al*, 2000). As well as varying with the age of the child, many other factors affect respiratory rate, and there can be a wide range of breathing patterns and respiratory signs to consider. Normal respiratory rates are given in *Box 6.3*.

Box 6.3: Normal paediatric respiratory rates at rest (APLSG, 2005)

Infant <1 year	30–40 breaths per minute
Infant 1–2 years	25–35 breaths per minute
Child 2–5 years	25–30 breaths per minute
Child 5–12 years	20–25 breaths per minute
Child >12 years	15–20 breaths per minute

Factors affecting respiratory rate (Milner and Greenough, 2004)

- Age
- Anxiety
- Fever
- Shock
- Recent physical activity
- Gender
- Sleep
- Conscious level

Signs to watch out for (Aylott, 2006b)

- Stridor (on inspiration: indicative of partial upper airway obstruction)
- Wheezing (on expiration: indicative of lower airway narrowing)
- Crackling
- Coughing
- Nasal flaring
- Tracheal tugging
- Head 'bobbing'
- Subcostal and intercostal recession
- Abnormal chest shape (eg. barrel-shape, due to hyperinflation)
- Unequal chest movements
- Difficulty speaking or hoarse voice
- Cyanosis
- Abdominothoracic asynchrony ('see-saw' breathing)
- Deterioration in conscious level or mental status

Patterns of respiration

- Apnoea (cessation of breathing for 20 seconds)
- Bradypnoea (Abnormally slow rate of breathing))
- Dyspnoea (difficulty in breathing)
- Head bobbing (the sternocleidomastoid and accessory muscles are being used and the head bobs up and down with each breath)
- Hypercapnia (increased levels of carbon dioxide)
- Hyperventilation (increased rate and depth of respirations)
- Hypoventilation (decreased depth of respirations)
- Hypoxia (low level of oxygenation)

- See-saw respiration (paradoxical movement of the abdomen during inspiration; the abdomen expands and the chest wall retracts during contraction of the diaphragm)
- Tachypnoea (abnormally fast rate of breathing)

Monitoring respirations

Reasons for the procedure

- To identify a baseline to enable future comparison
- To assess improvement or deterioration

Pre-procedure

Equipment required

- Watch with second hand
- Observation chart to record results
- Stethoscope cleaned with alcohol-impregnated swab (Hudson, 2003)

Specific patient preparation

- Ensure the environment is child friendly, provide toys and a quiet area and ensure privacy and dignity is maintained
- Explain all the procedures and care in an age/developmentally appropriate way to both the child and family. Encourage parental participation to promote child cooperation and understanding (NPSA, 2004)
- Obtain consent prior to the procedure. The child, or their carer, may give consent so long as they are informed of the implications, potential side-effects and alternatives. If they are competent, seek informed consent directly from the child (British Medical Association, 2001; Department of Health, 2001)
- Before approaching the child, consider his or her age when selecting most appropriate method to use (Lockwood *et al*, 2004)

During the procedure

- In infants and young children, respirations are often difficult to assess because of their inability to cooperate and anxiety caused by being in an unfamiliar environment
- Try to ensure the child is relaxed and has not carried out any physical activity in last 20 minutes (if appropriate), for example baseline observations prior to elective surgery

- Where possible, carry out observation without the child being aware to ensure an accurate assessment is made (Lockwood *et al*, 2004)
- Count the respiratory rate for a full minute – one breath is counted as one 'inspiration plus one expiration'
- Infants have irregular breathing patterns so it is important to count for a full minute (Panitch, 2005)
- As well as monitoring respiratory rate, you should also carry out an assessment of the child's chest and the work of breathing (Aylott, 2006b) and observe for (Aylott, 2007a):
  - Depth of respiration
  - Use of accessory muscles
  - Difficulty in speaking
  - Poor feeding (in infants)
  - Asymmetry of chest movements
- Auscultate for wheeze, crackles, equal breath sounds, and bronchial breath sounds (Aylott, 2007b)

Post-procedure

- Record on the appropriate documentation (NMC, 2004)
- Ensure the patient is comfortable
- Report any significant changes (>10% difference from the expected norm) or concerns to a medical practitioner for further review if necessary

Oxygen saturation

Pulse oximetry is the non-invasive monitoring technique used to estimate the measurement of arterial oxygen saturation (SaO_2) of haemoglobin (Schutz, 2001) The reading, obtained through pulse oximetry, uses a light sensor containing two sources of light (red and infrared) that are absorbed by haemoglobin and transmitted through the peripheral tissues to a photodetector (*Figure 6.3*). The amount of light transmitted through the tissues is then converted to a digital value representing the percentage of haemoglobin saturated with oxygen blood. Saturation probe sites on the hand and foot are shown in *Figure 6.4*.

Oxygen saturation values obtained from pulse oximetry (SpO_2) are expressed as a percentage. SpO_2 monitoring is just *one* part of a complete assessment of the child's oxygenation status and not a substitute for measurement of arterial partial pressure of oxygen (PaO_2) or of ventilation. Pulse oximetry offers a useful an adjunct to the assessment and monitoring process and should be used in conjunction with direct observation of the child or young person and the monitoring of other parameters (Bloxham, 2007). Normal parameters are shown in *Box 6.4*.

NB: Oxygen saturation does NOT reflect the child's ability to ventilate.

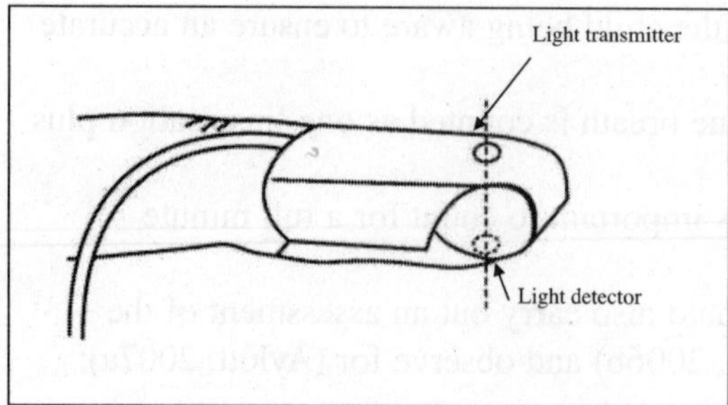

Figure 6.3: A saturation probe

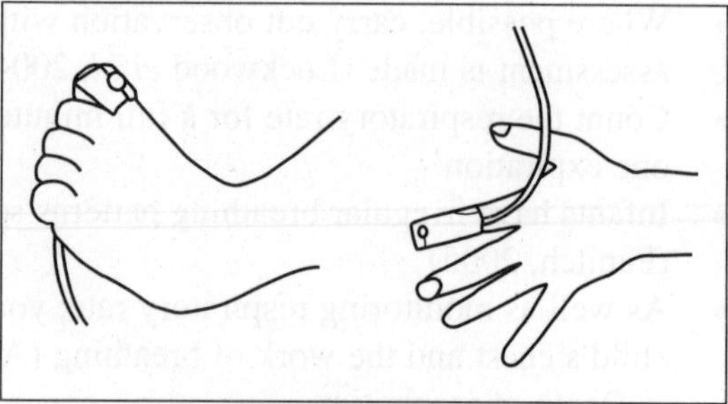

Figure 6.4: Saturation probe sites

Useful definitions

- **SaO_2** is the percentage of arterial haemoglobin saturated with oxygen
- **SpO_2** is the percentage of peripheral haemoglobin saturated with oxygen
- **FiO_2** is the percentage of inspired oxygen

Box 6.4: Normal paediatric oxygen saturations

Neonates (premature)	Upper limits about 95% Until 'due date' is reached (to avoid retinal fibrosis and reduced vision) (Chandler, 2000)
Children	In air >92% With supplemental oxygen >95% (British Thoracic Society, 2005)

Sites for SpO_2 probes

In infants

- Finger or big toe, using a finger probe or self-adhesive probe
- Earlobe, using a non-disposable clip probe

In young children

- Finger or big toe, using an adhesive wrap around the probe
- Across the palm of the hand, ensuring that the probe is situated close to the joint of the little finger
- Around the foot, with the probe sited close to the joint of the little toe (Chandler, 2000)

Accuracy of measurements

The accuracy of measurements can be affected by the following factors (Hoo, 2004):

- Haemoglobin level
- Arterial blood flow to the vascular bed
- Temperature of digit or the area where the oximetry sensor is located
- Oxygenation ability of the child (eg. in carbon monoxide poisoning, the sensor is unable to differentiate between oxygen and other gases such as carbon monoxide in the haemoglobin molecules)
- Excessive movements of the child
- Amount of ambient light seen by the sensor
- Nail-varnished nails
- Intravenous dyes

Signs and symptoms of a decreased ability to oxygenate

- Cyanosis
- Dyspnoea
- Tachypnoea
- Decreased level of consciousness
- Increased work of breathing
- Loss of protective airway

Measurement of oxygen saturation

Reasons for the procedure

- To anticipate conditions in which hypoxia could be present, allowing early intervention before unfavourable deterioration occurs
- To detect signs and symptoms of decreased ability to oxygenate

Pre-procedure

Equipment required

- Observation chart to record results
- Pulse oximeter with charged battery or mains supply

- Saturation probe appropriate to the site of recording and size of child

Specific patient preparation

- Ensure the environment is child friendly, provide toys and a quiet area and ensure privacy and dignity is maintained
- Explain the need for determining oxygen saturation with pulse oximetry and what it entails in an age/developmentally appropriate way to both the child and family. Encourage parental participation to promote child cooperation and understanding and decrease anxiety (NPSA, 2004)
- Explain the equipment to the child in an age/developmentally appropriate way to facilitate their cooperation in maintaining sensor placement
- Explain the need for an audible alarm system for determining oxygen saturation values below a set acceptable limit and demonstrate the alarm system. This alerts the child and family to the possibility of alarms, including causes of false alarms. It helps the child and family understand the values seen
- Obtain consent prior to the procedure. The child, or their carer, may give consent so long as they are informed of the implications, potential side-effects and alternatives. If they are competent, seek informed consent directly from the child (British Medical Association, 2001; Department of Health, 2001)
- Before approaching the child, consider his or her age when selecting most appropriate sensor for the area, including size with the best pulsatile vascular bed to be sampled. Use of the correct sensor optimises signal capture and minimises artefact-related difficulties (Lockwood *et al*, 2004)

During the procedure

- Use the monitor used in accordance with manufacturer's instructions, including setting the upper and lower limits as monitors are often set with a low alarm default limit of 75% (Medical Devices Agency [MDA], 1996). Turn monitor on and allow 30 seconds for self-testing procedures
- Ensure that the child and family understands the pre-procedural teaching
- Wash your hands to reduce the transmission of micro-organisms (standard precautions)
- Determine the site with the best pulsatile vascular bed. Finger probes have been found to produce the best results compared to other sites (Robertson and Kaplan, 1991). Avoid sites that are distal to indwelling arterial lines, blood pressure cuffs, arteriovenous fistulas and blood transfusions
- Adequate arterial pulse strength is necessary for obtaining accurate SpO_2 measurements. Therefore, it is important to determine the conditions of the extremity (digit) or area where the sensor will be placed, including the following (which may affect the accuracy of measurements):
  - Decreased peripheral pulses
  - Peripheral cyanosis

  - Decreased peripheral temperature
  - Exposure to excessive environmental light sources for example examination lights, phototherapy lights
  - Excessive movement or tremor in the digit
  - Dark nail polish
  - Bruising under the nail
  - Dirty digits (Schutz, 2001)
- To properly determine a pulse oximetry value, the light sensors must be in opposing positions directly over the area of sample (Grap, 1998). Apply the sensor so that the light source is directly opposite the light detector
- Secure the probe to the site appropriately. Take care not to attach too tightly as this is uncomfortable and can lead to development of pressure ulcers. Moreover, a tightly applied sensor will restrict site arterial flow and venous return and the pulse oximeter will be unable to distinguish between arterial and venous pulsations, giving falsely low readings (Wahr *et al*, 1995)
- Light from other sources (such as examination lights and phototherapy lights) can cause falsely elevated oximetry values (Hanowell *et al*, 1987); therefore the probe site must be shielded from excessive ambient light with a towel or blanket or commercially available shield
- Determine the accuracy of detected waveform by comparing the numeric heart rate value to that of the monitored heart rate or an apical heart rate. If there is insufficient arterial blood flow through the sensor, the heart rate and SpO_2 values will vary significantly. If the pulse oximeter pulse rate does not correlate with the child's heart rate; move the sensor to another site
- Set appropriate alarm limits according to the child's condition. It is recommended that oxygen saturation limits are 5% less than the child-acceptable baseline (MDA, 1996)

Post-procedure

- If continuous monitoring is necessary, assess the skin and tissues under the probe site every 3-4 hours in order to identify skin breakdown or loss of vascular flow. Change the probe site at least every 3-4 hours to promote skin integrity and prevent pressure ulcer damage to the skin
- When reading a result of the monitor, check signal strength to ensure accuracy. Also, compare and monitor the actual heart rate with the pulse rate value from the oximeter to determine accuracy of values. The two values should correlate closely
- When taking one-off readings, it is good practice to monitor the child for a minimum of 10 minutes (Schutz, 2001)
- Report any abnormalities whereby SpO_2 falls below 92% in air or below 95% in prescribed oxygen
- SpO_2 values are just *one* part of a complete evaluation of oxygenation and supplemental oxygenation therapy. It is also vital to carry out a full respiratory assessment as described above (Monaghan, 2005)

- Monitor the site for excessive movement as this can result in unreliable SpO_2 values. Move the sensor to a less 'active' site to reduce motion artefacts and encourage the child to rest the monitored digit
- It is important to remember that pulse oximetry is NOT a replacement for manual pulse taking – the oximeter does not take a real-time reading, but an *average* of sensed pulsatile flow over 5–20 seconds (Hill, 2000), and it cannot determine pulse volume
- Maintain documentation (NMC, 2004), which should include the following:
  - Child and family education
  - Indications for pulse oximetry
  - Child's pulse with SpO_2 measurements
  - FiO_2 delivered (if oxygen is being delivered to the child)
  - Skin assessment at sensor site
  - Simultaneous arterial blood gases (if available)
  - Recent haemoglobin measurement (if available)
  - Alarm settings
  - Events precipitating acute desaturation
  - Nursing interventions

Be cautious about interpreting values where there had been an instantaneous change in saturation (for example, 99% falling suddenly to 85%). This is physiologically not possible (Hill, 2000).

Blood pressure

Blood pressure is a physiological variable. It is not constant throughout the day and varies every time the heart squeezes and relaxes. It increases before waking and decreases with sleep. Normal parameters are shown in *Box 6.5*. The level of blood pressure is regulated by the kidneys, brain, heart, endocrine glands and blood vessels. Pressure developed in the artery depends on the blood being pumped into it, the *cardiac output*, the resistance to blood flowing out of the arteries, and the peripheral resistance (Noble *et al*, 2005). Arterial blood pressure provides the driving force to perfuse the tissues of the body with blood. This is why the measurement is more significant when recorded alongside other signs.

Blood pressure is the force exerted by circulating blood on the walls of blood vessels.
Systolic pressure is the peak pressure in the arteries (near the beginning of the cardiac cycle).
Diastolic pressure is the lowest pressure (at the resting phase of the cardiac cycle).
The cardiac cycle consists of both the contraction and relaxation phase of the heart:
- The contraction phase is termed *systole*
- The relaxation phase is termed *diastole*

The *sinoatrial node* stimulates the atria, the atria contract, and force blood into the ventricles. A period of relaxation allows the right atrium to fill with blood from the inferior and superior vena cava and the left atrium to fill from the pulmonary veins. Ventricular contraction occurs at the same time as atrial relaxation. The *atrioventricular node*, stimulated by atrial contraction, sends impulses to the ventricles to contract. Pressure in the ventricles increases rapidly, thus exceeding atrial pressure. The high pressure causes the mitral and tricuspid valves to close and the pulmonary and aortic valves to open, forcing blood into the pulmonary artery and aorta (Boxwell *et al*, 2001). The average pressure throughout the cardiac cycle is reported as *mean arterial pressure*, which reflects the difference between the maximum and minimum pressures measured.

Box 6.5: Normal paediatric systolic and diastolic blood pressures (Resuscitation Council UK, 2004)

Age	Systolic BP	Diąstolic BP	Mean
Newborn (premature) <1 kg	39–59	16–36	24–43
Newborn 3 kg	50–70	25–45	33–53
Newborn 4 days	60–90	20–60	33–70
Infant 6 months	87–105	53–66	64–79
Child 2 years	95–105	53–66	67–79
Child 7 years	97–112	57–71	70–84
Adolescent	112–128	66–80	81–96

Manual blood pressure recording

Manual sphygmomanometers seem to be in less frequent use than in previous years, possible due to safety hazards associated with mercury in the glass tube (O'Brien, 2002; Pickering, 2003) – there are already impositions on usage in countries such as the Netherlands and Sweden (cited in Tholl *et al,* 2004). It is important to know how to take blood pressure this way in case the electronic devices fail, or if you are working in an area where the method is still used. It is important to know what sounds you are listening for on auscultation, and what they mean in relation to what you are recording.

Manual blood pressure recording is dependent on Korotkoff sounds. In 1905, a Russian surgeon called Korotkoff developed the ausculatory method of recording blood pressure. The sounds made within the artery are relevant for identifying systolic and diastolic measurements. Blood flow in the artery generates vibrations on the vessel wall, and this is what you hear on auscultation. The turbulent flow is known as Korotkoff sounds (Noble *et al*, 2005) and these are differentiated as shown in *Box 6.6*.

Box 6.6: Korotkoff sounds

Phase I	The first faint, clear tapping sounds are heard (which increase as the cuff is deflated) – the systolic recording point
Phase II	A murmur or swishing sound is heard (during cuff deflation)
Phase III	Sounds become crisper and increase in intensity
Phase IV	A distinct, abrupt, muffling sound is heard
Phase V	The final sound is heard (disappearance of the sound) – the diastolic recording point

It is sometimes difficult to take a blood pressure reading from a child who is not still. Giving clear explanations to an older child can alleviate their anxiety but if the procedure causes distress the measurement won't be an accurate reflection of their blood pressure. In children who are still and quiet this procedure is more accurate and should be taken into consideration with other observations such as pulse, respiration rate, pulse oximetry and capillary refill time to give an overall view of the child's condition.

More reliable blood pressures are taken when the infant is quiet, still and not crying. Movement can cause artefacts and cause inaccurate results. Choose an appropriate site, usually the infant's upper arm. Check the integrity of the skin prior to applying a cuff and check that the cuff fits properly (see below). Avoid a limb that has a cannula *in situ* (Strebor, 2005).

Correct cuff sizes in children

Always follow the manufacturer's advice on cuff and bladder size, and remember:
- A cuff that is *too narrow* over-estimates blood pressure
- A cuff that is *too wide* under-estimates blood pressure (Lockwood *et al*, 2004)

For neonates choose a cuff with:
- Width: 50% of the arm circumference
- Length: the cuff must not extend over the elbow joint

For children choose a cuff with:
- Width: 40% of the arm circumference
- Length: 80% of the arm circumference

Blood pressure measurement

Reasons for the procedure

- To assess baseline blood pressure
- To record a trend and monitor treatment accordingly (eg. when antihypertensive medication is being prescribed)
- To monitor a condition and treat accordingly (eg. in postoperative children in whom the blood pressure may indicate a requirement for fluid replacement). This observation will be recorded in conjunction with other observations such as heart rate, pulse oximetry and capillary refill

Pre-procedure

Equipment required

- Stethoscope
- Sphygmomanometer or automated blood pressure device (analyses pressure pulses by oscillometric principles; Tholl *et al*, 2004)
- Appropriately sized cuff as per manufacturer's advice
  - A cuff that is **too narrow** over-estimates blood pressure
  - A cuff that is **too wide** under-estimates blood pressure (Lockwood *et al*, 2004)

Specific patient preparation

- Ensure equipment is in working order (mercury moves freely up and down the glass tubing). Adequate maintenance of equipment ensures the reliability of the reading
- Ensure the cuff is the appropriate size for the child (the bladder should have a length that is 80% of the child's arm circumference and a width that is 40%)
- Check the inflatable bulb allows air in and out freely before commencing procedure
- Inform the child of the procedure to alleviate any anxiety, and obtain informed consent
- Ensure the child is sitting or lying comfortably prior to the procedure, ideally with their arm horizontally supported at the level of their heart (gives the most accurate results)

During the procedure

Using manual sphygmomanometer

- Apply the cuff to the arm above the elbow
- Place the sphygmomanometer next to the child at the level of their heart, if able. Ensure the palm of their hand is facing upwards so you can easily palpate the radial and brachial arteries

- Inflate the cuff, palpating the radial artery as you do so. As soon as the pulse is no longer felt, deflate the cuff, remembering the number on the sphygmomanometer at that point (this is the point at which the artery has been compressed and you can use it as a reference point to inflate the cuff for your next measurement; Hall and Grim, 1991)
- Re-inflate the cuff above the reference point just obtained –20 to 30 mmHg above the measurement
- Place the bell of the stethoscope over the previously located brachial artery; the bell is specifically designed to amplify low frequency sounds (Hall and Grim, 1991)
- Deflate the cuff slowly, 2 mmHg at a time, to ensure you hear the Korotkoff sounds (see *Box 6.6*)

Using an automated device

In newborns and infants

- Wash your hands to reduce the risk of infection
- Ensure you use an appropriately sized blood pressure cuff as recommended by manufacturers – in neonates the cuff width should be 50% of the arm circumference, and it should not extend over the elbow joint. Ensure it is clean and used only for this patient to reduce infection risk and cross-contamination
- Make sure the baby is held securely in a comfortable position to prevent unnecessary discomfort and movement, so that the cuff inflates smoothly and quickly (increased activity affects the recording)
- Set the cuff pressure on the machine appropriately for this age group (often they default to adult pressure settings)
- Take the middle of three separate readings

In older children and adolescents

- Ensure clear explanations are given to alleviate any anxiety as this may raise the blood pressure unnecessarily
- Wash your hands to reduce the risk of infection between patients
- Ensure an appropriately sized blood pressure cuff is used, as variations can cause inaccurate measurements as described above
- Apply the blood pressure cuff to the upper arm and secure in place
- Ensure the child is sitting or resting with their arm supported, and at the level of their heart
- Check the machine is set to the appropriate pressure for this age group
- Ask the child to keep their arm still and explain it will take less time if they are still as the cuff will pump up and release without faltering. The procedure may need to done again if they move during the procedure, causing unnecessary discomfort
- Take the middle of three separate readings

Post-procedure

- Ensure the cuff is removed and the child comfortable. If the cuff is to be left *in situ* then ensure the site is rotated and regularly inspected to prevent pressure areas or skin marking
- Record your findings and report any abnormal findings to medical staff further review if necessary (or repeat the procedure to check)
- Be aware of normal parameters and possible reasons for increased blood pressure (eg. movement, crying or ill-fitting cuff)
- Repeat as necessary or as the child's condition dictates, and record findings to identify a trend

Capillary refill time (CRT)

Oxygen, which is critical to the survival of tissue, is carried to various parts of the body by the blood (vascular) system. Capillary refill time (CRT) attempts to measure how well the vascular system is functioning in the body's extremities (hands and feet) or skin tissues that are the parts of the body farthest from the heart. Children maintain perfusion to vital organs by an increase in heart rate and constriction of the peripheral blood vessels (Marieb, 2004). If a child is dehydrated, or tissue perfusion is blocked by other means, this quick test can alert you to the possibility that care needs to be taken to restore normal vascular flow. CRT is, therefore, an indication of peripheral perfusion and should not be thought of as an indicator of blood pressure. It is the rate at which blood returns to the capillary bed after it has been compressed digitally. Normal values are shown in *Box 6.7*.

Box 6.7: Normal paediatric capillary refill times

Neonate	≤ 3 seconds
Child	≤ 2 seconds

CRT is used primarily in the assessment of prepubertal children. It is not considered as accurate in adults due to differences in circulation from medications and various other factors (Bumke and Maconochie, 2001). Contrary to myth, skin pigmentation does not hide changes in the skin's underlying colour (Ball, 2004).

CRT has become universally used in paediatrics (APLSG, 2005); it does, however, have a number of limitations as a marker of peripheral perfusion. These limitations include the effects of ambient temperature and environmental lighting conditions, as well as different values being recorded at different sites of assessment. All these factors have been shown to have a bearing on the value obtained. With regards to the age continuum from newborns to young adults, its range varies from 2 seconds to 4 seconds (Raju, 1999). But despite its limitations, CRT does have a role as **one** of the physiological assessments of peripheral perfusion, to be used in combination with other markers such as heart rate, respiratory rate and level of consciousness (Leonard and Beattie, 2004).

Measurement of CRT

Reasons for the procedure

- To evaluate the ability of the circulatory system to restore blood to the capillary system (perfusion)

Pre-procedure

Specific patient preparation

- Ensure the environment is child friendly, provide toys and a quiet area and ensure privacy and dignity is maintained
- Explain all procedures and care in an age/developmentally appropriate way to both the child and family. Encourage parental participation to promote child cooperation and understanding (NPSA, 2004)
- Obtain consent prior to the procedure. The child, or their carer, may give consent so long as they are informed of the implications, potential side-effects and alternatives. If they are competent, seek informed consent directly from the child (British Medical Association, 2001; Department of Health, 2001)
- Consider the age of child and the effects of ambient temperature and environmental lighting on the site of CRT and the reliability of the result (for example, exposure of small hands to a cool ambient temperature will falsely lengthen the CRT time)

During the procedure

- Wash your hands to ensure there is reduced risk of infection (Department of Health, 2003)
- Ensure you explain the forthcoming procedure to reduce the child's anxiety
- Determine the site with the best pulsatile vascular bed – avoid sites distal to indwelling arterial lines, blood pressure cuffs, arteriovenous fistulas and blood transfusions, as these will restrict pulsatile flow and lengthen CRT time
- If the child has been in a warm ambient temperature for over 30 minutes, place your thumb on the sole of their foot (*Figure 6.5*) or fleshy part of the hand (*Figure 6.6*). If the child has been in a cool ambient temperature for over 30 minutes, place your thumb on their sternum

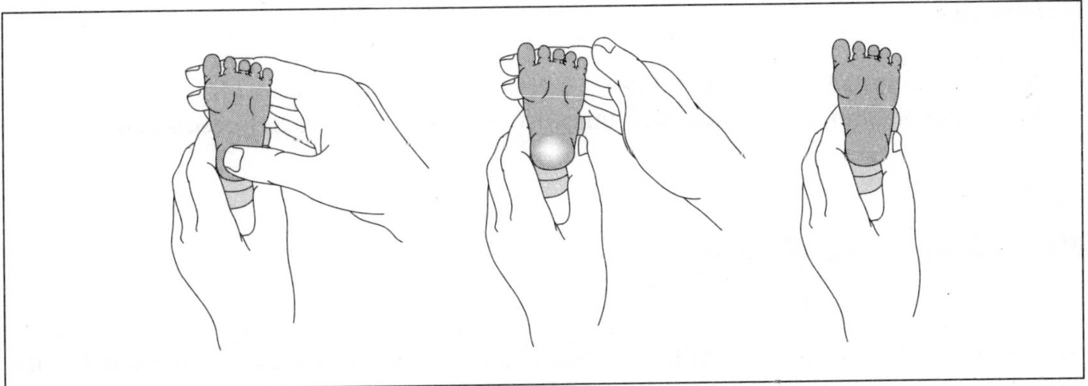

Figure 6.5: Testing capillary refill time on the sole of the foot. Press the sole firmly (left), release (middle) and count as the colour returns to the blanched tissue (right)

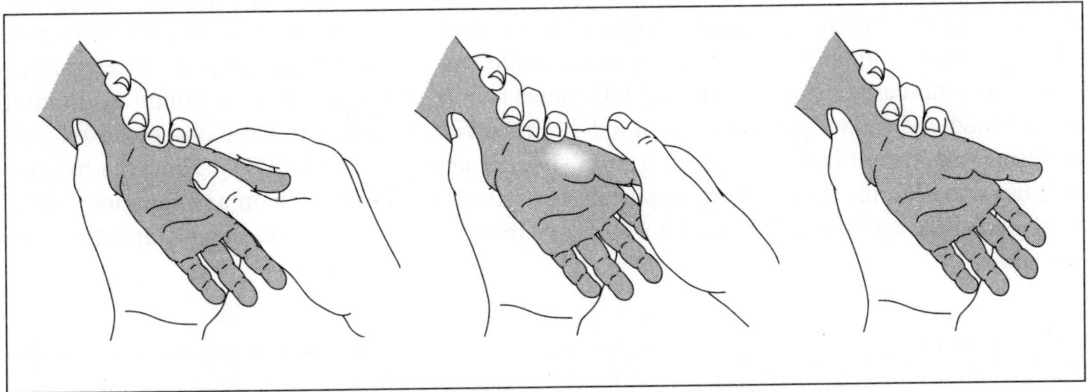

Figure 6.6: Testing capillary refill time on the palm of the hand. Press the fleshy part of hand firmly (left), release (middle) and count as the colour returns to the blanched tissue (right)

- Gently compress with sufficient pressure to cause the skin to blanche (go white), indicating that blood has been forced out of the capillaries in the tissue (blanching). Do this for 5 seconds to standardise the process (APLSG, 2005)
- Release the pressure and count in seconds (one million…two million…three million…') as you observe the skin return to its normal colour
- As the capillaries refill, the nail bed returns to a normal deep pink colour. Capillary refill should be both prompt and pink
- Colour should be restored in about the time it takes to say 'capillary refill', that is within:
  - 3 seconds in neonates
  - 2 seconds in children
- Prolonged CRT is due to vasoconstriction, which may be caused by hypovolaemia, hypothermia, fear or pain
- Wash your hands (Department of Health, 2003)

Post-procedure

- Maintain documentation (NMC, 2004).
- Report abnormalities to medical staff immediately as part of an overall assessment

Monitoring blood glucose

Glucose is a simple sugar that provides an immediate energy source for cell metabolism. It is the preferred source of energy for brain cells, which rely on adequate supplies as the brain has very limited glycogen stores. Glucose is derived from carbohydrates, which are digested in the gut to produce glucose as the end product. Together with oxygen, glucose is used by cells to synthesise adenosine triphosphate (ATP), a high-energy molecule that provides the chemical energy for effective cellular function (Kanneh, 2006). Glucose is the major substrate of brain metabolism – ketone bodies, although easily used by brain tissue, are normally found in low concentrations which only increase during fasting; and fatty acids cannot be used as they are bound to albumin in the blood and cannot penetrate the blood–brain barrier. A decline in the blood glucose level, therefore, may result in neurological injury (Theorell and Degenhart, 2003). Thus, the balance of glucose within the body is very important for effective cell metabolism and function, and it is of particular importance to children with metabolic disorders. Normal levels are shown in *Box 6.8.*

Box 6.8: Normal paediatric blood glucoses levels

Neonate	2.6 mmol/L (Aynsley-Green, 1989)
Child	3.3–7 mmol/L (Hanas, 2004)

Point-of-care testing (POCT)

POCT is defined as any analytical test performed outside the conventional laboratory setting (MDA, 2002). Among these are:

- Near-patient testing (NPT)
- Bedside testing
- Extra-laboratory testing
- Disseminated laboratory testing

Prior to undertaking POCT it is important that those carrying out the tests are aware of the Medical Devices Agency recommendations (MDA, 1996) to ensure safety. You must be aware of all these factors:

- The manufacturer's instructions and any contraindications for use (discrepancies have arisen when they were not followed; Roche Advantage, 2007)
- The intended purpose of the device
- Interpretation of the results (especially important because a suspect test result may result in inappropriate patient management
- Limitations of use (within manufacturer's guidelines)
- Sample requirements and type
- Storage of reagents
- Expiry dates
- Quality-assurance procedures (including daily checking of device and record keeping)
- Health and safety issues (including safe disposal of sharps and prevention of needlestick injuries) (MDA, 2001)

Contraindications to extra-laboratory blood glucose measurement

According to the Medical Devices Agency (MDA, 1996) blood glucose testing should not be conducted in the following cases:

- **Peripheral circulatory failure** (eg. severe dehydration, hyperglycaemic-hyperosmolar state with or without ketosis, hypotension, shock, peripheral vascular disease)
- **Severe dehydration** (eg. vomiting or diarrhoea, prescription drugs (such as diuretics), inability to recognise or respond to 'thirst' sensations, sustained uncontrolled diabetes)
- **Variations in blood oxygen tension** (eg. patients receiving intensive oxygen therapy)
- **High concentrations of non-glucose-reducing substances in the blood** (eg. intravenous infusion of ascorbic acid can depress readings)
- **High bilirubin values** (eg. jaundice, above 0.43 mmol/L can increase readings)
- **Extremes of haematocrit** (eg. neonatal blood samples)
- **Dialysis treatment** (eg. may elevate readings)
- **Hyperlipaemia** (eg. containing abnormal fat concentrations (for example, cholesterol above 5.6 mmol/L may elevate readings))

Sites for blood glucose testing

It is common practice to carry out the procedure on the outer side of a finger. Other sites are available but are not often used in practice (eg. the forearm, palm or thigh). New lancing devices allow a shallow skin puncture to be performed at these alternative sites, but research has shown that rapid changes in blood glucose levels may be detected at fingertip sites before the forearm (Ellison *et al*, 2002). Moreover, such alternative sites are not all the same; routine testing on an un-rubbed forearm, upper arm, thigh or calf gives a test result that is 20–30 minutes old, which is the same as the conventional finger-site test.

The National Committee for Clinical Laboratory Standards (1992) identified that capillary punctures should not be performed at or through the following sites:

- The posterior curvature of the heel (the device may puncture the bone or calluses may form on it)
- The fingers of neonates (risk of nerve damage)
- Previous puncture sites
- Inflamed, swollen or oedematous tissues
- Cyanotic or poorly perfused tissues
- Localised areas of infection
- Peripheral arteries

The Medical Devices Agency (2002) outlines the risk of the misleading results obtained from POCT and the need for adequate training.

Blood glucose measurement

Reasons for the procedure

- To provide a guide for baseline measurement of capillary blood glucose at the time of the test (BNFc, 2006)
- To provide serial measurements to guide clinical management and allow change in treatment as per hospital protocol (Bayer Diagnostics, 2007); treatment is also based on laboratory results
- To detect high (hyperglycaemia) and low (hypoglycaemia) blood glucose
- Be aware of manufacturer's contraindications (as shown above)

Pre-procedure

Equipment required

- Glucometer and testing strips
- Lancet device
- Sterile gauze/cotton wool
- Gloves
- Apron
- Sharps container

Specific patient preparation

- Ensure a quality control test has been carried out on the glucometer and the results recorded, to ensure the equipment is accurate prior to testing (MDA, 1996)
- Ensure testing strips are in date and the machine is calibrated according to the manufacturer's instructions
- Ensure a new lancet used each time to prevent contamination, infection or risk of needlestick injury (MDA, 2001)

During the procedure

- Obtain consent from the child and parent when able
- Give a full explanation of the procedure, to promote understanding, cooperation and trust and to allow a partnership in care
- Check that the site is clean because there may be contamination from sugary substances which can interfere with the result (Cowan, 1997). If necessary, wash the child's hand or clean the located site with soap and water. Dry thoroughly with cotton-wool or gauze. Do *not* use alcohol wipes; they may give a false reading and toughen the skin if used repeatedly (Roche Advantage, 2007; Bayer Diagnostics, 2007)
- Practice standard precautions to lower the risk of cross infection and contamination; wash your hands and put on gloves
- If the child's hand is cold then allow it to warm up before trying to obtain a blood sample (washing hands in warm water is a useful way to do this)
- The side of the finger is less painful as it has fewer nerve endings; it is also easier to apply the drop of blood to the test pad from here. Avoid using the index finger and thumb as these are the more commonly used digits (*Figure 6.7*)
- Prick the side of the finger with the lancet device. Promote blood flow to the site using gravity by allowing the arm to hang down by the child's side if possible
- Dispose of the lancet device or lancet section of the device directly into a sharps bin to reduce the risk of needlestick injury
- About 5 seconds after pricking the finger, gently 'milk' the blood from the finger. Do *not* squeeze the finger as this will cause the capillaries to contract and prevent blood flow, and tissue fluid may contaminate the sample
- Ensure that the test strip is covered
- Apply gentle pressure to the puncture site with sterile gauze to prevent haematoma formation and bleeding

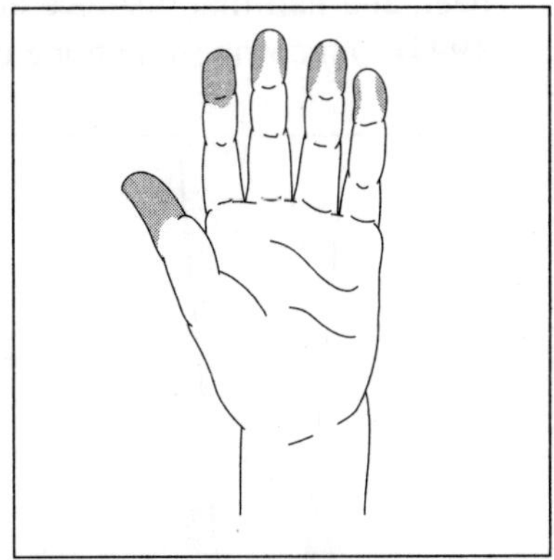

Figure 6.7: Areas on the hand that should not be pricked for taking glucose measurements

Special considerations in the neonate and infant under 6 months

- Assess the need for the baby to have this test carried out. It may be more appropriate to time it with venous blood sampling
- Fundamentally the procedure is the same but there are several differences
- Position the baby in a semi-lateral/supine position with the cot tilted or on a parent's knee
- Facilitate self-regulatory behaviour through hands to mouth position/non-nutritive sucking/ sucking at the breast
- Allowing a tilt on the cot or on the parent's knee means the baby's foot hangs lower than the torso, improving blood flow
- Snuggle or position the baby to maintain a neutral flexed position, which helps to facilitate self-regulatory behaviour and helps the infant cope with the painful procedure (McIntosh *et al,* 1994)
- Ensure the heel of the foot is warm (either with a commercially available heel-warming device or by placing the heel on a latex glove filled with warm water at <42°C for 5–10 minutes) to increase blood flow, thereby reducing haemolysis and bruising (Barker *et al*, 1996)
- Place a towel under the heel to prevent blood spillage on the cot clothing (leading to unnecessary handling of infant)
- Grasp the heel firmly but gently with the index finger wrapped around the foot supporting the arch, and the thumb wrapped around the ankle and below the proposed safe puncture site (this reduces the risk of the baby moving, which would lead to the inadvertent puncture of the wrong area of the heel or needlestick injury to the person carrying out the test)
- Raise the foot above the baby's heart level and select the site to be punctured (avoiding any oedematous area or previous puncture sites)
- Identify a 'safe' area to lance the heel. Remember, the calcaneus bone of the preterm baby may be as little as 2.4 mm below the surface of the plantar surface (bottom) of the heel, and half that distance at the posterior curvature (back) of the heel (Barker *et al*, 1994); puncturing this bone can cause painful osteomyelitis or bone infection as well as

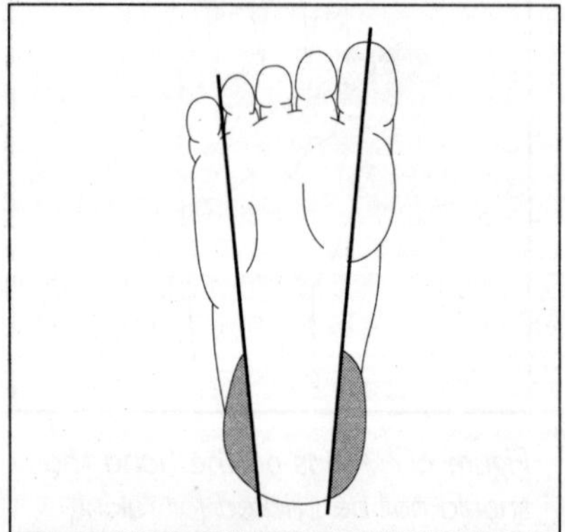

Figure 6.8: Safe sites for lancing or puncturing the infant heel

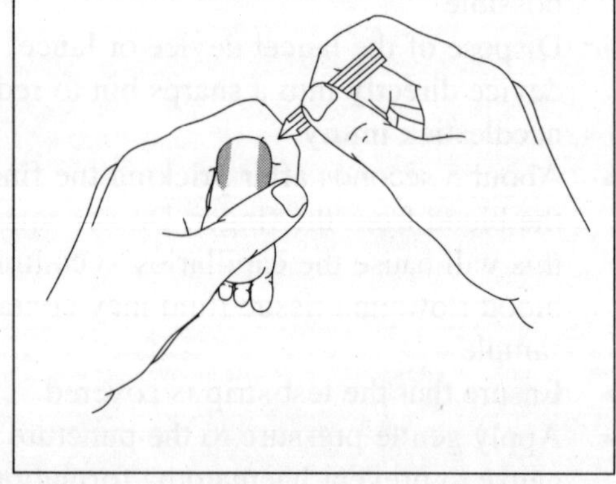

Figure 6.9: Holding and lancing the infant heel

osteochondritis, inflammation of the bone and cartilage. There are two safe areas (*Figure 6.8*):
  - One lies at the bottom of a line that extends posteriorly from a point between the fourth and fifth toes and runs parallel to the lateral aspect of the heel
  - One lies at the bottom of a line that extends posteriorly from the middle of the great toe and runs parallel to the medial aspect of the heel
- Puncture the site (*Figure 6.9*) within the safe area shown, avoiding previous puncture sites (puncturing a previously used site may spread infection) (Meehan, 1998)

Post-procedure

- Apply gentle pressure to the puncture site because neonates, particularly those born prematurely, have prolonged clotting times (Boxwell, 2001)
- Wash your hands
- Maintain documentation (NMC, 2004)
- Report abnormalities to medical staff immediately as part of an overall assessment

References

Advanced Paediatric Life Support Group (2005) *Advanced Paediatric Life Support: The Practical Approach*, 4th edn. BMJ Books: Blackwell Publishing, London

Aynsley-Green A (1989) Hypoglycaemia. In: Brook CGD (ed) *Clinical Paediatric Endocrinology*, 2nd edn. Blackwell Scientific, Oxford

Aylott M (2006a) Life threatening illness and the family. In: Glasper EA, Richardson J (eds). *A Textbook for Children's and Young People's Nursing*. Elsevier, Edinburgh

Aylott M (2006b) Developing rigour in observation of the sick child: Part 1. *Paediatr Nurs* **18**(8): 38–44

Aylott M (2007a) Observing the sick child: Part 2b Respiratory palpation. *Paediatr Nurs* **19**(1): 38–44

Aylott M (2007b) Observing the sick child: Part 2b Respiratory auscultation. *Paediatr Nurs* **19**(3): 38–45

Ball TM (2004) Review: capillary refill time, abnormal skin turgor, and abnormal respiratory pattern help to detect dehydration in children. *Arch Dis Child Ed Pract* **291:** 2746–54

Barber J. Campbell A, Morgan L (eds) (2000) *Clinical Care Manual For Children's Nursing. The Birmingham Children's Hospital NHS Trust*. Quay Books, Wiltshire

Bayer Diagnostics (2007) *Technical information bulletin: Finger Pricking for Capillary Blood Collection and Testing*. Bayer, Berkshire

Barker DP, Latly BW, Ruuer N (1994) Heel blood sampling in preterm infant: which technique? *Arch Dis Child Fetal Neonat Edn* **74**(2): 206–08

Barker DP, Willets B, Cappendijk VC, Rutter N (1996) Capillary blood sampling: should the heel be warmed? *Arch Dis Child Fetal Neonat Edn* **71:** F139–F140

Bloxham N (2007) Pulse oximetry. In: Glasper A, McEwing G, Richardson J. *Oxford Handbook of Children's and Young People's Nursing*. Oxford University Press, Oxford

Boxwell G (2001) *Neonatal Intensive Care Nursing*. Routledge, London

British Medical Association (2001) *Consent, Rights and Choices in Health Care for Children and Young People*. BMJ Books, London

British National Formulary for Children (BNFc) (2007) *British National Formulary*. BNF/BMJ, London

British Thoracic Society (2005) *British Guideline on the Management of Asthma. A National Clinical Guideline*. British Thoracic Society , London

Brown A (2007) Assessing a child's temperature. In: Glasper A, McEwing G, Richardson J (eds) *Oxford Handbook of Children's and Young People's Nursing*. Oxford University Press, Oxford

Bumke K, Maconochie I (2001) Paediatric capillary refill times. *Trauma* **3**(4): 212–20

Chandler T (2000) Oxygen saturation monitoring. *Paediatr Nurs* **12**(8): 37–42

Childs C, Harrison R, Hodkinson C (1999) Tympanic membrane temperature as a measure of core temperature. *Arch Dis Child* **80**(3): 262–67

Cowan T (1997) Blood glucose monitoring devices. *Profess Nurs* **12**(8): 503–96, 599

Craig JV, Lancaster GA, Taylor S, Williamson PR, Smyth RL (2003) *BMJ* **326**(7380): 60

Department of Health DOH) (2001) *Seeking Consent: Working with Children*. The Stationary Office, London

Department of Health (DOH) (2003) *Winning Ways: Working Together to Reduce Healthcare Associated Infection in England*. DH, London

Ellison JM, Stegman JM, Culner SL, Sharma MK, Ervin KR, Horwitz DL, Michael RH (2002) *Rapid changes in postprandial blood glucose produces concentration differences at finger, forearm and thigh sampling sites*. Diabet Care **25**(6): 961–64

European Resuscitation Council (2004) *European Paediatric Life Support Course Provider Manual for use in the UK,* 1st edn. European Resuscitation Council and Resuscitation council (UK) , London

Grap MJ (1998) Pulse oximetry. *Crit Care Nurs* **18:** 94–99

Hall MN, Grim CM (1991) How to take a precise blood pressure. *Am J Nurs* **41**(2): 38–42

Hanas R (2004) *Type 1 Diabetes in children, Adolescents and Young Adults,* 2nd edn. Class Publishing, Sweden

Hanowell L, Eisele JH, Downs D (1987) Ambient light affects pulse oximeters. *Anesthesiology* **67:** 864–65

Harrison M (2007) Care of a child with raised body temperature. In: Glasper EA, McEwing G, Richardson J (eds) *Oxford Handbook of Children's and Young People's Nursing*. Oxford University Press, Oxford

Hill E (2000) *Practical applications of pulse oximetry*. Update in Anaesthesia www.nda.ox.ac.uk/wfsa/html/u11/u1104_01.htm

Hoo A (2004) The respiratory system in infancy and early childhood. In: Neill S, Knowles H (eds) *The Biology of Child Health. Palgrave Macmillan, Basingstoke*

Hudson H (2003) Stethoscopes and infection control: a study into the use of stethoscopes in a paediatric ward and their possible contamination. J Child Hlth Care **7**(2): 142–3; discussion p. 144

Hwu YJ, Coates VE, Lin FY (2000) A study of the effectiveness of different measuring times and counting methods of human radial pulse rates. *J Clin Nurs* **9**: 146–52

Kanneh AB (2006) Caring for children with body fluid and electrolyte imbalance. In: Glasper A, Richardson J (eds) *A Textbook of Children's and Young People's Nursing*. Churchill Livingstone, Edinburgh

Leonard PA, Beattie TF (2004) Is measurement of capillary refill time useful as part of the initial assessment of children? *Eur J Emerg Med* **11**(3): 158–63

Lockwood C, Conroy-Hiller T, Page T (2004) *Systematic Review: Vital Signs*. Joanna Briggs Centre for Evidence-Based Nursing, Adelaide

Marieb EN (2004) *Human Anatomy and Physiology*, 6th edn. Addison-Wesley, San Francisco

Mcintosh N, Van Veen L, Braymeyer H (1994) Alleviation of the pain of heel prick in preterm infants. *Arch Dis Child* **70:** F177–F181

Medical Devices Agency (1996) *Safety notice 16: Extra Laboratory Use of Blood Glucose Meters and Test Strips: Contraindications, Training and Advice to Users*. MDA, London

Medical Devices Agency (2001) *Safety Notice 19: The Safe Use and Disposal of Sharps*. MDA, London

Medical Devices Agency (2002) *Management of IVD Point of Care Test Devices DB 2002 (3)*. MDA, London

Meehan RM (1998) Heel sticks in neonates for capillary blood sampling. *Neonat Net* **17**(1): 17–24

Milner AD, Greenough A (2004) Applied respiratory physiology. *Curr Paed*, **12:** 51–56

Noble A, Johnson R, Thomas A, Bass P (2005) Arterial blood pressure. In: Noble R, Johnson R (eds) *The Cardiovascular System Basic Science and Clinical Conditions*. Churchill Livingstone, Edinburgh

Monaghan A (2005) Detecting and managing deterioration in children. *Paediatr Nurs* **17**(1): 32–35

National Committee for Clinical Laboratory Standards (1992) *Procedures for the Collection of Diagnostic Blood Specimens by Skin Puncture*, 3rd edn. NCCLS, Villanova PA

National Patient Safety Agency (2004) *Right Patient- Right Care*. NPSA, London

Neill S, Knowles H (2004) *The Biology of Child Health: A Reader in Development and Assessment*. Palgrave Macmillan, Basingstoke

National Institute for Clinical Excellence (2006) *Feverish Illness in Children*. NICE, London

O'Brien E (2002) Has conventional sphygmomanometry ended with the banning of mercury? *Blood Press Monit* **7:** 37–40

Panitch HB (2005) *Pediatric Pulmonology: The Requisites in Pediatrics*. Elsevier Mosby, Philadelphia

Pickering TG (2003) What will replace the mercury sphygmomanometer? *Blood Press Monit* **8:** 23–25

Pickersgill J, Fowler H, Bootham J, Thompson K (2003) Temperature taking: children's preferences. *Paediatr Nurs* **15**(2): 22–26

Raju V (1999) Capillary refill time in the hands and feet of normal newborn infants. *Clin Pediatr* **38**(3): 139–44

Robertson RE, Kaplan RE (1991) Another site for the pulse oximeter probe. *Anesthesiology* **74:** 198

Roche Advantage (2007) *Blood Glucose Monitor: User's Manual*. Roche, Indianapolis

Rudolf M, Levene M (2006) *Paediatrics and Child Health*, 2nd edn. Blackwell Publishing, Oxford

Rush M, Wetherall A (2003) Temperature measurement: Practice guidelines. *Paediatr Nurs* **15**(9): 25–28

Schutz SL (2001) Oxygen saturation monitoring by pulse oximetry. *AACN Procedure Manual for Critical Care*, 4th edn. WB Saunders, New York

Smith SF, Duell DJ, Martin BC (2005) *Clinical Nursing Skills: Basic To Advanced*, 6th edn. Pearson Prentice Hall, New Jersey

Strebor AD (2005) Basic principles of non-invasive blood pressure measurement in infants. *Adv Neonat Care* **5**(5): 252–61

Taylor C (2006) Primary care nursing. Managing infants with pyrexia. *Nurs Times* **102**(39): 42–43

Theorell C, Degenhart M (2003) Assessment and management of the metabolic system. In: Kenner C, Wright Lott J (eds) *Comprehensive Neonatal Nursing: A Physiologic Perspective*, 3rd edn. Elsevier Science, London

Tholl U, Forstner K, Anlauf M (2004) Measuring blood pressure: Pitfalls and recommendations. *Nephrol Dialysis Transplant* **19**(4): 766–70

Tortora GJ (2005) *Principles of Human Anatomy*, 10th edn. Wiley, Danvers

Tortora GJ, Derrickson B (2007) *Introduction to the Human Body: The Essentials of Anatomy and Physiology*, 7th edn. Wiley, Danvers

Wahr JA, Tremper KK, Dlab M (1995) Pulse oximetry. *Respir Care Clin N Am* **1:** 77–105

Further reading

British National Formulary for Children (2006) *Blood Glucose Monitoring*. BMJ/RPS/RCPCH Publishing, London

Candy D, Davies G, Ross E (2001) *Clinical Paediatrics and Child Health*. WB Saunders, Edinburgh

Kelsey J, McEwing G (2006) Respiratory illness in children. In: Glasper A, Richardson J (eds) *A Textbook of Children's and Young People's Nursing*. Churchill Livingstone, Edinburgh

Useful websites

Accu-Check
www.accu-check.co.uk

BD Diabetes Education
www.bddiabetes.com

Up-to-date Patient Information
www.patients.uptodate.com

Chapter 7

Fundamental aspects to safe administration of medicine

Gary Barrett, Terri Fletcher and Tiffany Russell

Administration of medicines

Most medications are prescribed, dispensed and administered safely and effectively. However, since humans are involved there is always a risk of error, and mistakes occasionally occur (Cousins, 2006). Medicine administration is the most common therapeutic intervention carried out in the National Health Service and is an essential area of responsibility for the nurse. Indeed, the nurse is often the last checker in the process and is pivotal in preventing serious harm to patients (Audit Commission, 2001). Children are especially vulnerable to medication errors (Conroy *et al*, 2007).

Risk areas have been identified in the following areas:

- Calculation checking procedures
- Failure to follow double-checking procedures
- Failure to follow patient-identity checking procedures
- Poor administration technique
- Poor documentation

A medicine may be defined as any substance or combination of substances used to prevent or treat disease, and the administration of a medicine is a term used to define the act of putting into effect a medicine, either by introduction into the body or by external application (Department of Health [DH], 1999). In order to comply with legislation, national and local protocols should be followed when administering medications.

There are a number of guiding principles for children's nurses when undertaking the administration of medicines. The National Service Framework for Children (Department of Health, 2004) clearly outlines that the administration of medicines must be based on the best available evidence to underpin practice. The Guidelines for the Administration of Medicines (Nursing and Midwifery Council [NMC], 2004a) states that:

> *"The administration of medicines is an important aspect of the professional practice of persons whose names are on the Council's register. It is not solely a mechanistic task to be performed in strict compliance with the written prescription of a medical practitioner. It requires thought and the exercise of professional judgement..."*

As a nurse, you are accountable for all medications that you administer. To ensure safe administration of medicines to children, nurses require knowledge and a comprehensive understanding of the medications being taken by children in their care (Royal College of Paediatrics and Child Health, 1999; British National Formulary for Children [BNFC], 2005).

REMEMBER, in the administration of any medication you should always refer to local policies.

All prescriptions should be written legibly and should include the following:

- The child's name, date of birth and identification number
- The child's weight in kilograms
- Allergies documented (awareness of the constituents of medications is essential, for example co-amoxiclav contains both amoxicillin and clavulanic acid)
- The date that the prescription was written, the signature of the prescriber, and their printed name
- The medication and dosage, the route of administration, the time of administration and the duration of the treatment
- Only recognised abbreviations may be used

In recent years the use of Patient Group Directives (PGD) has grown. A PGD is a written direction relating to the supply and administration, or just administration, of a prescription-only medication by certain healthcare professionals (British National Formulary for Children, 2006). For children's nurses this means that a PGD signed by a doctor and agreed by a pharmacist can be used to supply and administer prescription-only medicines to children based on an individual assessment of the child's needs (Royal College of Nursing, 2004). Only nurses who have received appropriate training and have been deemed 'competent' following local NHS trust policy are able to administer medications under the guidance of a PGD. See *Table 7.1* for the main principles for safe administration of medicines.

Table 7.1: Key points to guide safe administration of medicines (adapted from Watt, 2003b)

Problem	Action
The prescription is illegible or ambiguous	Do not second guess and administer Inform the prescriber and ask for the prescription to be rewritten
The prescription is incomplete (eg. no route, mg/mL not defined)	Do not assume you know and administer Inform the prescriber and ask for the prescription to be rewritten
The prescription has been altered after it has been written	Do not use Ask for the prescription to be rewritten in full
Dose deviates from formulary guidance	Do not give Discuss with the prescriber but if doubt remains check with the pharmacist
Discrepancy in dose calculation	Do not be intimidated – you are accountable for your actions Re-check independently and then again with a third person if necessary
Identity of child not clear	If no parent is present and the child is unable to confirm their identity, do not administer If urgent, contact the parents/guardian
Medicine not signed for by nurse previously caring for child	Do not repeat Check with nurse concerned
Medicine previously prepared but no expiry date has been completed on label	Do not use Discard and start again

Checking procedures for safe administration of medications

The administration of medications should follow one of these schemes of safe practice – the five principles embodied by the '5Rs' and the '5Cs'.

The 5Rs (recommended by Parboteeah, 2002)

- Right medication
- Right amount

- Right patient
- Right time
- Right route

The 5Cs (identified by Watt, 2003b)

- Correct child
- Correct medicine
- Correct dose
- Correct time
- Correct route

Just as nurses know the 5Rs or the 5Cs of medicine administration, they should also know what rights they have when administering medications. These '6 rights' for the nurse – that is *your* six rights – in administering medications offer further guidance in caring and maintaining a safe environment.

The 6 rights of nurses

- The right to a complete and clearly written prescription form
- The right to have the correct medication dose and medication for the route dispensed
- The right to have access to medication information
- The right to have written policies on medication administration
- The right to administer medications safely and to identify problems in the system
- The right to stop, think and be vigilant when administering medications

Medication errors

Your first responsibility is *to ensure the safety of the child first*. The ward, unit or area manager must be informed immediately of any instances of a missed dose or error in the medication process. Medical advice must be sought immediately. Such an 'adverse event' must be reported by completing an incident form (Royal College of Nursing, 2005a). A medication error can be defined as any preventable event that may cause or lead to inappropriate medication use or patient harm, while the medication is in the control of the healthcare professional. Such events may be related to:

- Professional malpractice
- Healthcare products, procedures and systems, including:
  - Prescribing
  - Product labelling
  - Packaging and nomenclature
  - Compounding

- Dispensing
- Distribution
- Administration
- Education
- Monitoring
- Use

This is then reported by the trust, institution or service to the Medicines and Healthcare Related Agency (MHRA) via the yellow card system.

Calculation of medicine doses

There is a significant amount of research that indicates that calculation errors in paediatrics are an ongoing problem. Calliari (1995) demonstrated a correlation of nurses failing calculation tests and subsequent drug errors. Lerwill (1999) found that in qualified staff only 59% scored more than 50% in calculation tests. Barrett (2007) demonstrated that out of 206 second-year student nurses undertaking child branch, the average score was only 53.3% in a simple scenario-structured calculation test. It has also been reported that calculation errors have resulted in fatal consequences where Incorrect placement of the decimal point during the calculation resulted in 10 times the prescribed dose of digoxin being administered (Stephenson, 2005). There are a growing number of incidents which result in iatrogenic disease, many of which can be attributed to prescribed medical treatment (Ross *et al*, 2000; Watt, 2003a).

Many medicines administered to children require complex calculations (Cohen, 2000) and errors are more significant where small volumes are involved (Smith, 2004). It is your responsibility as a nurse to minimise the risk of such errors and there is no substitute for arithmetical knowledge or conscientious practice (Nursing and Midwifery Council, 2004a).

In order to calculate medications accurately you must understand some of the standard mathematical calculations. A useful summary of information is provided in *Box 7.1*.

Box 7.1: Standard mathematical calculations

Base units

Weight	Gram (g)
Volume	Litre (L)
Amount of substance	Mole (mol)

Prefixes used in clinical practice

Mega- (M)	A million units
Kilo- (k)	A thousand units
Deci- (d)	A tenth of a unit
Centi- (c)	A hundredth of a unit
Milli- (m)	A thousandth of a unit
Micro- (μ)*	A millionth of a unit
Nano- (n)	A thousand millionth of a unit

Units used in clinical practice

1 kilogram (kg)	1000 grams (g)
1 gram (g)	1000 milligrams (mg)
1 milligram (mg)	1000 micrograms (μg/mcg)
1 microgram (μg)*	1000 nanograms (ng)
1 litre (L)	1000 millilitres (mL)
1 mole (mol)	1000 millimoles (mmol)
1 millimole (mmol)	1000 micromoles (μmol)

*The abbreviation commonly used for microgram is mcg.

Conversion of units

It is quite likely that you will need to convert metric units in order to be able to accurately calculate the dose of the drug required. For example, a doctor may have prescribed 0.125 mg of digoxin (a cardiac drug). Digoxin is provided as 250 μg (mcg) in 5 mL solution. Here you are working with two different metric units – mg and μg. To ensure that you administer the correct dose to the patient, you need to work in the same metric unit to reduce calculation errors.

Throughout the following calculations we will use the abbreviation mcg for the unit μg.

Conversion of one unit to another

Normally to convert from a LARGER unit to a SMALLER unit, you multiply by 1000 (move the decimal point three places to the right).

- 0.125 mg to mcg = 0.125 mg × 1000 = 125 mcg
- Note that the larger unit (mg) is multiplied by 1000 to get the smaller unit (mcg) that you wish to work with in your calculation

Normally to convert from a SMALLER unit to a LARGER unit, you divide by 1000 (move the decimal point three places to the left).

For example:

- 2000 g to kg = 2000 g ÷ 1000 = 2 kg
- Note that the decimal point moves three to the left, so that 2000 g becomes 2.000 kg

This conversion is crucially important in paediatrics, given that we often work in elixir and fluids, and failure to convert to the same metric units when calculating can result in over- or under-dosing the child.

REMEMBER

- 1 gram (g) = 1000 milligrams (mg)
- 1 milligram (mg) = 1000 micrograms (mcg)
- 1 litre (L) = 1000 millilitres (mL)

The conversion rules

To convert between grams and milligrams:

mg	to	**g**	*divide by*	1000
g	to	**mg**	*multiply by*	1000

To convert between micrograms and milligrams:

mcg(μg)	to	**mg**	*divide by*	1000
mg	to	**mcg(μg)**	*multiply by*	1000

Calculating the volume of drug to administer

The amount of drug prescribed is often different from the strength of the drug available to you. It is therefore essential that you can work out the required dose using the following standard calculation formula for administering drugs.

The formula

$$\frac{\text{WHAT YOU WANT}}{\text{WHAT YOU'VE GOT}} \times \frac{\text{WHAT IT'S IN}}{1}$$

Where:
What you want = the dose of medicine prescribed by the doctor/nurse
What you've got = the amount of substance/drug you have
What it's in = the volume of solution that the amount of substance is in

For example:

- The doctor prescribes 60 mg of paracetamol suspension (*What you want*)
- The drug comes in a bottle of 120 mg (*What you've got*) in 5 mL (*What it's in*)

Thus:

$$\frac{60}{120} \times \frac{5}{1} \quad \begin{array}{l}\textit{(Top numbers)}\\ \textit{(Bottom numbers)}\end{array}$$

REMEMBER when using this formula that you MUST obey the rules of the formula for a correct calculation:

- You can only multiply the 60 and 5 together and only multiply the 120 and 1 together – never multiply a *top* number with a *bottom* number
- You can only divide a top and bottom number together – never divide the 60 with the 5 or the 120 with the 1

Until you are familiar with this format you can write the formula as below to remind you of the basic rules of this formula:

$$\frac{60 \times 5}{120 \times 1}$$

Therefore:

$$\frac{60 \times 5}{120 \times 1} = \frac{300}{120}$$

We can simplify this calculation by looking for a common denominator to reduce the size of the numbers. The common denominator is a number that goes into the number above and the number below the division line. If you have numbers above and below the line that end in a 0 you can remove the 0 (providing you remove an equal number of 0s from above and below the division line). For example:

$$\frac{300}{120} = \frac{30\emptyset}{12\emptyset} = \frac{30}{12}$$

This can be further reduced by using another common denominator – the number 2 – whereby both 30 and 12 can be divided by 2. REMEMBER what you do above the division line you must also do below. Therefore:

$$\frac{30}{12} = \frac{15}{6}$$

This can be reduced yet further with another common denominator – the number 3 – whereby both 15 and 6 can be divided by 3. Remember what you do above the division line you must also do below:

$$\frac{15}{6} = \frac{5}{2}$$

There are no other common denominators of the numbers 5 and 2, so the remaining numbers must be divided to arrive at a final calculation. Some people get confused at this point, about whether to divide the 5 by the 2 or divide 2 by 5. This is crucially important as obviously these two sums have *very* different answers! For example:

5 divided by 2 is 2.5 mL
2 divided by 5 is 0.4 mL

As you can see this can lead to a significantly wrong dose being administered to the child. A simple way to remember the correct approach to this final part of the calculation is to read the sum as you do words on the page of a book – from top to bottom! Thus:

$\frac{5}{2}$ *reads as 5 divided by 2 (ie. 2.5 mL)*

As you become more familiar with the calculation formula you can start to take shortcuts to safely speed up the process. For example:

$$\frac{60}{120} \times \frac{5}{1}$$

This can be reduced before you commence your calculation, using the rule mentioned above.

$$\frac{60}{120} \times \frac{5}{1} = \frac{6\not{0}}{12\not{0}} \times \frac{5}{1} = \frac{6}{12} \times \frac{5}{1}$$

It can still be reduced by using a common denominator, this time 3, which goes into 6 twice and into 12 four times.

$$\frac{6}{12} \times \frac{5}{1} = \frac{2}{4} \times \frac{5}{1}$$

Now you can do one further reduction before performing the calculation:

$$\frac{2}{4} \times \frac{5}{1} = \frac{1}{2} \times \frac{5}{1} = \frac{5}{2}$$

Therefore:

$$5 \text{ divided by } 2 \text{ (or } 2\overline{)5}\text{) } = 2.5\,\text{mL}$$

The GEC system

An additional safety mechanism to reduce the likelihood of calculation errors is to adopt the GEC system (Barrett, 2007). This is a triple-checking system that reduces the chance of getting an answer with the decimal point in the wrong place – ordinarily the most common calculation error in paediatrics (Cohen, 2000). The GEC system should be used for every calculation and is a simple 'belt and braces' mechanism.

The letters GEC stand for *Guesstimate*, *Estimate* and *Calculate*.

1. Guesstimate

First, guess the volume of medication to be administered, for example the doctor or nurse has prescribed 50 mg of liquid paracetamol. It comes in a solution of 120 mg in 5 mL. We know that

50 mg is less than 120 mg so we can see that we require less than 5 mL volume. Any subsequent calculation that gives an answer greater than 5 mL will alert you to a potential error.

2. Estimate

Second, estimate the volume of medication to be administered. Using the same example, we can see that if we have 120 mg in 5 mL, half of the dose would be 60 mg and that would be in half of the volume, 2.5 mL. If we halve the dose again we have 30 mg in half that volume, 1.25 mL, and so on. What we need is 50 mg, and from our estimates we see that we would get this from a volume of drug of less than 2.5 mL but greater than 1.25 mL (50 mg falls between 30 mg and 60 mg). Any calculation outside that range would alert you to a potential calculation error.

3. Calculate

Third, perform the calculation to obtain a precise answer, using the formula above. In this example, we get 50 mg divided by 120 mg multiplied by 5, which comes to 2.08 mL. The *Guesstimate* and *Estimate* suggested a volume of between 1.25 and 2.5 mL, so we would be happy to administer this volume of medication.

Student skill laboratory activity

Now try these examples, using the GEC system before performing the calculation:

- ✓ A child is prescribed ibuprofen 25 mg, and the stock preparation is 100 mg/5 mL
- ✓ A child is prescribed cefotaxime 700 mg, and the stock preparation is 2 g in 10 mL
- ✓ A child is prescribed spironolactone 10 mg, and the stock preparation is 100 mg in 5 mL
- ✓ A child is prescribed ondansetron 2 mg, and the stock preparation is 4 mg in 5 mL
- ✓ A child is prescribed morphine sulphate 600 mcg, and the stock preparation is 10 mg in 1 mL

(Answers are given at the end of this chapter)

Routes of administration

Medicines can be administered by many different routes (Royal College of Paediatrics and Child Health [RCPCH], 2003) as shown in *Table 7.2*. Choosing the most appropriate route optimises the effectiveness of the treatment and aims to maximise the action of the drug, while reducing the side-effects (John and Stevenson, 1995).

Table 7.2: Forms of medicine and their routes of administration

Oral (by mouth)	Liquids – solutions, suspensions, syrups, elixirs, emulsions, oils Solids – tablets, capsules, granules, lozenges, beads, chewing gum, sublingual tablets (rarely)
Gastric (nasogastric/ oropharyngeal tubes)	Solutions, suspensions, syrups, elixirs, emulsions, oils
Inhalational (into the lungs)	Metered-dose inhalers, powder devices, compressed-air nebulisers, sterile liquids
Injection	Water solutions, suspensions, emulsions, dilutions (depending on route) – subcutaneous (under the skin) – intramuscular (into the muscle) – intravenous (into the vein) – intracardiac (into the heart) – intrathecal (into the cerebrospinal fluid) – intraosseous (into the bone/bone marrow) – arterial (into the artery) – endotracheal (into endotracheal (artificial ventilation) tube to the lungs)
Intra-aural (into the ear)	Solutions, suspensions, drops
Intraocular (into the eye)	Solutions, suspensions, drops, ointments
Intravaginal (into the vagina)	Pessaries, liquids, solutions, ointments, creams, lotions
Nasal (into the nose)	Solutions, suspensions, drops, ointments, sprays
Topical (on the skin)	Solutions, suspensions, ointments, sprays, creams, lotions, pastes, powders, shampoos, soaps
Rectal (into the rectum)	Enemas (large and small), water solutions, suspensions, oils, suppositories, ointments

Standard abbreviations

Knowledge of the standard abbreviations used in medicine administration is an essential part of ensuring that you understand the instructions on a patient's prescription chart. The abbreviations in *Box 7.2* are commonly used for drug measurement, dosage forms, routes and times of administration.

Box 7.2: Standard abbreviation in administration of medicines

Drug and solution measurements

μg/mcg	microgram
mg	milligram
g	gram
kg	kilogram
mL	millilitre
L	litre

Drug dosage forms

Cap.	capsule
Elix.	elixir
Liq.	liquid
Sol.	solution
LA	long acting
SR	slow release

Routes of administration

ID	intradermal
SC	subcutaneous
IM	intramuscular
IV	intravenous
NG	nasogastric
PO	per oral
PV	per vagina
PR	per rectum
SL	sublingual (under the tongue)

Times of administration

a.c.	before food
p.c.	after food
mane	morning
nocte	night
p.r.n.	when required
b.i.d./b.d.	twice daily
t.i.d/t.d.s.	three times a day
q.i.d/q.d.s.	four times a day

Administration of medicines via the enteral route

The enteral route includes all routes via the alimentary tract:

- Oral
- Sublingual
- Rectal

Oral and rectal routes are discussed in detail here.

Glossary of terms used in reference to enteral administration

Appropriate manner	Slowly from a spoon, syringe or medicine pot for oral medication, without handling the drug
Aseptic	A method of handling sterile material employing techniques that minimise the risks of microbial contamination
Oral	The drug is swallowed and absorbed into the blood from the gut. Effects usually start 30–40 minutes after administration (NB in serious illness or injury, absorption may be delayed)
Rectal	The drug is absorbed from the wall of the rectum. Effects usually occur 5–15 minutes after administration
Non-touch	A technique which avoids touching areas where bacterial contamination may be introduced

Oral administration

Reasons for the procedure

To administer medicines by a route that is most convenient for children; it is less stressful for the child and is not associated with any discomfort or pain. If the child is 'nil by mouth' seek the advice of the prescriber as an alternative route may be required. Some medications may be administered with caution in this situation (RCPCH, 2003).

Risks of the procedure

- Incorrect dosage calculation
- Selection of the wrong drug

- Incorrect method of preparation
- Bacterial contamination

Pre–procedure

Equipment required

- Prescription chart
- Appropriate formulary
- Drugs trolley (if necessary)
- Medications
- Administration utensil
- Medicine pot (with measured volumes)
- Spoon (with measured graduations)
- Oral syringes (National Patient Safety Agency, 2007a)
- Appropriate oral fluid and container (if required)
- Water jug
- Drinking cup
- Disposable tray/receiver

Specific patient preparation

- Refer to local policy
- Discuss the procedure with the child and family as appropriate and obtain consent. Discuss any concerns or queries and respect the rights of the child/family (Watt, 2003a)
- Always adopt a calm and confident manner
- Infants and young children will feel less anxious with their parents, therefore encourage parental involvement and participation. It may be beneficial and more appropriate for the parents to administer the medication
- Ensure administration is at a time that suits child's normal routine if therapeutically possible
- Additional consideration must be given if medication is to be administered with or after food (preferably before feeds for infants unless otherwise indicated)
- Provide clear guidance, one direction at a time using age-appropriate language
- Encourage the child to take part if age/developmentally appropriate
- Be patient and allow the child to 'drink' at their own pace
- Play and distraction are often used; the use of a favoured toy can be invaluable (offer the medication to 'teddy')
- Infants should be held in a semi-reclining or seated position and the medication introduced slowly towards the side of the mouth, allowing time for the infant to swallow. Gentle stroking of the cheek and chin will encourage sucking and swallowing (Dyer *et al*, 2006)
- Avoid adding medications to food and drinks as there may be dosage and absorption problems (Watt, 2003a). In addition, food and drinks may be avoided or viewed with suspicion in the future

- Gather all equipment required on to a suitable clean surface and ensure (as far as is reasonable) that the working area is clear, quiet and uncluttered
- Clean the surface where preparation is to take place using an appropriate cleaning agent as recommended in local policy
- Wash hands as directed by local policy to reduce the risk of cross infection (Royal College of Nursing, 2005b)
- Check that the prescription form is the child's and check it against the child's identity bracelet. Check that the medication is correctly prescribed with regards to the child's age and weight (Preston, 2004)
- Read all relevant information leaflets and note any specific safety or handling and administration instructions such as 'with food'
- Check drug, dose and route against the prescription and product information (that is the 5Rs and 5Cs, remembering 'Your 6 rights')
- Check medication expiry date and integrity of all packaging (Cousins, 2006)
- Observe medication at all stages of preparation for signs of contamination
- Check that the medicine has not already been given
- Ensure that administration of the medicine is commenced immediately following preparation

The practice of crushing or dividing tablets and capsules is NOT recommended as there may be problems associated with calculation of the dose, the stability and efficacy of the medication (James, 2004). ALWAYS seek the advice of a pharmacist in this situation. Under NO circumstances should 'slow release' or 'enteric coated' tablets ever be divided or crushed (RCPCH, 2003).

During the procedure

- Shake suspensions, elixirs or syrups to ensure thorough mixing of medication so that the correct dose is administered
- Dispense medications using a non-touch method; empty the required dose into a medicine pot or spoon or draw up into an oral syringe
- Volumes of less than 0.5 mL should be drawn up in 1 mL oral syringes to ensure accuracy (Department of Health, 2006)
- If a tablet is dropped or liquid is spilled prior to administration, then replace using fresh medication
- Take the medications and the prescription chart to the child
- Check and confirm the child's identity and the drug to be given (5Rs or 5Cs)
- Administer the medication in an 'appropriate manner'
- Offer water to drink (sterile water for infants) to reduce risk of damage to gums and teeth from medication or sucrose (using 'sugar free' medications whenever possible)
- Ensure medication has been taken
- If a child refuses medication then this should be clearly recorded on the prescription chart, in the nursing and medical notes. Every encouragement should be given to ensure that the

medication is taken. However, the child must not be forced to take medication. If a child refuses medication, medical advice must be sort

- If medication is spat out immediately and the tablet, capsule or liquid is recovered unspoiled (caught by a vigilant nurse or parent in the medicine pot or spoon) then re-administer it. If a liquid medication is spat out and it is unclear whether any of the initial dose has been swallowed, or the child has vomited within 30 minutes of administration, the medication should not be re-administered and medical advice must be sought at the earliest opportunity

Post–procedure

- Dispose of equipment as appropriate
- Wash hands
- Record in the prescription chart that the medication has been given and complete other relevant documentation (Nursing and Midwifery Council, 2004b)

For administration of medication via a nasogastric or gastrostomy tube, please refer to Chapter 10.

Rectal administration

The rectal route is indicated if the oral route is not available or a local effect is required. A careful explanation is essential for both the child and the parents as both may find this distressing, embarrassing and difficult. There is a taboo surrounding this route, perhaps owing to child protection and cultural or sexual taboos (Dyer *et al,* 2006). The nurse must exercise great sensitivity and understanding.

- Medications for administration via the rectal route include enemas and suppositories:
  - An enema is a quantity of fluid infused into the rectum through a tube passed into the anus
  - A suppository is a solid, bullet-shaped preparation designed for easy insertion into the anus
- Rectal medications can be used to alleviate constipation, to clean the lower bowel and rectum before surgery, for therapeutic purposes, and to prevent complications of nausea and vomiting often associated with the oral route (Shepherd, 2002)
- Rectal administration of medications is contraindicated in cases of abdominal pain, bowel obstruction, lower bowel surgery and infection

Administering an enema

Reasons for the procedure

- To remove faeces from the bowel or intestine, when normal bowel activity is not adequate. Constipation in children should not be repeatedly treated with enemas, but approached through exercise, diet and laxatives (Kannah, 2003a)

Risks associated with the procedure

- Abdominal discomfort
- Distress
- Loose stools

Pre-procedure

Equipment required

- Incontinence sheets and tissues
- Potty, toilet or commode nearby
- Lubricant gel
- Gloves and apron
- Sterile container if sample required

Specific patient preparation

- Inform the child of the procedure to ensure that it is understood and valid consent is obtained (Nursing and Midwifery Council, 2004)
- Advise the child to try to clench their buttocks and hang onto to the enema fluid if possible
- Ask the child to try to remain calm and help with their procedure. Consider play specialists to help with distraction techniques as appropriate. In relation to adolescents, adopt a cool, matter-of-fact style

During the procedure

- Select the appropriate enema and check it against the prescription in the usual manner, paying attention to the 5Rs and/or the 5Cs and 'Your 6 rights' to maintain safety, so that the child is given the correct drug in the prescribed dose and by the correct route (Watt, 2003a)
- Wash your hands and put on gloves to minimise the risk of cross infection

- Position or help the child to position themselves either face down with their knees bent up and buttocks raised, or lying on their left side with the left leg remaining straight and the right leg bent up and resting comfortably (Kannah, 2003b)
- Lubricate the tip of the enema to facilitate insertion of the suppository and ensure the child's comfort (Watt, 2003b)
- Gently insert into the child's rectum to the marked distance. It may be helpful to ask the child to yawn or blow bubbles, relaxation techniques that bring about anal relaxation and distraction (Watt, 2003b)
- Squeeze contents into the rectum – a little will remain in the container
- Remove the tip
- Ask the child to clench their buttocks and keep the liquid in for as long as possible before sitting on the toilet or commode
- If the child is too young, hold his or her buttocks together for a couple of minutes
- Wipe away any excess lubricating jelly from the perineal area with a gauze swab or tissues to promote the child's comfort
- Praise the child for doing well during the procedure

Post-procedure

- Remove gloves and dispense of soiled items in appropriate waste receptacle
- Wash hands to reduce the risk of cross infection
- Document outcome of procedure on the stool chart, noting nature and volume. It is a legal requirement for patient safety to maintain accurate records, provide a point of reference in the event of any queries and prevent any duplication of treatment (Nursing and Midwifery Council, 2002)
- Ensure the child is comfortable and not distressed or in pain

Administering a suppository

Reasons for the procedure

- To remove faeces from the bowel or intestine, when normal bowel activity is not adequate
- To administer medication when the oral route is contraindicated

Risks associated with the procedure

- Abdominal discomfort
- Distress

Pre-procedure

Equipment required

- Incontinence sheets or protective disposable sheets and tissues
- Potty, toilet or commode nearby
- Lubricant gel
- Gloves and apron
- Sterile container, if sample required

Specific patient preparation

- Inform the child of the procedure to ensure that it is understood and valid consent is obtained (Nursing and Midwifery Council, 2002)
- Advise the child to try to clench his or her buttocks and hang onto to suppository if possible
- Ask the child to try to remain calm and to help with procedure

During the procedure

- Select the appropriate suppository and check it against the prescription in the usual manner, paying attention to the 5Rs and/or 5Cs and 'Your 6 rights' to maintain safety, so that the child is given the correct drug in the prescribed dose and by the correct route (Watt, 2003a)
- Wash your hands and put on gloves to minimise the risk of cross infection
- Position or help the child to position themselves either face down with their knees bent up and their buttocks raised or lying on their left side with their left leg remaining straight and their right leg bent up and resting comfortably to facilitate correct insertion of the suppository (Kannah, 2003b)
- Lubricate the suppository to facilitate insertion and to ensure the child's comfort
- Gently insert into the child's rectum. It may be helpful to ask the child to yawn or blow bubbles to bring about anal relaxation and distraction (Watt, 2003b)
- Ask the child to clench their buttocks and keep the suppository in for as long as possible before sitting on the toilet or commode
- If the child is too young, hold their buttocks together for a couple of minutes
- Wipe away any excess lubricating jelly from the perineal area with a gauze swab or tissues to promote the child's comfort
- Praise the child for doing well during the procedure

Post-procedure

- Remove gloves and dispense of soiled items in appropriate waste receptacle
- Wash hands to reduce the risk of cross infection

- Document the outcome of the procedure on the stool chart, noting nature and volume. It is a legal requirement for patient safety to maintain accurate records, provide a point of reference in the event of any queries and prevent any duplication of treatment (Nursing and Midwifery Council, 2004)
- Ensure the child is comfortable and not distressed or in pain

Administration of medicines via the parenteral route

The parenteral routes include:

- Intravenous (IV)
- Intramuscular (IM)
- Subcutaneous (SC)
- Nebulisation (Neb.)
- Endotracheal (ET)
- Intraosseous (IO)
- Intracardiac (IC)

Nebulisation is covered in detail in *Chapter 8*, but endotracheal, intraosseous and intracardiac routes are not covered specifically in this book.

Glossary of terms used in reference to parenteral administration

Aseptic	A method of handling sterile material employing techniques that minimise the risks of microbial contamination
Bolus	Administration of a small volume of a medicine directly into tissue or vein by manual means using a syringe, as a single dose given over a short period of time
Displacement value	The volume occupied by the powder in a vial when a suitable diluent is added during reconstitution
Endotracheal	Administration of drug through an endotracheal tube, which facilitates rapid absorption of drugs from the bronchial tree
Infusion	Administration of a large volume of fluid or solution of a medicine directly into tissue or vein by means of gravity or a pump system, given over a relatively long period of time
Intracardiac	A rigid needle is inserted directly into the cardiac muscle. Resuscitation drugs may be administered by this route. Absorption is quicker than the intravenous route

cont./..

Intramuscular	Injection of the drug into muscle, which is then absorbed into the blood. Absorption may be decreased in poor perfusion states
Intraosseous	A rigid needle inserted directly into the bone marrow. Resuscitation drugs and fluid replacement may be administered by this route. Absorption is as quick as the intravenous route
Intravenous	Direct introduction of the drug into the cardiovascular system, normally delivering the drug to the target organs very quickly
Nebulisation	Liquid drugs agitated in a stream of oxygen which create fine droplets that are absorbed rapidly from the lungs
Non-touch	A technique that avoids touching areas where bacterial contamination may be introduced
Parenteral	Administered by injection or infusion into the body
Preparation	Manipulation of ingredients and components to make a final product
Ready-to-administer	Medication that requires no further dilution or reconstitution before it is transferred to the administration device ready for administration or connection to a needle or giving set
Ready-to-use	Medication that requires no further dilution or reconstitution before it is transferred to the administration device for example a liquid in an ampoule, of the required concentration, that requires only to be drawn up into a syringe
Reconstitution	Addition of a diluent to a freeze-dried (powder) medicine for administration as a liquid solution
Subcutaneous	Injection of the drug into subcutaneous tissue, with a slower rate of absorption than the intramuscular route

Medications administered by injection

Medicines for injection via the intravenous (most commonly), subcutaneous (less commonly), and intramuscular (rarely) routes are not always available from the manufacturer in a ready-to-use form. Therefore, many injections need to be prepared before they can be administered. This process of preparation may be straightforward, such as a simple dilution, or complicated, involving several calculations and manipulations involving a number of risks, as shown below. Therefore, medicines should only be given by injection when no other route is suitable (Clinical Resource and Audit Group [CRAG], 2002). Furthermore, the preparation of injections should be carried out by suitably instructed children or their parents or healthcare practitioner who has completed a competency-based training and update programme, in a suitable environment, using safe procedures.

Risks associated with procedure

- Incorrect dosage calculation
- Selection of the wrong drug and/or diluent
- Incorrect method of preparation
- Incompatibility of constituents
- Instability of final product
- Microbial contamination
- Particulate contamination
- Health and safety risk to the practitioner and/or the environment

Reasons for the procedure

- The condition of the child does not allow administration by another route (oral, nasogastric, rectal)
- The condition of the child requires the medicine to be administered by injection to achieve immediate affect and/or therapeutic levels
- The medicine (or equivalent) is unavailable by any other route
- Administration by injection is in the best interests of the child

Pre-procedure

Equipment required

- Medication
- Disposable tray/receiver
- Glass ampoule opener (if required)
- Alcohol swab if necessary
- Gloves
- Sharps bin
- Diluent (if necessary)
- 23 G needle for drawing up medicine
- Appropriate needle (length and gauge) for route and site of administration (if required)
- Syringe of appropriate size (volumes of less than 0.5 mL should be drawn up in 1 mL syringes to ensure accuracy (Department of Health, 2006)
- Sterile hub cap (if required)

Specific patient preparation

- Refer to local policy
- Discuss the procedure with the child and family as appropriate and obtain consent. Discuss any concerns or queries and respect the rights of the child and family

- Gather all equipment required onto a suitable clean surface and ensure (as far as is reasonable) that the working area is clear, quiet and uncluttered
- Clean the surface where preparation is to take place using an appropriate cleaning agent as recommended in local policy
- Wash hands as directed by local policy to reduce the risk of cross infection (Royal College of Nursing, 2000)
- Put on gloves if required (eg. in antibiotic preparation) to prevent unnecessary exposure and potential future antibiotic resistance
- Select the appropriate medication and check it against the prescription in the usual manner, paying attention to the 5Rs and/or 5Cs and 'Your 6 rights' to maintain safety, so that the child is given the correct drug in the prescribed dose and by the correct route (Watt, 2003a)
- Read all relevant information leaflets and note any specific safety or handling/ reconstitution instructions
- Check the drug, the dose and diluent against the prescription and product information
- Check the medication expiry date and integrity of all packaging
- Observe the medication at all stages of preparation for signs of discolouration, precipitation and contamination (Department of Health, 2006; Health Protection Agency, 2006) – *NB: Some forms of medicines and diluents are similar (eg. ampoules and nebules)*
- Ensure that administration of injection is commenced immediately following preparation as far as possible bearing stability factors in mind

During the procedure

- Use a non-touch aseptic technique throughout to keep the injection free from microbial contamination (CRAG, 2002)
- Peel wrappers from needles and syringes. Do *not* push through wrappers as this will result in heavy particulate contamination. Volumes of less than 0.5 mL should be drawn up in 1 mL syringes to ensure accuracy (Department of Health, 2006)

Withdrawing liquid medication from an ampoule into a syringe

- Gently tap the upper area of the ampoule to release any medication trapped at the top of the ampoule
- Swab the neck of the ampoule using an alcohol wipe and allow to dry
- Snap open the neck of the ampoule using an 'ampoule breaker'
- Peel wrappers from needles and syringes. Do *not* push through wrappers as this will result in heavy particulate contamination. Volumes of less than 0.5 mL should be drawn up in 1 mL syringes to ensure accuracy (Department of Health, 2006)
- Using a 'non-touch' technique, carefully withdraw the required dose using a blue needle (23 G) if using a glass ampoule (Nichols, 2000). The blue needle gauge is sufficiently small enough to filter any tiny shards of glass from opening the vial (MDA,2006)
- Tilt the ampoule if necessary so that the required contents can be removed
- Do *not* tap the barrel of the syringe in an effort to dislodge any air bubbles; this causes tiny

splinters in the syringe plastic leading to particulate contamination of the medication. Hold the syringe with the needle upright and swirl it using a wrist action to create a cyclone effect which will expel the air (MDA,2006)

- Remove and immediately dispose of the needle into the sharps bin (May and Brewer, 2001; MHRA, 2001). This reduces the risk of infection, avoids contamination of superficial tissues, reduces the risk of sharps injury and ensures that the correct needle is used for injection. If a needle is not required, fit a sterile blind hub/protective cap to the syringe to maintain medication sterility

Withdrawing medication from a vial into a syringe

- Remove the tamper-evident seal, swab the top of the vial with an alcohol wipe and allow to dry
- Peel wrappers from the blue needle and syringe. Don't push them through the wrappers as this will result in heavy particulate contamination
- Keeping the blue needle cover on, draw the syringe plunger back to the desired volume
- Remove the needle cover and insert the needle into the rubber bung
- Invert the vial, keeping the needle end in the liquid and slowly depress the plunger pushing air into the vial. If a large volume is required, you may need to use a 'push and pull' technique, adding the air in exchange for liquid by small amounts at a time to prevent pressure from building up and the inherent risk of aerosol spray (Nichols, 2000)
- Release the plunger so that the liquid enters the syringe (Parboteeah, 2002)
- Do not tap the barrel of the syringe in an effort to dislodge any air bubbles (they can cause tiny splinters in the syringe plastic, leading to particulate contamination of the medication). Hold the syringe with the needle upright and swirl it using a wrist action to create a cyclone effect that expels the air
- Remove and immediately dispose of the needle into the sharps bin (May and Brewer, 2001) to reduce the risk of infection, avoid contamination of superficial tissues, reduce the risk of sharps injury, and ensure that the correct needle is used for injection. If a needle is not required, fit a sterile blind hub/protective cap to the syringe to maintain medication sterility

Reconstituting and withdrawing a powdered medication into a syringe

Ideally, hospital and private institution pharmacies should be seeking to provide IV drugs in a reconstituted form. However, there are occasions when drugs, most commonly antibiotics, need to be reconstituted from a dry powder with an appropriate diluent, using a needle and syringe. Further dilution, by adding the reconstituted antibiotic to an infusion bag via the injection port, is necessary for some antibiotics.

Risks associated with the procedure

- Microbiological or particulate contamination
- Septicaemia
- Phlebitis
- Hazard to staff (repeated exposure to aerosolised antibiotic and possible increase in antibiotic resistance; Turner *et al,* 2003)
- Needlestick injury
- Errors including
  - Incorrect selection of drug
  - Incorrect selection of diluent; the diluent must be compatible with drug
  - Incorrect diluent (see *Displacement value* below)
  - Preparation of an incorrect dose
  - Incorrect method of administration
  - Incorrect rate of administration

Displacement value

This is the volume occupied by the powder in a vial when a suitable diluent is added during reconstitution. For example, the displacement value of amoxicillin 250 mg is 0.2 mL. Therefore if 4.8 mL of diluent is added to a 250 mg vial, the resulting volume is 5 mL – that is, amoxicillin 250 mg in 5 mL. The displacement value is important because the dose used in children constitutes only a proportion of the vial content (Khoo and Bolton, 2003). *Note that displacement values of the same drug can differ between brands.*

During the procedure

- Swab the vial top or ampoule neck with an alcohol wipe and allow to dry
- Peel wrappers from needles and syringes, but do NOT push through wrappers (causes heavy particulate contamination). Volumes of less than 0.5 mL should be drawn up in 1 mL syringes to ensure accuracy (Department of Health, 2006)
- Follow the procedure described above in *Withdrawing liquid medication from an ampoule into a syringe*. Draw the required amount of diluent as recommended by the manufacturer to maintain drug concentration
- Inject this slowly down the wall of the vial. The syringe will fill with air that has been displaced by the liquid added to the vial (unless the vial has been vacuum filled). If a large volume of liquid is required use a 'push and pull' technique, adding the liquid in exchange for air mL by mL, to avoid pressure building up and the risk of aerosol spray (Nichols, 2000)
- With the needle and syringe still attached to the vial, shake the contents of the vial carefully to dissolve the powder, unless otherwise indicated by manufacturers' instructions (CRAG, 2002)
- Remove the needle and syringe and dispose of in the sharps bin

- Inspect the vial for cloudiness or precipitation. If present, follow local policy regarding disposal and reporting
- Fit a new needle and syringe and draw up the required volume of medication using the procedure above *Withdrawing medication from a vial into a syringe* (CRAG, 2002). Remember to peel wrappers from needles and syringes. Do NOT push through wrappers because that may cause heavy particulate contamination
- Also, remember that volumes of less than 0.5 mL should be drawn up in 1 mL syringes to ensure accuracy (Department of Health, 2006)

Medications administered by subcutaneous injection

Risks of the procedure

- Local and systemic allergic reaction
- Tissue fibrosis
- Infection

Pre-procedure

Equipment required

- 23–25 G needle of 16 mm length
- Syringe
- Gloves
- Disposable receiver or tray
- Sharps bin
- Plaster or small dressing

Specific patient preparation

- Ensure that the child and parents are prepared for the procedure, including discussion of safety issues. There are many techniques for helping children cope with the discomfort and fear associated with injections (eg. breathing techniques such as blowing bubbles and balloons, guided imagery) (Gaskell *et al*, 2005)
- Gain informed consent for the procedure from child and/or parents as appropriate
- Infants and young children should be seated comfortably in a position optimum for the procedure, on their parents lap, ensuring that they are held gently but securely so that they feel safe but not restrained (Gaskell *et al*, 2005)
  - *If using the anterolateral site* encourage the parent to cuddle the child close to them with the child's nearest arm around their back. The parent then places one arm over the child's other arm, holding both of the child's legs firmly above the knee

– *If using the deltoid site* (if willing) encourage the parent to hold the child's arm that is to be injected close to the child's body and to tuck the child's other arm behind their own back. The child's legs are tucked between the parent's legs or the parent holds them firmly (Health Protection Agency, 2006)

During the procedure

- Wash hands and put on gloves
- Select the appropriate medication and check it against the prescription in the usual manner, paying attention to the 5Rs and/or 5Cs and 'Your 6 rights' to maintain safety, so that the child is given the correct drug in the prescribed dose and by the correct route (Watt, 2003a)
- Prepare the needle and syringe on a tray as recommended by the manufacturer
- Peel wrappers from needles and syringes (do *not* push through wrappers, which can result in heavy particulate contamination)
- Volumes of less than 0.5 mL should be drawn up in 1 mL syringes to ensure accuracy (Department of Health, 2006)
- Withdraw the appropriate amount of solution in relation to the prescribed dose; refer to guidelines above depending on whether you are withdrawing medication from a vial or an ampoule into a syringe
- For injection, use a short orange (25 G) needle unless supplied with a pre-filled, pre-assembled syringes or pens. Expose the site for injection while maintaining the child's privacy and dignity
- Identify the desired site for injections. These are given beneath the dermis into the fat and connective tissue underlying the skin and are used for a slow sustained absorption of medication (Workman, 1999). The most suitable sites are shown in *Figure 7.1* with the abdomen and thigh areas being the most easily accessible for self-administration

REMEMBER repeated injections in one site can cause fibrosis of the subcutaneous layer and may affect the absorption of the drug. If a site is already used frequently or is to be used frequently (eg. in a child with insulin-dependent diabetes) the injection site must be rotated. Furthermore, the anatomical site, the particular site of injection, must be at least one finger's breadth away from the last one (King, 2003).

- Assess the site for skin damage and for fibrosis as these affect the rate of absorption of the drug (Workman, 1999). Do not use a site where there is evidence of skin damage and/or fibrosis (document and report to medical staff)

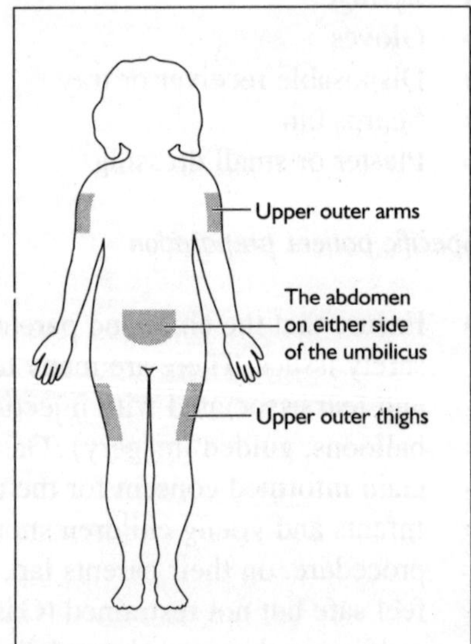

Figure 7.1: Injection sites for subcutaneous injections (shaded)

- Skin cleansing is not thought to be necessary if the skin is visibly clean (RCPCH/Royal College of Nursing, 2002; Pratt *et al*, 2005) especially in the case of repeated subcutaneous injections. Repeated alcohol swabbing predisposes the skin to harden and may inactivate the medication (Workman, 1999). If the skin is visibly soiled, wash it with soap and water and dry
- For a subcutaneous injection, *either*:
  - inject at an angle of 90° without bunching up the skin *or*
  - inject at an angle of 45° while bunching up the skin. Do this if you calculate that the needle is likely to go beyond the subcutaneous layer because the child is underweight. 'Bunching' up the skin lifts adipose tissue from the underlying muscle, especially in underweight children (King, 2003). Avoid squeezing the skin tightly as injecting medication into compressed tissue irritates the nerve endings, causing unnecessary pain
- Administer the medicine slowly and once complete release the skin. Ideally wait for 10 seconds before withdrawing the needle to allow dissipation of the medication (might be more risky than beneficial in a wriggly child)
- Dispose of the syringe and needle directly into the sharps bin (Royal College of Nursing, 2005b). Do NOT re-sheath (MHRA, 2001)
- Praise the child
- If any bleeding is noted, apply gentle pressure to prevent haematoma formation and apply a small dressing such as a plaster if necessary
- Dispose of equipment as per hospital policy and wash hands

Post-procedure

- Document on the prescription chart accordingly
- Inspect the injection site 2–4 hours after the injection for signs of adverse reaction, excessive bruising and/or signs of inflammation (Beyea and Nicoll, 1995; Workman, 1999)

Medications administered by intramuscular injection

Risks of the procedure

- Nerve injury
- Septic and sterile abscess formation
- Muscle fibrosis and contracture
- Necrosis and gangrene
- Intramuscular haemorrhage
- Local and systemic allergic reaction (Hemsworth, 2000)

Pre-procedure

Equipment required

- Needle
- Syringe
- Gloves
- Disposable receiver or tray
- Sharps bin
- Tissue
- Sterile gauze squares

Specific patient preparation

- Ensure that the child and parent are prepared for the procedure including discussion of safety issues. There are many techniques for helping children cope with the discomfort and fear associated with injections (breathing techniques such as blowing bubbles and balloons, guided imagery) (Gaskell *et al*, 2005)
- Gain informed consent for the procedure from the child and parents
- Where possible consider using topical local anaesthetics, prescribed and applied in advance of administering IM injections (eg. EMLA, Ametop gel, ethyl chloride spray) (Dyer *et al*, 2006)
- Select an appropriate site for the injection and assess the site for muscle mass, blood supply, skin damage and for fibrosis (all of which affect the rate of absorption of the drug) (Pratt *et al*, 2005) and apply topical local anaesthetic as prescribed. If the skin is visibly soiled, wash it with soap and water and dry first (RCPCH/Royal College of Nursing, 2002). Do NOT cleanse with alcohol as this inactivates some drugs if it is not completely dried and hardens the skin over time, leading to greater pain on injection
- There are a limited number of recommended sites for IM injection for children as compared to adults, namely the deltoid muscle, the anterolateral thigh, and the dorsogluteal muscle
- **Deltoid muscle** is primarily used for older children (RCPCH/Royal College of Nursing, 2002). It can be located in the lateral aspect of the upper arm (*Figure 7.2*). The injection site is located two fingerbreadths (2 cm) below the acromion process, but above the axilla (deltoid groove) (Health Protection Agency, 2006). The injection should be given into the densest part of the muscle and the needle inserted at an angle of 90° angle (Hemsworth, 2000). Due to its limited surface area, the number and volume of injections that can be given should be limited as appropriate (Cook and Murtagh, 2005)

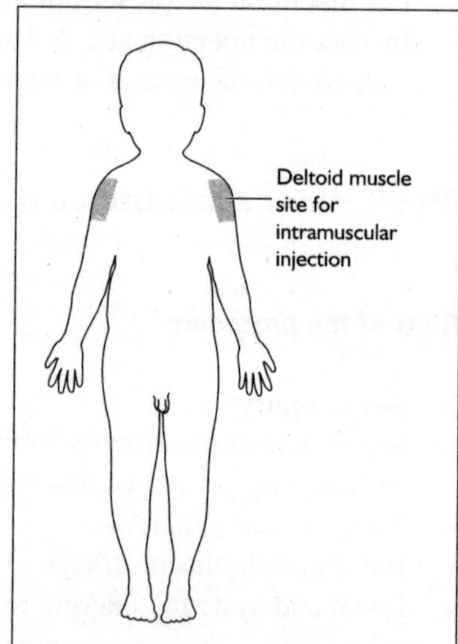

Figure 7.2: Deltoid muscle site for intramuscular injection (shaded)

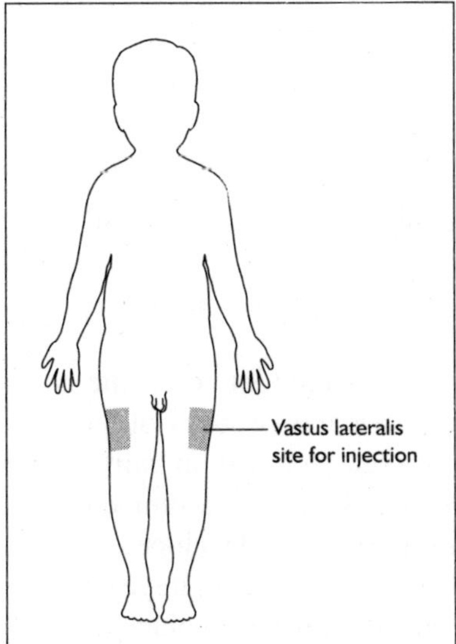

Figure 7.3: Anterolateral thigh site (vastus lateralis) for intramuscular injection (shaded)

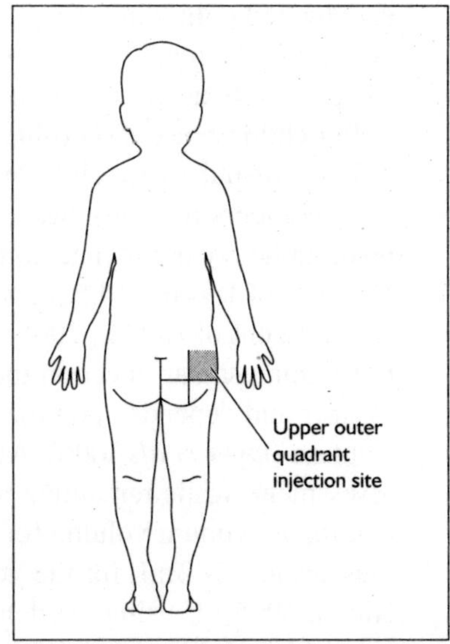

Figure 7.4: Dorsogluteal site (gluteus maximus) for intramuscular injection (shaded)

- **Anterolateral thigh (vastus lateralis)** is a quadriceps femoris muscle located along the anterior lateral aspect of the thigh. The target area is the midpoint between the greater trochanter of the femur and the lateral femoral condyle of the knee (Cook and Murtagh, 2005) as shown in *Figure 7.3*. This is the most appropriate site for infants (Department of Health, 2006). It is preferable to other sites because:
  - It is easily accessible
  - There are no major blood vessels or nerves in the area
  - There is generally a large muscle mass
- **Dorsogluteal (gluteus maximus)** muscle is identified by dividing the buttock into four equal quadrants with imaginary lines bisecting it vertically and horizontally; the injection is placed into the upper outer quadrant (*Figure 7.4*). Alternatively, locate the correct site by identifying the posterior superior iliac spine and the greater trochanter; inject laterally and superior to the midpoint of an imaginary line joining the two points (Rodgers and King, 2000). The children's nurse must be fully cognizant of the landmarks and boundaries, taking care to locate the injection site accurately (Small, 2004)
  - This site is not recommended for general use in children following reports of injury to the sciatic nerve or superior gluteal artery which lie close to the injection site (Kozier *et al*, 2000)
  - This site is contraindicated in the infant and young children for at least a year after they have started to walk because the muscle is underdeveloped until this time (Small, 2004; Department of Health, 2006)
- The needle you select needs to be sufficiently long to ensure that the medicine is injected into the muscle, but not so long that underlying neurovascular structures or bone are

endangered (Chiodini, 2000). The needle's gauge should be as small as possible while delivering the medicine safely:
  - For infants use 16 G (orange 16 mm)
  - For children use 23 G (blue 25 mm)
  - For post-pubescent children use 21 G (green 38 mm)
- Peel wrappers from needles and syringes (do NOT push through wrappers as this will result in heavy particulate contamination)
- Volumes of less than 0.5 mL should be drawn up in 1 mL syringes to ensure accuracy (Department of Health, 2006)
- For intramuscular injection the precise volume that can be administered into each site is unclear and depends upon the size of muscle, the medication used and viscosity of the solution (Dyer *et al*, 2006). All decisions regarding volume should be based on individual assessment, while remaining within existing guidelines (Small, 2004). It is recommended that the maximum volume for a child post-puberty is 4–5 mL into a well-developed muscles and 1–2 mL for the younger child with less-well-developed muscles (Beyea and Nicoll, 1995). If using the deltoid, 0.5–1 mL is the recommended maximum volume at once. Always, check manufacturer's instructions for medication-specific recommendations regarding volume and needle length and gauge
- Consider administering a large volume in divided doses (John and Stephenson, 1995) in order to:
  - Avoid pain
  - Allow appropriate absorption
  - Reduce the risk of neurovascular and muscle injuries

During the procedure

- Wash hands and put on gloves
- Select the appropriate medication and check it against the prescription in the usual manner, paying attention to the 5Rs and/or 5Cs and 'Your 6 rights' to maintain safety, so that the child is given the correct drug in the prescribed dose and by the correct route (Watt, 2003a)
- Prepare the prescribed medication using the guidelines above, depending on whether you are withdrawing medication from a vial or an ampoule into a syringe
- Infants and young children should be seated comfortably in a position optimum for the procedure, on their parents lap, ensuring that they are held gently but securely and making them feel safe rather than restrained (Gaskell *et al*, 2005)
  - *Anterolateral site*: ask the parent to cuddle the child close to them with the child's nearest arm around their back. The parent then places one arm over the child's other arm, holding both of the child's legs firmly above the knee
  - *Deltoid site* (if willing): encourage the parent to hold the child's arm that is to be injected close to the child's body and to tuck the child's other arm behind their own back. The parent can tuck the child's legs between their own legs or hold their child's legs firmly (Health Protection Agency, 2006)

- Expose the site for injection while maintaining the child's privacy and dignity and wipe away topical cream with a tissue if applicable
- Remove the sheath from the needle and place the sheath in the injection tray
- To reduce the child's discomfort and anxiety ask the parent, play specialist or colleague to use the distraction techniques discussed prior to the procedure
- Using your non-dominant hand either to isolate and stretch the skin over the injection site or to bunch the skin and underlying tissue (Hemsworth, 2000)
- Hold the syringe in your dominant hand and insert the needle quickly at an angle of 90° to the skin (*Figure 7.5*). Ensure that it is inserted to a depth that gives sufficient access to the muscle but avoids the bone (Cook and Murtagh, 2005)
  - If you are confident that the needle is accurately placed in the muscle, inject the medicine over a number of seconds
  - If you are *not* confident that the needle is in the muscle layer (perhaps you are unsure as the child is either obese or emaciated) aspirate and pull back on the syringe plunger for 5 seconds to ensure that a blood vessel has been avoided. If you are unable to aspirate any fluid, go ahead and inject slowly. However, if you aspirate blood into the syringe, remove the needle and discard of this syringe needle and medicine directly into a sharps bin. You will need to start all over again if blood is in the syringe (RCPCH, 2003). *This issue remains controversial*
- Withdraw the needle slowly, maintaining the angle of 90°
- Apply gentle pressure using sterile gauze

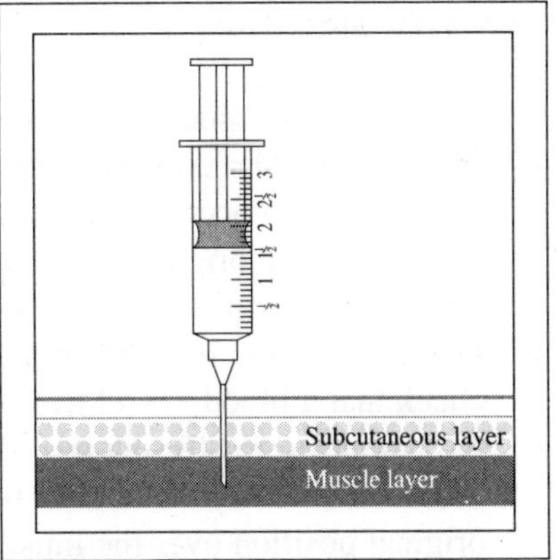

Figure 7.5: Angle and depth of intramuscular injections

Post-procedure

- Document on the prescription chart accordingly
- Inspect the injection site 2–4 hours after the injection for signs of adverse reaction; excessive bruising and/or signs of inflammation (Beyea and Nicoll, 1995; Workman, 1999)

Administering intramuscular medication using the Z-track technique

Reason for the procedure

- To administer drugs that would stain the skin and subcutaneous tissues
- To administer drugs that are particularly irritant

During the procedure

- Place the ulnar side of your non-dominant hand distal to the chosen injection site
- Draw the child's skin laterally away from the injection site, and this pulling action draws the skin and subcutaneous tissues away from the muscle, which remains static. Take care to ensure that the original site is landmarked, therefore aim for the underlying muscle – not a mark on the skin (Workman, 1999)
- Insert the needle into the skin at the original site while the skin is still held taut, aspirate to check that a blood vessel has not been punctured and inject the medication slowly
- After waiting for 10 seconds, withdraw the needle quickly and release the taut skin
- When skin and subcutaneous tissue are released after the injection they return to their original position over the muscle, thus breaking the medication track and therefore decreasing leakage of the drug into the subcutaneous tissues, and subsequent pain and irritation to the tissues (Hemsworth, 2000)

Post-procedure

- Document on the prescription chart accordingly
- Inspect the injection site 2–4 hours after the injection for signs of adverse reaction, excessive bruising and/or signs of inflammation (Beyea and Nicoll, 1995; Workman, 1999)

Administering intravenous medication

Intravenous (IV) is the term used to describe the administration of sterile preparations directly into the blood stream via a vein. IV administration is most commonly achieved by addition of the medication to an infusion reservoir, by injection via an established venous access point (for example, IV cannula), or by infusion with the assistance of a volumetric or peristaltic infusion device. IV medication can therefore be given as a continuous infusion or a bolus injection

The intravenous route for children is now commonplace in both hospital and community settings (Royal College of Nursing, 2005c). Practitioners administering intravenous medication must have undertaken suitable education and training in the theory and practice of the skill and be deemed competent in all aspects of intravenous therapy (Finlay, 2004; Royal College of Nursing, 2005c)

Reasons for the procedure

- To avoid pain (once venous access is established, medication can be administered painlessly – unlike with intramuscular or subcutaneous injections)
- To allow rapid speed of action
- To maintain consistent plasma levels of medications

- To allow close therapeutic control and titration of medications
- To allow delivery of large volumes of medication (RCPCH, 2003; Watt, 2003b)

Risks of the procedure

- Extravasation (commonly referred to 'tissuing')
- Phlebitis
- Thrombophlebitis
- Embolism
- Bacterial contamination
- Particulate contamination
- Incompatibility
- Allergic reactions
- Medication overload/overdose

(For more information on these risks, please refer to *Chapter 15*.)

Administration of medication by bolus injection

Reasons for the procedure

- To administer a small volume of medicine directly into an IV cannula

Pre-procedure

Equipment required

- Ampoule 0.9% NaCl for injection (to flush)
- Disposable receiver or tray
- Needles and syringes
- Alcohol swab
- Gloves
- Sharps bin

Specific patient preparation

- Ensure that the child and parent are fully informed and prepared for the procedure
- Check any infusion in progress
- Check the prescription chart to ensure that the medication is correctly prescribed

- Select the appropriate medication and check it against the prescription in the usual manner, paying attention to the 5Rs and/or 5Cs and 'Your 6 rights' to maintain safety, so that the child is given the correct drug in the prescribed dose and by the correct route (Watt, 2003a)

During the procedure

- Wash hands, put on gloves and assemble necessary equipment
- Prepare the medication for injection using an appropriate procedure from those described previously:
  - *Withdrawing liquid medication from an ampoule into a syringe*
  - *Withdrawing medication from a vial into a syringe*
  - *Reconstituting and withdrawing a powdered medication into a syringe*
- Follow the manufacturer's instructions. Maintain an aseptic technique and observe universal precautions throughout (Royal College of Nursing, 2005a; Royal College of Nursing, 2005b)
- Prepare a syringe containing at least 2 mL 0.9% NaCl for injection as a 'flush', using an appropriate procedure from those described previously:
  - *Withdrawing liquid medication from an ampoule into a syringe*
  - *Withdrawing medication from a vial into a syringe*
- Withdraw the appropriate amount of solution in relation to the prescribed dose. Dispose of the needle safely (Royal College of Nursing, 2005a). Many systems are now needle-free, in which case needles are not required for introduction of the medication. If needles are required select one with an appropriate gauge
- Re-check and confirm child's identity
- Expose and inspect the insertion site. Ensure that it is secured correctly. Check the IV cannula site for signs of infection, infiltration, phlebitis and if any of these are present, do not proceed (Royal College of Nursing, 2005a) and report to medical staff
- Clean the injection port using an alcohol wipe and allow to dry
- If using a needle, remove the sheath from the needle and place the sheath in the injection tray
- If using a cannula that already has an infusion in progress, stop the infusion (if appropriate) while you administer the bolus medication. Be sure not to cause any disruption to the child's therapy by (a) using this line, and (b) stopping the infusion for a brief period
- Flush the IV cannula with 0.5–1 mL 0.9% NaCl to ensure patency, as evidenced by the following (Ingram and Lavery, 2005):
  - very little resistance of the cannula to a slow flush
  - no pain or discomfort for the child
  - no blanching of tissue around the cannula site
  - no redness of tissue around the cannula site
  - no leakage of fluid around the cannula site
- If you suspect a problem, or you are in some doubt, do not use the cannula and inform medical staff

- Inject medication via the injection port – slowly and smoothly in the direction of flow at the rate as advised by manufacturer/drug formulary. While instilling medication and flushing continuously, observe the insertion site and, if able, ask the child in age-appropriate language to tell you if they feel any discomfort or pain
- Flush between medications if more than one is to be administered to avoid incompatibility of solutions and following the last medication given
- Re-start the infusion (if appropriate) at the prescribed rate
- Dispose of needles and syringes directly after use, during the procedure, into a sharps bin. *Never* re-sheath a needle (MHRA, 2001)
- Check the cannula is secure, comfortable and re-apply any bandage as needed

Post-procedure

- Document on the prescription chart accordingly (Nursing and Midwifery Council, 2004)

Administration of medication via intermittent infusion

Reasons for the procedure

- To allow medication to be administered as a stat dose or repeated at specific time intervals
- To allow slow administration to avoid toxicity

These medicines are usually given over a period of 20 minutes to 2 hours.

Pre-procedure

Equipment required

- 0.9% NaCl to flush
- Clean tray
- Needles and syringes
- Alcohol swab
- Gloves
- Sharps bin
- Giving sets
- Infusion pump or syringe driver as necessary
- Label showing drug additive, date and time

Specific patient preparation

- Ensure that the child and parents are fully informed and prepared for the procedure
- Check any infusion in progress
- Check the prescription chart, to ensure that the medication is correctly prescribed
- Select the appropriate medication and check it against the prescription in the usual manner, paying attention to the 5Rs and/or 5Cs and 'Your 6 rights' to maintain safety, so that the child is given the correct drug in the prescribed dose and by the correct route (Watt, 2003a)
- Prepare additive label according to local policy

During the procedure

- Wash hands, put on gloves and assemble necessary equipment
- Prepare the medication for infusion using an appropriate procedure from those described previously:
  - *Withdrawing liquid medication from an ampoule into a syringe*
  - *Withdrawing medication from a vial into a syringe*
  - *Reconstituting and withdrawing a powdered medication into a syringe*
- Follow the manufacturer's instructions. Maintain an aseptic technique and observe universal precautions as you add the prepared medication to the prescribed amount and type of infusion fluid as prescribed, according to manufacturer's instructions (Royal College of Nursing, 2005a; Royal College of Nursing, 2005b)
- Prime the IV administration/giving set with the infusion mixture and close the control valve
- Prepare a syringe containing at least 2 mL 0.9% NaCl for injection to use as a 'flush' using an appropriate procedure from those described previously:
  - Withdrawing liquid medication from an ampoule into a syringe
  - Withdrawing medication from a vial into a syringe
- Place the flush, the infusion admixture and connected giving set in the disposable tray and proceed to the child
- Re-check and confirm child's identity and medication to be given
- Expose and inspect the insertion site of the cannula. Ensure that the cannula is secured correctly. Check the IV cannula site for signs of infection, infiltration, phlebitis and, if present, do not use (Royal College of Nursing, 2005a) and report to medical staff
- Remove the cap from the cannula at the same time as applying digital pressure above the cannula tip to prevent fluid/blood leakage
- Inject gently 0.5–2 mL 0.9% NaCl flush into the cannula to ensure patency, as evidenced by the following (Ingram and Covery, 2005):
  - very little resistance of the cannula to a slow flush
  - no pain or discomfort for the child
  - NO blanching of tissue around the cannula site
  - no redness of tissue around the cannula site
  - no swelling is evident
  - no leakage of fluid from around the cannula site

- If you suspect a problem, or you are in some doubt, do not use the cannula and inform medical staff
- Connect the giving set using a sterile non-touch technique
- Load the infusion device as appropriate and as trained to do so (Medical Devices Agency , 2006; Amore and Ingram, 2003) and set the infusion to run at the rate prescribed
- Dispose of needles and syringes directly after use, during the procedure, into a sharps bin. *Never* re-sheathe the needle (MHRA, 2001)
- Dispose of all equipment appropriately and wash hands
- Once the infusion is completed, wash hands and put on gloves
- Disconnect the infusion set and flush the cannula with 0.9% NaCl 0.5–2 mL and check for patency as before
- Dispose of needles and syringes directly after use during the procedure into a sharps bin, and *never* re-sheathe the needle (MHRA, 2001)
- Check the cannula is secure, comfortable and re-apply any bandage as needed

Post-procedure

- Document on the prescription chart and fluid balance chart accordingly
- Ensure the child is comfortable

Administration of medication via continuous infusion

Reasons for the procedure

- To administer large or small volumes of fluids or medications at a set rate over a period of time (hours or days)
- To allow slow administration to avoid toxicity

Ideally, pre-prepared solutions should be used where possible. Only one additive should be added to one bag or syringe unless stability is confirmed by pharmacy (Cousins, 2006).

Pre-procedure

Equipment required

- 0.9% NaCl to flush
- Clean tray
- Needles and syringes
- Alcohol swab
- Gloves

- Sharps bin
- Giving sets
- Infusion pump or syringe driver as necessary
- Label showing drug additive, date and time

Specific patient preparation

- Ensure that the child and parent are fully informed and prepared for the procedure
- Check any infusion in progress
- Check the prescription chart, to ensure that the medication is correctly prescribed
- Select the appropriate medication and check it against the prescription in the usual manner, paying attention to the 5Rs and/or 5Cs and 'Your 6 rights' to maintain safety, so that the child is given the correct drug in the prescribed dose and by the correct route (Watt, 2003a)
- Prepare the additive label according to local policy if unable to use a pre-prepared solution

During the procedure

- Wash hands, put on gloves and assemble necessary equipment
- If not able to use a pre-prepared solution: Prepare the infusion using an appropriate procedure from those described previously:
  – *Withdrawing liquid medication from an ampoule into a syringe*
  – *Withdrawing medication from a vial into a syringe*
  – *Reconstituting and withdrawing a powdered medication into a syringe*
- Follow the manufacturer's instructions. Maintain an aseptic technique and observe universal precautions as you add the prepared medication to the prescribed amount and type of infusion fluid as prescribed, according to manufacturer's instructions (Royal College of Nursing, 2005a; Royal College of Nursing, 2005b). If injecting an infusion bag with medication, first swab the injection port with alcohol wipe and allow it to dry. Add the medication using a 23 G needle
- Invert the container a number of times to ensure thorough mixing of the medication and solute (as layering may occur and the child will inadvertently receive a concentrated bolus)
- Check the additive solution now for discolouration and/or precipitation – this can even happen when a mixture is theoretically compatible! Vigilance is essential (Cousins, 2006)
- Complete the additive label and fix to infusion container
- Prime the IV administration/giving set with the infusion mixture and close the control valve
- Prepare a syringe containing at least 2 mL 0.9% NaCl for injection to use as a 'flush' using an appropriate procedure from those described previously:
  – *Withdrawing liquid medication from an ampoule into a syringe*
  – *Withdrawing medication from a vial into a syringe*
- Place the flush, the infusion admixture and connected giving set in the disposable tray and proceed to the child
- Re-check and confirm child's identity and medication to be given

- Expose and inspect the insertion site of the cannula. Ensure that the cannula is secured correctly. Check the IV cannula site for signs of infection, infiltration, phlebitis and if present do not use (Royal College of Nursing, 2005a) and report to medical staff
- Remove the cap from the cannula at the same time as applying digital pressure above the cannula tip to prevent fluid/blood leakage
- Inject gently 0.5–2 mL 0.9% NaCl flush into the cannula to ensure patency, as evidenced by the following (Ingram and Covery, 2005):
  - very little resistance of the cannula to a slow flush
  - no pain or discomfort for the child
  - NO blanching of tissue around the cannula site
  - no redness of tissue around the cannula site
  - no swelling is evident
  - no leakage of fluid from around the cannula site
- If you suspect a problem, or you are in some doubt, do not use the cannula and inform medical staff (Royal College of Nursing, 2003)
- Connect the giving set using a sterile non-touch technique
- Load the infusion device as appropriate and as trained to do so (Medical Devices Agency, 2000; Amore and Ingram, 2003) and set the infusion the prescribed rate
- Dispose of needles and syringes directly after use during the procedure into a sharps bin. *Never* re-sheathe the needle (MHRA, 2001)
- Dispose of all equipment appropriately and wash hands

Post-procedure

- Document on the prescription chart and fluid balance chart accordingly
- Ensure the child is comfortable
- Monitor the infusion at least hourly for discolouration or the presence of particles
- Monitor the IV cannula site at least hourly. Observe for signs of redness or swelling, pain or discomfort. If in doubt stop infusion and seek further guidance and as necessary (for example if the child's complains of discomfort)
- Maintain infusion and fluid balance records
- Solutions must be discarded a maximum of 24 hours after being added (British Medical Association, 2006; National Patient Safety Agency, 2007b). Always check the manufacturer's guidance, appropriate formulary and pharmacist regarding the appropriate solution and length of stability of medication
- Observe the child for signs of discomfort or more serious complications (such as anaphylaxis)
- Monitor the infusion hourly and record the volume infused, the rate, and venous pressure of the pumps used
- Ensure the child is comfortable; use splinting and appropriate bandaging as required

Administering eye medication

Medications used to treat eye disorders are available in liquid, gel or ointment form so that they can be applied easily to the eye without causing any damage to the delicate cornea. The gel and ointment formulations keep the drug in contact with the eye surface for longer, whereas liquid eye drops may run off the eye too quickly and not be absorbed adequately to produce any beneficial effect. Ocular drugs are almost always used for their local effects.

The cooperation of the child is essential for administration of medicines by this route to be successful. In some instances, minimal, gentle restraint by the parent may be necessary. As with other routes of administration, patience and parental participation is essential. The child and parent should be carefully prepared for the administration of these medications because they may cause a considerable level of discomfort.

Pre-procedure

Equipment required

- Eye medication
- Container of warm water at 32°C to pre-warm medication
- Separate bottles for left and right eyes
- Prescription chart
- Eye toilet pack
- Normal saline
- Swabs or tissues as necessary
- Eye pads or eye protection and adhesive tape as necessary

Specific patient preparation

- Inform the child of the procedure to ensure that it is understood and valid consent is obtained (Nursing and Midwifery Council, 2004)
- If a fluid is being applied, explain to the child that they may feel some of it run into their nose (via the punctum of the eye into the nasal cavity), and that they may be able to taste the drug (as it drains into the nasopharynx)
- Provide privacy to maintain dignity
- Wash hands to reduce the risk of cross infection
- Select the appropriate medication and check it against the prescription in the usual manner, paying attention to the 5Rs and/or 5Cs and 'Your 6 rights' to maintain safety, so that the child is given the correct drug in the prescribed dose and by the correct route (Watt, 2003a)

During the procedure

- Provide eye care as necessary to remove any discharges
- Ensure the best position for instillation of the drops, that allows easy access to the eyes and that promotes comfort and compliance:
  - Negotiate with children their preferred position, either lying on their back or sitting in a chair, with their head tilted backwards and their chin upwards
  - Carefully position infants on a parent's lap or in a cot supported by a blanket, with their head tilted backwards and their chin upwards

Separate tubes or bottles should always be used for the left and right eyes.

Eye drops

- Warm to body temperature, if allowed, to reduce potential discomfort
- Ask the child to look up as far as possible or use play to encourage the child to look up in the direction wanted (for ease of access)
- Hold the dropper as close as possible without touching either the lids or cornea to avoid trauma
- Rest the hand that is instilling the medicine on the child's forehead to enable accurate instillation
- Gently pull down on the lower eyelid to instil the drops just inside the inner corner of the eyelid, into the upper rim of the inferior fornix so that the medication reaches the area requiring therapy (the conjunctiva in this area is less sensitive than the overlying cornea so discomfort is minimal, and the drops will run into the pocket of the inferior fornix rather than being lost immediately into the lacrimal drainage system)
- Replace the cap on the container
- Gently wipe away any excess medication to promote comfort
- Wash your hands to reduce the risk of cross infection

Eye ointment

- Hold the tube as close to the eye as possible without touching either the lids or cornea and rest the hand that is instilling the medicine on the child's forehead
- Gently pull down on the lower eyelid and gently squeezing a 1 cm line of ointment along the inside of the lower lid, from the angle near the nose (the inner canthus) towards the ear. Avoid touching the eye with the sharp nozzle
- Hold a cotton-wool ball or tissue at the corner of the eye, and ask the child to close the eye or eyelid (do it on the child's behalf if appropriate). Ask the child to move the eye around (to 'roll' it) to ensure that the medication reaches the area requiring therapy
- Warn the child that the ointment can cause 'blurriness' or 'fuzzy vision' until it melts
- Replace the cap on the container
- Gently wipe away any excess medication to promote comfort
- Wash your hands to reduce the risk of cross infection

Post-procedure

- Praise the child and advise them not to rub or squeeze the eye
- Document administration on the drug chart as this is a legal requirement for patient safety, maintains accurate records, and provides a point of reference in the event of any queries and prevent any duplication of treatment

Consider the implications of instilling eye drops when neurological observations are being recorded.

Administering ear drops

Although these cause no pain on administration there may some unpleasant sensations, and it is important that the child and parent are informed of these

Pre-procedure

Equipment required

- Prescription chart
- Ear drops – ensure they are in date as they have a very short life once opened
- Container of warm water 32°C to pre-warm medication
- Dressing pack to clean and dry ear as necessary

Specific patient preparation

- Inform the child of the procedure to ensure that it is understood and valid consent is obtained (Nursing and Midwifery Council, 2004)
- Provide privacy to maintain dignity
- Wash hands to reduce the risk of cross infection
- Select the appropriate medication and check it against the prescription in the usual manner, paying attention to the 5Rs and/or 5Cs and 'Your 6 rights' to maintain safety, so that the child is given the correct drug in the prescribed dose and by the correct route (Watt, 2003a)

During the procedure

- Provide aural toilet as necessary to remove any discharges and dry the ear canal
- Ensure the best position for instillation of the drops:
  - Negotiate with the child their preferred position, either lying on their side with the

  affected ear facing upwards, with their head tipped sideways or sitting in a chair with their head tilted away from where the side the medication is to be applied
  - Carefully position infants on the parent's lap or in a cot supported by a blanket, with their head tilted to the side away from where medication is to be applied
- Warm the drops to body temperature, if allowed, to reduce potential discomfort
- Prepare the auditory meatus for instillation of the drops:
  - In children aged >8 years pull the ear up and back
  - In children aged <8 years pull the ear down and back
- To ensure that the medication reaches the area requiring therapy allow each drop to fall in the direction of the external canal onto the side of the ear canal (avoid dropping it directly down the ear canal which can 'stun' the child). Instil the number of prescribed drops into the ear canal
- Gently massage the area immediately in front of the ear to aid passage of medication and relax the child
- Replace the cap on the container
- To allow the medication to reach the ear drum and be absorbed encourage the child to wait 5 minutes with their ear upwards (use cotton-wool to help the medication stay in place in children who cannot be persuaded to wait)
- Apply as above to the other ear after 5 minutes
- Gently wipe away any excess medication to promote comfort
- Wash your hands to reduce the risk of cross infection

Post-procedure

- Praise the child for helping
- Advise the child and parent not to insert objects such as 'cotton buds' into the ear canal – 'Put nothing smaller than your elbow in your ear!'
- Inform the child and parent that there may be some temporary hearing disturbance in the affected ear
- Document administration on the drug chart (a legal requirement for patient safety, to maintain accurate records, and provide a point of reference in the event of any queries and prevent any duplication of treatment)

Administering nasal medication

Medications for administration via the nose are available in the form of drops, nasal sprays or inhalers

Pre-procedure

Equipment required

- Prescription chart
- Medication as prescribed
- Test nasal inhaler/spray to ensure that the system is working and also that there is sufficient drug in the container

Specific patient preparation

- Inform the child of the procedure to ensure that it is understood and valid consent is obtained (Nursing and Midwifery Council, 2004)
- Warn the child that some of the medications may trickle down the nasopharynx
- Provide privacy to maintain dignity
- Wash hands to reduce the risk of cross infection
- Select the appropriate medication and check it against the prescription in the usual manner, paying attention to the 5Rs and/or 5Cs and 'Your 6 rights' to maintain safety, so that the child is given the correct drug in the prescribed dose and by the correct route (Watt, 2003a)

During the procedure

- Ensure the best position for instillation of the drops:
  - Negotiate with the child their preferred position, either lying supine with a pillow under their shoulders to support their head, neck and shoulders throughout the procedure, or sitting in a chair with their head tilted back and their chin upwards
  - Carefully position infants on their parent's lap or in a cot supported by a blanket, with their head tilted backwards
- Ensure maximum penetration of the medication, if appropriate, immediately prior to instillation, by asking the child to blow their nose gently to clear the nostrils and wipe any nasal secretions with a soft tissue; if the child is unable to do this for themselves, clean the child's nasal passages with damp tissues. Make sure you have paper tissues available to wipe away secretions and/or medication and maintain dignity
- Warm the drops to body temperature if allowed to reduce potential discomfort, or ensure that the inhaler or spray device has been stored at room temperature
- To obtain a safe optimum position for insertion of the medication, ask the child to tilt their head backwards
- To avoid the child's discomfort and to prevent sneezing, place the tip of applicator into the nostril and avoid touching the external nares with the dropper
- Ask the child to breathe in through the nostril while squeezing the spray container or pressing the inhaler. If the child can taste the spray this indicates that it has been sniffed straight through too quickly for the drug to permeate the nasal passages (Hopkinson and Powell, 2003)

- Deliver the prescribed amount of drops/puffs/sprays
- Encourage the child to keep their head back for 3–5 minutes so that medication is fully absorbed into the sinuses
- Rinse the dropper tip with hot water and replace the cap on the container (Walker, 2003)
- Gently wipe away any excess medication to promote comfort
- Wash your hands to reduce the risk of cross infection
- Repeat the procedure in the other nostril as instructed

Post-procedure

- Praise the child for cooperating
- Advise the child and parent not to insert objects up their nose
- Document administration on the drug chart as a legal requirement for patient safety, to maintain accurate records, provide a point of reference in the event of any queries and prevent any duplication of treatment

Fundamental aspects of pain assessment in childhood

Pain is a common complaint in childhood, therefore it is essential that healthcare professionals have a thorough understanding of pain assessment and its management (Franck, 2003). Despite misconceptions that infants do not experience pain in the same way as adults, scientific evidence clearly indicates that both infants and adults perceive pain in the same way (Andrews, 2003). A child's perception of pain is affected by their past pain experiences, cognitive development, age, culture, learning ability and personality (Royal College of Nursing, 2002). It is important for healthcare professionals to understand how a child's development relates to his or her understanding of pain (Franck, 2003).

Choosing and using pain assessment tools

It is vital that a child's pain is assessed, because without regular assessment pain is often left untreated leading to increased morbidity and psychological problems (Twycross *et al*, 1998). Upon admission to the ward, a thorough pain history should be undertaken and the child's usual response to pain should be recorded, the words they use, any behavioural changes, and their usual pain coping strategies, for example. Pain should be assessed using a valid and reliable assessment tool (Royal College of Nursing, 2002) that provides an accurate representation of the child's pain. When deciding which tool to use it is imperative to consider the child's age, cognitive development, emotional development and medical condition. If appropriate the tool should be explained to the child to ensure that they understand how to use it. Ensure that the child's parents have adequate support and information so that they can participate in pain assessment. This is very important because parents are the experts in reading their own child's behaviour (Simons *et al*, 2001). Four commonly used tools for pain assessment are the Faces, VAS, FLACC, and CRIES.

Faces (Bieri et al, 1990)

- Consists of a series of faces (usually three to six) with expressions ranging from happy to sad
- Child points to the face that best depicts how much pain they are feeling
- Commonly used with verbal children aged over 5 years

VAS (visual analogue scale) (Scott and Huskisson, 1979)

- Consists of a single straight line with the words 'No pain' at one end and 'Worst imaginable pain' at the other
- Child points to a place along the line that best describes their pain level
- Commonly used with older children (over 5 years of age)

FLACC (Merkel et al, 1997)

- Consists of five categories of observation (Face, Legs, Activity, Crying, Consolability)
- Each category is given a value between 0 and 2 and scores are totalled
- A higher score indicates a higher pain level
- Commonly used with younger children (under 3 years of age) and those who are non-verbal

CRIES (Krechel and Bildner, 1995)

- Consists of five categories of observation (Cries, Requires increased oxygen saturation, Increased vital signs, Expression and Sleepiness)
- Each category is given a value between 0 and 2 and scores are totalled
- A higher score indicates a higher pain level
- Commonly used with neonates

Limitations of pain tools

Rarely does a single pain assessment tool encompass all factors associated with pain. Therefore it is important when assessing a child's pain to adopt a holistic approach and use a combination of assessment tools, physiological indicators and behavioural measures (Moor, 2001).

Physiological indicators of pain (Royal College of Nursing, 2002)

- increase in heart rate

- increase in respiratory rate
- increase in blood pressure
- decrease in oxygen saturation levels

There is controversy surrounding the reliability of such physiological parameters as indicators of pain because children may have any of these symptoms for other reasons, for example tachycardia may be due to fluid depletion. It is important, therefore, not to rely on physiological symptoms solely as an indicator of pain.

Behavioural indicators of pain (Chambers et al, 1996)

- Facial expressions
- Head banging
- Curling up on one side
- A change from normal behaviour

Of course, behaviour can be influenced by many things other than pain, so relying on behavioural indicators alone can be misleading (Tesler *et al*, 1998). They should be together with other methods of pain assessment.

Healthcare professionals should document any changes in the child's behavioural and vital signs as the child may not be able to, or may not want to, report their pain. Once a child's pain has been assessed, the pain score should be documented and pharmacological and non-pharmacological pain-relieving interventions should be considered. Pain should be re-assessed on a regular basis to evaluate the effectiveness of the pain-relieving interventions.

The only reason to assess pain is to *take action* in order to relieve pain.

Administration of Entonox

Entonox is a gaseous mixture of 50% nitrous oxide and 50% oxygen. It is widely used for the control of relatively short-term or procedural pain. It is quick acting, with its rapid-onset analgesic and anaesthetic effects being felt within the first 2 minutes of inhalation. It has a short duration of action and is quick to wear off after inhalation has ceased (British Oxygen Company, 2001).

It is a highly effective analgesic, with the benefits of being patient-controlled and entirely non-invasive. It is thought that its analgesic and anaesthetic properties relate to the activation of descending noradrenergic pathways (Maze and Fujinaga, 2000). It has few documented side-effects, of which dizziness and nausea are the most common. However, the incidence of side-effects like nausea and vomiting is reduced compared to opiates. Entonox also helps children, and therefore their families, by minimising feelings of apprehension, pain and anxiety associated with procedures such as venous cannulation, changes of wound dressings, stabilisation of fractures, and removal of wound drains. The 50% oxygen concentration is valuable in medical and trauma conditions.

Administration of Entonox should always be in conjunction with pain score assessment and monitoring.

Reasons for the procedure

- To produce rapid analgesic effect with minimal side-effects
- To prevent symptoms being masked post inhalation (because of its short duration of action)
- To give the child some degree of control through self-administration
- To provide-effective analgesia when supplemented with stronger agents such as opiates

Pre-procedure

Equipment required

- A room that is suitable for both the procedure and the use of Entonox, well ventilated to prevent build up of gas within room, and with easy access to all basic life support equipment including oxygen and suction
- Prescription for administration of Entonox
- Cylinder of Entonox containing sufficient gas to complete the procedure (stored at or above 6° because at lower temperatures the gas splits and is less clinically effective)
- Single-patient use mouthpiece or facemask (a mouthpiece is preferable as it allows gas delivery to be entirely patient controlled)
- Filter for use within the delivery circuit (to prevent risks of cross infection)
- Administration circuit (should be primed before use)
- Connect up circuit to filter and cylinder

Specific patient preparation

- Explain the procedure to the child and family and any options available for management of pain or distress during procedure
- Consider using distraction techniques and a play specialist at the earliest possible moment
- Assess the child's need for analgesia during the procedure. If required, other analgesics should be given at an appropriate time beforehand to ensure the required analgesic level is reached
- Consider the child's suitability for use of Entonox regarding contraindications (see below) and ability and desire to self-administer the gas. If it is used, explain both the benefits and potential side-effects of the gas in an age/child appropriate manner, and make sure the child understands how it will make them feel
- Show the child the Entonox circuit and demonstrate the noise associated with inhalation
- Choose a mouthpiece or facemask as appropriate in discussion with child and family
- Explain to parents the need for the Entonox to be solely self-administered because it reduces the risk of over-sedation (the child cannot hold the mouthpiece or make a seal with

his or her lips when sleepy)
- Turn cylinder 'on' and ensure gas flow is present by pressing the demand valve test button
- Allow the child a few practice inhalations to ensure that he or she can activate the demand valve and feel comfortable in its use
- Lie the child down on a suitable trolley or bed, ensuring they are comfortable and in a relaxed in position

If Entonox is to be used frequently (more than every 4 days) a full blood count should be checked to observe for any signs of megaloblastic changes in red cells and hypersegmentation of neutrophils (British Oxygen Company, 1995). The use of alternative methods should be considered.

During the procedure

- Ask the child to breath normally throughout the procedure, holding the mask over mouth and nose, or placing the mouthpiece between teeth and sealing lips around it
- Allow the child to inhale gas for approximately 2 minutes prior to commencing to ensure full anaesthetic and analgesic effect
- Continuously assess the child, observing skin colour, ability to obey commands, respiratory rate and any signs of pain or distress
- Observe the child for any side-effects (see below), reassuring them as appropriate as they continue inhalation. Consider discontinuing the use of Entonox and stopping the procedure until the side-effects lessen

Remember that Entonox should be self-administered, via a facemask or mouth piece after suitable age and developmentally appropriate instruction. Entonox is safe to use with children provided that they are capable of following administration instructions.

Contraindications to the use of Entonox

- Pneumothorax (spontaneous, traumatic or artificial)
- Air embolism
- Maxillofacial injuries preventing appropriate inhalation of gas
- Head injuries with impaired consciousness
- Alcohol or drug intoxication
- Middle-ear occlusion
- Gross abdominal distension
- Decompression sickness
- Following air encephalography
- Following a recent underwater dive

Side-effects associated with Entonox

- Dizziness
- Nausea
- Excitation
- Numbness
- Light-headedness
- Dry mouth
- Tingling in the fingers

Post-procedure

- Switch off the cylinder
- Ensure the child is comfortable and discuss any elements of the procedure with them as required
- Document the procedure, including use of analgesics or distraction methods and their efficacy, the period of time over which the gas was used and any side-effects experienced
- Ensure equipment is stored correctly for next use
- Dispose of the mouthpiece as per hospital policy
- Clean the circuit as per hospital policy

Acknowledgement

Tiffany Russell is currently studying towards a PGDip (Child) at the University of Southampton.

References

Amore J, Ingram P (2003) Learning from adverse incidents involving medical devices. *Nurs Stand* **17**(20): 41–46

Andrews K (2003) Human developmental neurophysiology of pain. In: Schechter NL, Berde CB, Yaster M (eds) *Pain in Infants, Children and Adolescents*, 2nd edn. Lippincott, Williams & Wilkins, Philadelphia

Audit Commission (2001) *A Spoonful of Sugar: Medicines Management In the NHS Hospitals*. London: Audit Commission

Barrett G (2007) Improving student nurses' ability to perform drug calculations: guesstimate, estimate, calculate. *J Child Young People Nurs* **1**(1): 29–35

Beyea SC, Nicoll LH (1995) Administration of medicines via the intramuscular route: An integrative review of the literature and research-based protocol for the procedure. *Appl Nurs Res* **8**(1): 23–33

Bieri D Reeve RA, Champion GD (1990) The faces pain scale for self assessment of the severity of pain experienced by children: development, initial validation and preliminary investigation for ratio scale properties. *Pain* **41:** 139–50

Blood Transfusion Service (2005) *Guidelines for the Blood Transfusion Services in the UK*, 7th edn. Blood Transfusion Service, London

British Medical Association (2006) *British National Formulary*. BMA, London

British National Formulary for Children (2005) *British National Formulary*. BMJ/RPS/RCPCH, London

British National Formulary for Children (2006) *British National Formulary*. BMJ/RPS/RCPCH, London

British Oxygen Company (1995) *Entonox® Data Sheet*. BOC Group, Guildford

British Oxygen Company (2001) *Entonox® Controlled Pain Relief. Reference Guide*. BOC Group, Guildford

British Oxygen Company (2004) *Entonox® Reference Guide*. BOC Group, Guildford

Calliari D (1995) The relationship between a calculator test given in nursing orientation and medication errors. *J Cont Edu Nurs* **26**(1) 11–14

Chambers CT, Reid GJ, McGrath PJ, Finley GA (1996) Development and preliminary validation of a postoperative pain measure for parents. *Pain* **68:** 307–313

Chiodini. J (2001) Best practice in vaccine administration. *Nurs Stand* **16**(7): 35–38

Clinical Resource and Audit Group (2002) Good Practice Statement for the Preparation of Injections in Near-Patient Areas, including Clinical and Home Environments. Scottish Executive, Edinburgh

Cohen M (2000) *Medication Errors: Cause, Prevention and Risk Management*. Jones and Bartlett, London

Conroy S, Appleby K, Bostock D, Unsworth V, Cousins D (2007) Medication errors in a children's hospital. *Paediatr Perinat Drug Ther* **8**(1): 18–25

Cook IF, Murtagh J (2005) Optimal technique for intramuscular injection of infants and toddlers: a randomised control trial. Med J Australia **183**(2): 60–63

Cousins D (2006) Safe medication initiatives: sustaining good practice. *Hosp Pharm* **13:** 215–18

Department of Health (1999) *Review of Prescribing, Supply and Administration of Medicines: Final Report*. The Stationary Office, London

Department of Health (2004) *National Service Framework for Children, Young People and Maternity Services: Medicines for Children and Young People: Standard 10*. The Stationary Office, London

Department of Health (2006) *Immunisation Against Infectious Disease*. Green Book TSO, London

Dyer L, Furze C, Maddox C, Sales R (2006) Administration of Medicines. In: Trigg E, Mohammed TA (eds) *Practices in Children's Nursing*. Guidelines for Hospital and Community. Churchill Livingstone, Edinburgh

Finlay T (2004) *Intravenous Therapy*. Blackwell, London

Franck LS (2003) Nursing management of children's pain: current evidence and future directions for research, *NT Res* **8**(5): 330–53

Gaskell S, Binns F, Heyhoe M, Jackson B (2005) Taking the sting out of needles: education for staff in primary care. *Paediatr Nurs* **17**(4): 24–28

Health Protection Agency (HPA) (2006) *Correct administration of vaccines. Core Topic 9. Immunization training resources*. Available at: www.hpa.org.uk/infections/topics_az/vaccination/slides.htm

Hemsworth S (2000) Intramuscular (IM) injection technique. *Paediatr Nurs* **12**(9): 17–20

Hopkinson K, Powell P (2003) Management of allergic rhinitis. *Nurs Stand* **17**(40): 47–52

Ingram P, Lavery I (2005) Peripheral intravenous therapy: key risks and implications for practice. *Nurs Stand* **19**(46): 55–64

James A (2004) The legal and clinical implications of crushing tablet medication. *Nurs Times* **100**(50): 28–29

John A, Stevenson T (1995) A basic guide to the principles of drug therapy. *Brit J Nurs* **4**(20): 1194–98

Kannah A (2003a) Paediatric pharmacological principles: an update. Part 1: Drug development and pharmacodynamics. *Paediatr Nurs* **14**(8): 36–42

Kannah A (2003b) Paediatric pharmacological principles: an update. Part 2: Absorption and distribution. *Paediatr Nurs* **14**(9): 36–42

Khoo GP, Bolton O (2003) Neonatal and paediatric intensive care. *Hosp Pharm* **10:** 10–17

King L (2003) Subcutaneous insulin injection technique. *Nurs Stand* **17**(34): 45–52

Kozier B, Erb G, Berman AJ, Burke K (2000) Cited in: Small SP (2004) Preventing sciatic injury from intramuscular injections: Literature review. *J Adv Nurs* **47**(3): 287–96

Krechel SW, Bildner J (1995) CRIES: a new neonatal postoperative pain measurement score. *Paediatr Anaesth* **5:** 53–61

Lerwill C (1999) Ability and attitudes to mathematics of post-registration health-care professionals. *Nurs Edu Today* **19**(4) 319–22

May D, Brewer S (2001) Sharps injury: prevention and management. *Nurs Stand* **15**(32): 45–52

Maze M, Fujinaga M (2000) Recent advances in understanding the actions and toxicity of nitrous oxide. *Anaesthesia* **5**(4): 311–14

McClelland DBL (2001) *Handbook of Transfusion Medicine*, 3rd edn. HMSO, London

Medical Devices Agency (2000) *Equipped to Care: The Safe Use of Medical Devices in the 21st Century*. MDA, London

Medical Devices Agency (2006) *Drug Alerts*. MDA, London

Medicines and Healtcare products Regulatory Agency (2001) *Safe use and disposal of sharps. Medical Devices Alert SN2001(19)* www.mhra.gov.uk

Medicines and Healtcare Products Regulatory Agency (2001) Safe Use and Disposal of Sharps. Medical Devices Alert SN2001(19). Available at: www.mhra.gov.uk

Medicines and Healthcare Related Agency (2001) *Safety Notice 19: The safe use and disposal of sharps*. MHRA, London

Merkel S, Voepel-Lewis, T Shayevitz JR, Malviya S (1997) The FLACC: a behavioural scale for scoring post-operative pain in young children. *Paediatr Nurs* **23**(3): 293–97

Merkel S, Voepel-Lewis, T Shayevitz JR, Malviya S (1997) The FLACC: a behavioural scale for scoring post-operative pain in young children. *Paediatr Nurs* **23**(3): 293–97

Moor R (2001) Pain assessment in a children's A&E: A critical analysis. *Paediatr Nurs* **13**(2): 20–24

Moor R (2001) Pain assessment in a children's A&E: A critical analysis. *Paediatr Nurs* **13**(2): 20–24

National Patient Safety Agency (2007a) *Promoting safer measurement and administration of liquid medicines via oral and other enteral routes* www.npsa.nhs.uk/site/media/documents/2463_Oral_Liquid_Medicines_PSA_FINAL.pdf

National Patient Safety Agency (2007a) Promoting safer measurement and administration of liquid medicines via oral and other enteral routes. NPSA, London

National Patient Safety Agency (2007b) Promoting safer use of injectable medicines. NPSA multi-professional safer practice standard for injectable medicines. Available at: www.npsa.nhs.uk/display?contentId=5755

Nichols SN (2000) Evaluation of the Baxter Minibag Plus forward preparation of cefuroxime/metronidazole mixtures. *Hosp Pharm* **2**: 297–300

Nursing and Midwifery Council (2004a) *Guidelines for the Administration of Medicines*. NMC, London

Nursing and Midwifery Council (2004b) *Guidelines for Records and Record Keeping*. NMC, London

Parboteeah S (2002) Safety in practice. In: Hogston R, Simpson P (eds) *Foundations of Nursing Practice*. Macmillan, London

Preston R (2004) Drug errors and patient safety: the need for a change in practice. *Brit J Nurs* **13**(2): 72–78

Rodgers MA, King L (2000) Drawing up and administering intramuscular Injections: a review of the literature. *J Adv Nurs* **31**(3): 574–82

Ross LM, Wallace J, Paton JY, Stephenson T (2000) Medication errors in a paediatric teaching hospital in the UK: five years operational experience. *Arch Dis Child* **83:** 492–497

Royal College of Nurses (2004) *Informed Consent in Health and Social Care*. RCN, London

Royal College of Nursing (2000) *Good Practice in Infection Control. Guidance for Nursing Staff*. RCN, London

Royal College of Nursing (2001) *Administering Intravenous Therapy to Children in the Community Setting: Guidance for Nursing Staff.* RCN, London

Royal College of Nursing (2003) *UK Standards for Intravenous Therapy*. RCN, London

Royal College of Nursing (2004a) *Patient Group Directions. Guidance and Information for Nurses*. RCN, London

Royal College of Nursing (2004b) *Position Statement of Injection Technique*. RCN, London

Royal College of Nursing (2005a) *Standards for Infusion Therapy*. RCN, London

Royal College of Nursing (2005b) *Good Practice in Infection Control*. RCN, London

Royal College of Nursing (2005c) *Competencies: An Education and Training Framework for Administering Medicines Intravenously to Children and Young People*. RCN, London

Royal College of Nursing Institute (2002) *Clinical Practice Guidelines: The Recognition and Assessment of Acute Pain in Children: Recommendations*. RCN, London

Royal College of Paediatrics and Child Health (1999) *Medicines for Children*. RCPCH, London

Royal College of Paediatrics and Child Health (2003) *Medicines for Children*. RCPCH, London

Royal College of Paediatrics and Child Health and Royal College of Nursing (2002) *Position Statement on Injection Technique*. RCPCH/RCN, London

Scott J, Huskisson EC (1979) Graphical representation of pain. *Pain* **2:**175–84

Shepherd M (2002) Professional development. Medicines 3: Managing medicines. *Nurs Times* **98**(17): 43–46

Simons J, Franck L, Roberson E (2001) Parent involvement in children's pain care. *J Adv Nurs* **26**(4): 591–599

Small SP (2004) Preventing sciatic nerve injury from intramuscular injections: literature review. *J Adv Nurs* **47**(3): 297–96

Smith J (2004) *Building a Safer NHS for Patients: Improving Medication Safety*. The Stationary Office, London

Stephenson P (2005) Trust brings in maths test to reduce dosage errors. *Nurs Stand* **19**(38): 5

Tesler MD, Holzemer WL, Savedra MC (1998) Pain behaviours: post surgical responses of children and adolescents. *J Pediatr Nurs* **13**(1): 41–47

Turner D, Eggleton A, Cadman B (2003) An assessment of IV antibiotic reconstitution methods. *Hosp Pharm* **10:** 127–30

Twycross A, Moriarity A, Betts T (1998) *Paediatric Pain Management – A Multidisciplinary Approach*. Radcliffe Medical Press, Oxford

Walker S (2003) Management of allergic rhinitis. *Nurs Times* **99**(23): 60

Watt S (2003a) Safe administration of medicines to children: Part 1. *Paediatr Nurs* **15**(5): 4

Watt S (2003b) Safe administration of medicines to children: Part 2. *Paediatr Nurs* **15**(5): 40–44

Workman B (1999) Safe injection technique. *Nurs Stand* **13**(19): 47–53

Further reading

Addison R (2000) How to administer enemas and suppositories. *Nurs Times* **10**(96): S3–S4

Bruce E, Franck L (2000) Self-administered nitrous oxide for the management of procedural pain. *Paediatr Nurs* **12**(7): 15–19

Burden M (1994) A practical guide to insulin injections. *Nurs Stand* **8**(29): 25–29

Contreras M (ed) (2001) *ABC of Transfusion*, 3rd edn. BMJ Books, London

Department of Health (2000) *An Organisation with a Memory: Report of an Expert Group on Learning from Adverse Events in the NHS*. The Stationary Office, London

Department of Health (2001) *Building a Safer NHS for Patients: Implementing an Organisation with a Memory*. The Stationary Office, London

Department of Health (2002) *Better Blood Transfusion: Appropriate Use of Blood*. HSC 2002/009. Available at www.transfusionguidelines.org.uk

Kannah A (2003c) Paediatric pharmacological principles: an update. Part 3: Pharmacokinetics: Metabolism and excretion. *Paediatr Nurs* **14**(10): 36–42

Pratt RJ, Hoffman PN, Robb FF (2005) The need for skin preparation prior to injection: point–counterpoint. *Brit J Infect Cont* **6**(4): 16–20

Street D (2000) A practical guide to giving Entonox®. *Nurs Times* **96**(34): 47–48

Todd AAM (2002) Evidence-based use of blood products. *Curr Paediatr* **12:** 304–09

Useful websites

British National Formulary for Children
www.bnfc.org

Blood Transfusion Service
www.transfusionguidelines.org.uk

Health Protection Agency
www.hpa.org.uk

Medicines and Healthcare Products Regulatory Agency
www.mhra.gov.uk

National Patient Safety Agency
www.npsa.org

Answers to drug calculations

(1) *1.25 mL;* (2) *3.5 mL;* (3) *0.5 mL;* (4) *2.5 mL;* (5) *0.06 mL.*

Chapter 8

Fundamental aspects of respiratory care

Odette Rodda and Michelle Fuller

This chapter looks at the main treatment options and interventions for respiratory problems faced by children and young people, including the use of pulse oximetry, oxygen therapy, tracheostomy care, suctioning, inhalers and nebulisers and peak flow measurements. At the end of the chapter you will find a useful glossary of terms relating to respiratory care.

Pulse oximetry

Pulse oximetry is a frequently used, non-invasive tool used to measure capillary blood oxygen saturation (SpO_2) using an infrared light-emitting diode and a photodetector. It works on the principle that blood containing haemoglobin that is well saturated with oxygen is redder and more absorbent of red and infrared light than less-well saturated, bluer haemoglobin. It should always be used, where possible, alongside clinical assessments (see also *Chapter 6*), because such monitoring may give inaccurate results due to:

- Poor perfusion
- Movement
- Discoloured skin/nails including nail varnish
- Anaemia
- Carboxyhaemoglobinaemia
- Methaemoglobinaemia

Reasons for the procedure

Oxygen saturation monitoring is indicated for a variety of patient groups.

- To monitor oxygen saturation in children receiving oxygen therapy
- To monitor oxygen saturation in children with specific cardiac/respiratory conditions
- To monitor oxygen saturation during procedures in which sedation may be used
- To monitor oxygen saturation during and after general anaesthetic
- To monitor oxygen saturation in severely ill patients

Pre-procedure

Equipment required

- Oxygen saturation monitor
- Lead between machine and patient (as supplied with machine)
- Appropriately sized oxygen saturation probe, which may be:
  - a self-adhesive probe suitable for use in all ages
  - a finger clip
  - a clip suitable for use on an ear lobe
  - a light emitter and detector fastened to the patient by a disposable wrap

Specific patient preparation

- Explain the need for pulse oximetry to the child and the family in age-appropriate words
- Consider showing the child the use of the sensor on a family member, a cuddly toy or on yourself to help alleviate fears. Also consider involving a play specialist
- Choose an appropriate site. Those commonly used are a finger, a big toe, the palm of a hand (closest to the little finger), the outer aspect of the foot and the ear lobe. Ensure the chosen site is warm and well perfused. Remove any nail varnish or dirt from the fingernail or toenail if this is chosen area
- Explain to the child and the family that monitors frequently alarm and that this is not necessarily a cause for concern but may instead be due, for example, to motion, loss of the probe signal, disconnection of the probe, or cool peripheries. Explain to parents the best course of action to take if the machine does alarm

During the procedure

- Set up equipment as per the manufacturer's guidelines. Ensure all advice from the Medical Devices Agency (MDA) is followed and that all machinery is regularly checked by engineers for safety
- Secure the probe to the chosen area as appropriate with the light-emitting diode uppermost. Ensure that it is not fastened too tightly as this has been shown to be the major cause of burns and necrosis from saturation probes (MDA, 2000). Consider placing a sock or mitten over the probe to lessen the child's anxiety levels, maintain warmth and lessen the effects of ambient light
- Set the monitor alarm limits. Set the lower SpO_2 level as dictated by medical staff or hospital policy. The upper and lower limits of heart rate should also be set as appropriate for the individual child and age
- Ensure the monitor is clearly visible and alarm limits set sufficiently loud to be heard by staff

Post-procedure

- Re-position the probe at least 2-hourly or more frequently if indicated. If this is not carried out, tissue necrosis may occur due to excessive or prolonged pressure
- Check and document oxygen saturations at least hourly
- Check and document skin integrity in sites used for monitoring 4–6-hourly
- Clean the probe and machine as per the manufacturer's guidelines
- Monitor and record other respiratory observations as condition or medical instructions indicate. These may include respiratory rate and depth, signs of accessory muscle use, and respiratory noises. Inform medical staff if concerned that the child is exhibiting signs and symptoms of deterioration and/or exhaustion
- If the monitor alarms assess the child for colour and work of breathing. If recorded saturations are not consistent with assessment of the child, check the quality of the trace on display. Consider re-locating the probe if the trace is poor. If a good trace shows decreased SpO_2 readings inform the medical staff

Oxygen therapy

Oxygen is vital to all cells and tissues within the body for cellular metabolism. People are normally able to regulate and meet their own changing needs for oxygen through the inspiration of room air, which contains approximately 21% oxygen. However, at times, due to physiological and/or pathological problems, the respiratory system cannot achieve this and it is necessary to use supplemental oxygen therapy. The need is greater within the paediatric population than the adult population due to lower pulmonary reserves, which means there is greater risk of rapidly decompensating if the need for oxygen is not met.

Reasons for the procedure

- To support children showing signs of respiratory distress or insufficiency
- To correct a deficiency in arterial blood oxygen levels (hypoxaemia)
- To prevent insufficient oxygen supply to the body tissues (hypoxia)

Oxygen therapy is also indicated in the care of acutely unwell children in an emergency situation who are shocked or poorly perfused. If not treated, prolonged periods of hypoxia can result in cell death within 3 minutes (Bateman and Leach, 1998).

Pre-procedure

Equipment required

- A supply of oxygen; this may be piped, from an oxygen cylinder or oxygen concentrator
- A flow meter with controller
- An age/child-appropriate method of oxygen delivery (see *Box 8.1*) and any additional equipment for that method of delivery (as specified below)
- Oxygen tubing (if not integral with the delivery equipment)
- Humidification if required (see below)
- Oxygen saturation monitor, indicated for use in care of child requiring an acute period of oxygen therapy

As oxygen is a drug it is vital that it is prescribed. This should state what percentage is to be given, for what length of time, and when the prescription should be reviewed by an appropriately trained member of staff (BMA, 2004). In an emergency, oxygen administration should never be delayed while waiting for medical staff.

Box 8.1: Oxygen delivery devices (adapted from Pease, 2006)

Nasal cannula	May be used for only a low flow rate of under 2 litres per minute. Enables greater freedom of interaction/motion for a child or infant who does not require high-flow oxygen. Consider using colloid dressing between the tubing and skin to protect skin integrity before fastening with an adhesive dressing
Head box	Must be used in conjunction with an oxygen analyser. Allows delivery of high-flow oxygen with minimal distress. However it does limit interaction/movement of the child and if the oxygen is not humidified it may cool neonates and small infants. It allows for ease of observation. It is vital that the opening of the box is not blocked in any way as this may lead to build up of carbon dioxide
Simple oxygen mask	Used to deliver an increased oxygen percentage – dependent on achievable flow from the oxygen source. Facial masks are not always well tolerated by younger children
Non-re-breathe mask	Allows high concentrations of up to 99% oxygen to be delivered. Must have a flow rate of 10–15 litres per minute. The reservoir bag must be inflated prior to commencing therapy by occluding the valve at the base of the mask. Flow rate should not be below 10 litres per minute as this may allow carbon dioxide levels to build up in the reservoir bag

'Wafting' or 'blow-by'	Use only when other methods are excluded or not tolerated as it is hard to titrate to and measure the oxygen requirement. Oxygen tubing should be held within 10–20 cm of the child and point towards his or her face. At 5 cm from the patient, the delivered oxygen concentration is halved

Specific patient preparation

- Explain the need for oxygen therapy to the child and the family in appropriate terms for the situation and age of the child. The use of play therapy and distraction techniques should be considered to aid acceptability
- Sit the child upright in bed or in the parental lap, well supported by pillows, to assist effective lung expansion. In infants, where possible, tilt the head of the cot by 30°

During the procedure

- Set up desired equipment as per the manufacturer's guidelines. Ensure delivery device is working correctly and set to desired flow rate
- Commence oxygen therapy through chosen apparatus (set up as per *Box 8.1*)
- Include child and family to decrease distress and increase comfort

Post-procedure

- Children requiring an acute period of oxygen therapy should have their oxygen saturations monitored with a pulse oximeter (see *Chapter 6*). The oxygen flow should be increased or decreased to maintain the required oxygen saturations. This should be specified by medical staff, with the lower parameter generally being set at 92–94% unless otherwise specified by medical staff. During an emergency the intention of oxygen therapy is to raise the oxygen saturations as high as possible, thus lower parameters are irrelevant
- Observe the child for changes in respiratory status; monitor heart rate, respiratory rate and depth and observe for signs of accessory muscle use/respiratory noises. Inform medical staff if concerned that the child is deteriorating
- Document the time and date that oxygen therapy commenced. For an acute period of oxygen therapy the required oxygen flow rate and subsequent oxygen saturations should be recorded at least hourly
- Alert medical staff to any complications associated with the oxygen therapy
- Ensure child and family are kept fully informed of the need for oxygen therapy and its potential complications

- Monitor for pressure sores from the mask or nasal cannulae in areas such as the bridge of the nose, the ears and nostrils
- Ensure the oxygen delivery device is cleaned or changed regularly as the patient's condition, infection risk and local policy dictate

Humidification of air and oxygen therapy

The normal process of inspiration incorporates the warming and humidification of room air as it passes through the nose and upper airway. The oxygen delivered to patients as oxygen therapy does not contain the humidity normally present in room air. Prolonged or high-flow oxygen therapy can therefore rapidly dry the mucosa of the respiratory tract. Humidification is indicated for children who are likely to need oxygen for over 1 hour. Humidification is generally not indicated in emergency situations.

Reasons for the procedure

- To prevent the drying of respiratory mucosa, which could otherwise cause increased thickness of secretions that are difficult to clear from the chest by coughing or suctioning and may result in the blocking of smaller airways
- Active humidification warms the delivered air or oxygen as pumped gases can feel very cold, dry and uncomfortable for the child and may pose a thermoregulation risk for infants and small children

Pre-procedure

Cold 'humidity' or 'passive' systems may be used with patients who are able to effectively regulate their own body temperatures and who do not suffer from severe, chronic chest conditions.

Equipment required

- A bottle of sterile water for humidification
- A length of elephant tubing, sufficiently long to allow the child some freedom of movement
- An appropriate adaptor for the sterile water system
- Oxygen prescription

Specific patient preparation

- Explain the need for humidified oxygen therapy to the child and the family in age-appropriate words
- Explain to the child and the family the noise associated with the system

During the procedure

- Clean hands as per protocol
- Set up equipment as per the manufacturer's guidelines
- Connect adaptor to bottle of sterile water using a non-touch technique
- Connect adaptor to the oxygen supply (some adaptors allow for various percentages of oxygen to be set by turning a dial on the adaptor to the required percentage: the user must then set the oxygen flow rate as prescribed on the dial for the required oxygen percentage)
- Connect tubing to adaptor and chosen method of delivery (head box, mask or nasal prongs)
- Place chosen method of oxygen delivery on the child, making all efforts to include the child and the family to decrease distress and increase comfort
- Turn on oxygen flow to the desired rate

Post-procedure

- Record date and time that humidification commenced
- Change water bottle as required

'Active' humidification

The gold standard is an electronically heated or 'active' humidification system. This delivers warmed, humidified oxygen, and is indicated for use with all forms of invasive and non-invasive ventilation, in the care of children with chronic lung conditions such as cystic fibrosis, and in those with severe, acute conditions like bronchiolitis. Use of this is also recommended for infants receiving high-flow head-box oxygen, due to the cooling effect of high-flow unwarmed oxygen.

Equipment required

- An electronic heating humidification system or 'active' humidification system for respiratory humidification
- Bag of sterile water for humidification
- Dedicated disposable delivery circuit
- Prescription chart for water for humidification

Specific patient preparation

- Explain the need for humidified oxygen therapy to the child and the family in age-appropriate words

During the procedure

- Set up equipment as per the manufacturer's guidelines. Ensure that all machinery is regularly checked by engineers for safety
- Place the unit on a secure surface below the level of the bed and fit the chamber into position. This will prevent water build up in the circuit
- Connect bag of sterile water to the circuit using a non-touch technique and hang approximately 50 cm away from chamber of the unit
- Ensure the circuit is correctly connected with the heater wire and temperature sensors
- Turn on the humidifier. For optimal use this should be left unconnected for approximately 30 minutes to reach the set temperature. This is usually set at 34[°]C
- Place the chosen method of oxygen delivery on child, making all efforts to include the child and the family to decrease distress and increase comfort

Post-procedure

- Record the date and time that humidification commenced
- Check and document the temperature of the device at regular intervals to ensure it remains within set parameters
- Drain any condensation in the tubing back into the chamber at regular intervals
- Ensure that the complete circuit is changed at least every 7 days. Document this change
- If the child complains that oxygen delivery is too hot, check the temperature is as set and consider lengthening the circuit

Tracheostomy care

A tracheostomy is an artificial opening (stoma) in the anterior wall of the trachea, created by making an incision in the neck (Woodrow, 2002). This will allow air to enter the trachea and lungs and bypass the upper airway, which normally filters, warms and humidifies inspired air. A tracheostomy can be temporary or permanent and may be performed as an emergency procedure or as a routine operation. The main aim when caring for a child with a tracheostomy is to maintain patency of the tube, so ensuring a clear airway at all times (Aylott, 2006b). Parents should be encouraged to learn the necessary skills to enable them to care for their child at home as soon after the formation of a tracheostomy as possible.

Reasons for the procedure

- To clear an obstructed airway
- To assist breathing in children with:

- congenital abnormalities such as laryngeal haemangioma, choanal atresia, tracheo-oesophageal abnormalities, upper tracheal stenosis, vocal cord paralysis
- facial or neck tumours
- infections including acute epiglottitis and laryngotracheobronchitis

- To assist breathing in cases of trauma including subglottic stenosis, foreign body inhalation, emergency situations (eg. road traffic accidents)
- To aid children on long-term ventilation

Changing tracheostomy tapes and cleaning stoma site

Reasons for the procedure

- To ensure that the tracheostomy tube is secure
- To ensure that the stoma site remains free from infection

Skin care should be performed to prevent infection and skin breakdown and should be assessed on an individual, day-to-day basis depending on local policy and the child's condition. This process should performed by two people to maintain the child's safety. At least one of these two people should have performed the procedure before.

Pre-procedure

Equipment required

- Non-adhesive absorbent dressing (if required)
- Dressing pack (gauze and small sterile bowl)
- Sterile water or cleaning fluid as per local policy
- Gloves
- Scissors (if required)
- New tapes
- Emergency tracheostomy tube replacement kit (including a new tube of the same size and one a size below, tracheal dilators, new tapes)
- Apron and goggles
- Clinical waste bag and bin
- Suction and appropriate equipment in case of increased secretions
- Emergency equipment in case of need (oxygen, bag-valve mask device)

Specific patient preparation

- Assess the child's need to have the procedure undertaken
- Perform tracheostomy care before a feed or at least 2 hours after feeding

- Explain the need for tracheostomy tape change and cleaning of the stoma site to the child and the family in age-appropriate words. Consider showing the child the new tapes on a family member, a cuddly toy or on yourself to help alleviate fears. Also consider involving a play specialist
- Record baseline observations

During the procedure

- Position the child on his or her back with a small blanket or rolled towel under their shoulders. Some children may prefer to sit up for the procedure
- Open the dressing pack and set out equipment as for aseptic technique
- Wash hands (both people) and put on gloves
- The assistant should hold the tracheostomy tube in place throughout the procedure
- Either cut or untie the Velcro or tied tapes on one side and insert one side of the new tape
- Clean the skin around the tracheostomy tube with gauze dampened with cleaning fluid. Pat dry with a dry gauze square. Work from the centre outwards using four swabs, one for each quarter around the stoma. Do not allow any liquid to get into the tracheostomy tube or stoma area under the tube
- Feed new tape around the child's neck and secure the new ties before removing the old ones
- Secure the ties, allowing one finger gap between the child's neck and the ties
- Observe the skin for signs of infection or skin breakdown. If the stoma site is red, swollen, inflamed, warm to the touch or has a foul odour, inform the medical staff. Check the skin under the ties, especially on the back of the child's neck
- Apply a tracheostomy dressing flush to the skin if there is damage from the tracheostomy site or irritation from the tube rubbing on the skin

Post-procedure

- Praise the child
- Assess the child's respiratory status
- Record the procedure and observations made during and post tape change
- Ensure the child is comfortable and settled following the procedure

Tracheostomy suctioning

This process should performed by those with prior experience or by those under the direct supervision of experienced practitioners. Suctioning should be performed on an individually assessed basis and not routinely to reduce the risks of complications associated with the suctioning procedure (Aylott, 2006c).

Reasons for the procedure

- To assist the child in clearing their airway and to promote effective breathing

Pre-procedure

Equipment required

- Working suction set at 50–100 mmHg and appropriately sized suction catheters (a catheter with a diameter that is half the tracheostomy tube size, eg. for a size 3.0 tube use 6 Fr, and for a size 4.0 tube use 8 Fr)
- Gloves
- Tissues
- Water or alternative for cleaning suction equipment after use and a bowl
- Apron and goggles (if indicated by the child's condition or local policy)
- Clinical waste bag and bin
- Emergency tracheostomy tube replacement kit (including a new tube of the same size and one in a size below, tracheal dilators, new tapes)
- Emergency equipment in case of need (oxygen, bag-valve mask device)

Specific patient preparation

- Assess the child's need to have the procedure undertaken
- Explain the need for tracheostomy suction to the child and the family in age-appropriate words. Consider showing the child the use of the suction on a toy or using photo books to help alleviate fears. Also consider involving a play specialist
- Record baseline observations
- Select the correct size of catheter for the task with side ports and a finger-tip control valve (a catheter diameter that is half the tracheostomy tube size)
- Pre-measure the tracheostomy tube (see *Figure 8.1*) with a suction catheter so that is passes no more than 0.5 cm beyond the tip of the tube. Cut one to length and stick it on the child's bed or cot near to the suction equipment to aid correct selection of equipment required

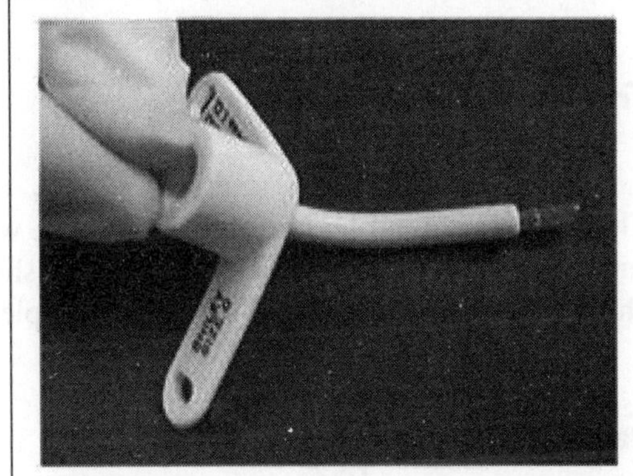

Figure 8.1: Pre-measuring the tracheostomy tube

During the procedure

- Wash hands and put gloves on

- Pre-oxygenate the child if clinically indicated necessary for 1 minute pre suction (usually recommended to be 10–20% above maintenance oxygen flow). This can be undertaken while you are getting the equipment ready
- Remove the suction catheter from the paper sheath ensuring that you do not touch the part of the catheter that is to be inserted into the tracheostomy tube. If you do touch it, discard and start again
- Gently insert the suction catheter into the tracheostomy tube to the pre-measured length without applying the suction
- Use finger-tip control to apply continuous suction while withdrawing the catheter. *Do NOT suction for more than 5 seconds*
- For tracheostomy tubes with cuffs, it may be necessary to deflate the cuff during suctioning
- Assess the child's respiratory status during and after the procedure
- Observe the colour, amount, consistency and odour of the secretions
- Dispose of the suction catheter by wrapping a hand around the catheter and pulling the glove over the catheter. Discard the glove with the catheter inside into the clinical waste bag
- Draw water from the bowl through the suction tubing
- Change the suction set regularly as per infection risks or local hospital policy

Post-procedure

- Let the child rest and breathe so that vital signs and oxygen saturations return to normal, then repeat suction procedure as needed. Be aware not to over suction the child as this may increase amount of secretions and distress the child
- Assess the child's respiratory status
- Praise the child
- Record the procedure and observations made during the suctioning, including colour, odour, amount and consistency of the secretions
- Ensure the child is comfortable and settled following therapy

Tracheostomy tube change

This process should be performed by those with prior experience or by those under the direct supervision of experienced practitioners. It should be performed by two people to maintain the child's safety. At least one of these two people should have performed the procedure before.

Reasons for the procedure

- To maintain a patent airway and to promote effective breathing

Pre-procedure

Equipment required

- Working suction set at 50–100 mmHg and appropriately sized suction catheters connected (with a catheter diameter half that of the tracheostomy tube size)
- Replacement sterile tracheostomy tubes (one of the same size and one of a size smaller)
- Tracheal dilators
- New tapes
- Scissors
- Gloves
- Hand towel (used rolled up under the child's neck)
- Tissues
- Apron and goggles (if indicated by the child's condition or local policy)
- Clinical waste bag and bin
- Emergency equipment in case of need (oxygen, bag-valve-mask device)

Specific patient preparation

- Assess the child's need to have the procedure undertaken. Tracheostomy tubes are usually changed between weekly and monthly depending on the manufacturer's guidelines to prevent mucous build up, maintain airway patency and to prevent infection
- Perform tracheostomy care before feeding or at least 2 hours after feeding to reduce the risk of aspiration
- Explain the need for the tracheostomy tube change to the child and the family in age-appropriate words. Consider showing the child the tracheostomy tube on a toy or using photo books to help alleviate fears. Also consider involving a play specialist
- Pre-oxygenate the child if clinically indicated necessary for 1 minute pre suction (usually recommended to be 10–20% above maintenance oxygen flow). This can be undertaken while you are getting your equipment ready
- Prepare all equipment needed to promote a safe procedure

During the procedure

- Open the dressing pack, and set out equipment as per aseptic dressing technique
- Wash hands (both people) and put gloves on
- Prepare the new tracheostomy tube by inserting one side of the new tapes and secure. Inspect the tube for signs of cracking, but avoid touching the end of the tube to prevent cross infection
- Position the child so that his or her neck is extended and the site is visible. Position the child on his or her back with a small blanket or rolled towel under the shoulders. This will hyperextend the child's neck and make access to the site easier. Some children may prefer to sit up for the procedure

- Consider swaddling an infant or holding a child firmly throughout the procedure. Comfort as necessary. Also consider involving the parents
- The assistant should hold the tube in place at all times throughout the procedure, to prevent accidental removal
- Cut the old tapes, gently remove the old tube and immediately insert the new tube using a smooth, curving action, directing the tip of the tube towards the back of the child's neck in a downward and inward arc. If the new tube is difficult to insert, try the size smaller
- Immediately remove the introducer, as the airway will be occluded while this is *in situ*. This is a good time to observe the stoma site for redness, swelling, excessive granulation around the stoma site, or odour. Remember to check the skin under the ties, especially on the back of the child's neck
- Feed the new tape around the child's neck and secure the new ties, allowing one finger gap between the child's neck and the ties
- Apply a tracheostomy dressing flush to the skin if there is damage from the tracheostomy site or irritation from the tube rubbing the skin
- Dispose of the dirty tracheostomy tube appropriately as indicated by the manufacturer

Post-procedure

- Let the child rest and breathe so that vital signs and oxygen saturations to return to normal, and assess the child's respiratory status
- Praise the child
- Record the procedure and observations made during the tube change
- Ensure the child is comfortable and settled following therapy

Suctioning and nasopharyngeal aspiration

Suctioning is the drawing of air out of a space to create a vacuum that will then suck in surrounding liquids (Griggs, 1998). It is a traumatic process and therefore it should be used with care for helping sick or disabled children where less invasive procedures are ineffective. Children and infants usually clear their airways by coughing, blowing their noses or sneezing. Increased production of mucous and secretions as a result of infection and inflammatory processes may make these mechanisms ineffective. In some childhood conditions and following surgery the coordination of the cough and gag reflexes may be compromised. Therefore suction may be required to maintain airway patency. Suctioning may be either oropharyngeal or nasopharyngeal. With either method, try not to suction for at least an hour after the child is fed.

Oropharyngeal (OP) suctioning involves the introduction of a fine catheter into the mouth, pharynx and trachea via an airway adjunct and application of suction to remove secretions. The technique involves advancing the catheter no further than the end of the hard palate to avoid trauma to the soft palate, triggering retching, or the possibility of a vasovagal response. Inserting the suction catheter may cause the child to become bradycardic by indirect vagal nerve stimulation through hypoxia or direct stimulation of the vagal nerve. The catheter should be advanced using direct visualisation.

Nasopharyngeal suctioning involves the introduction of a fine catheter into the nose, pharynx and trachea either directly through the nose or via an airway adjunct. If the suction catheter is to be passed further than the nose, pre-oxygenate the child if required. Measure the catheter length from the child's nose to ear. In babies, angle the catheter straight backwards and pass it carefully the measured length. *Never* force a catheter if resistance is felt (you may be more successful with the other nostril). NB: if an infant (aged over 6 months of age) has a nasogastric tube *in situ* remember that you will temporarily be occluding both nostrils while suctioning (babies are preferential nose breathers).

It has long been established that 'routine' suctioning is inappropriate and detrimental to the child's recovery. Establishing the need for suction is vital – to do this the whole picture of the child's respiratory status must be evaluated (Aylott, 2006a). The indications and contraindications of suctioning are listed in *Boxes 8.2* and *8.3* and complications of the procedure are given in *Box 8.4*. If secretions are dry and sticky, techniques to loosen them should be used – humidification (see below) or physiotherapy.

Box 8.2: Indications for oropharyngeal and nasopharyngeal suctioning

Suctioning may be required if the child demonstrates any of the following symptoms and their natural mechanisms are insufficient to maintain a clear airway (the frequency of suctioning must be tailored to individual needs).

Symptoms include:

- audible secretions that distress the child, or rattling, crackles or bubbling from the nose or mouth that can be heard with or without a stethoscope (these may be transmitted sounds from the upper respiratory tract)
- visible frothing or bubbling from the child's nose or mouth
- decreased oxygen saturations SpO_2 – make sure it is a good trace first!
- increased signs of respiratory distress such as tachypnoea, recession, nasal flare, tracheal tug, head 'bobbing', increased use of accessory muscles
- altered breathing sounds or difficulty breathing
- deterioration of arterial or capillary blood gases
- suspected aspiration

Suctioning is also indicated if:

- it is requested by the child
- the child is ventilated and the ventilator alarms indicating endotracheal tube occlusion
- the child is ventilated and secretions are audible on manual ventilation (bagging)

Box 8.3: Contraindications to oropharyngeal and nasopharyngeal suctioning

Suctioning should *not* be performed in children:

- over 1 year of age, who are alert and aware, able to cough or swallow secretions, and are not in respiratory distress
- with stridor
- with clotting disorders

Nasopharyngeal suctioning is normally contraindicated in children with severe intranasal disease and head injury (especially when there is cerebrospinal fluid leakage which often occurs with suspected basal skull fracture).

Reasons for the procedure

- To remove pulmonary secretions from the upper respiratory tract
- To maintain a patent airway
- To reduce child and parental stress

Pre-procedure

Good preparation helps to avoid the possible complications listed as well as reducing the amount of stress to the child and parents.

- Always establish a genuine need for suctioning the child
- Explain the procedure in an age-appropriate manner to the child to establish consent and cooperation. If present, explain the procedure to the parents to reduce anxiety and obtain their assistance
- Ensure that suction equipment is in good working order and is cleaned ready for use following local policy
- Ensure that you have ALL the appropriate equipment to hand BEFORE the procedure is commenced. Suctioning can be an emergency procedure, so equipment should ALWAYS be readily available

Equipment required

- An adequate supply of catheters of a size and style appropriate to the type of suction that you intend to perform. The size of the suction catheter is chosen according to the age of the child, size of the nostril or airway and/or the amount of secretions. If suctioning orally a larger sized catheter may be used. A small Yankauer catheter may make control of the suctioning less traumatic, but should be used with care

- A Yankauer or large-bore suction catheter (10 F) in case the child vomits
- A vacuum suction unit with pressures set within recommended parameters of 50–100 mmHg (6–12 kPa (the least applied pressure that is effective should be used, *within* these parameters)
- A supply of gloves (sterile gloves too, if likely to handle the catheter for practical purposes)
- Clinical waste bag
- Water or alternative for cleaning suction after use and a bowl
- An oxygen supply and associated equipment (bag-valve mask)
- Oxygen saturation monitor if available
- Another person to assist with resuscitation or to fetch help if necessary

Specific patient preparation

- Reassure the child and parent to reduce anxiety
- Wash your hands or use alcohol hand-rub to prevent cross infection
- Position the child on his or her side or a high-side lying position to reduce possible aspiration if the child should vomit. If suctioning a baby, and time allows, wrap the baby securely to enable swift intervention, boundaries and, therefore, less distress
- Pre-oxygenate the child if clinically indicated necessary for 1 minute pre suction (give extra oxygen to prevent hypoxia, usually recommended at 10–20% above maintenance)
- Identify the length of suction catheter needed – particularly for tracheotomy tubes – and clearly mark this close to the child's bed space. This is done by pre-determining the size and length of the suction catheter required, in relation to the size of the tracheostomy tube, so that it passes no more than 0.5 cm beyond the tip of the tube

During the procedure

- Select the correct size of catheter for the task with side ports and a finger-tip control valve
- Attach the catheter to the suction tubing
- Observe pre-suctioning saturation and heart rate, and pre-oxygenate (give extra oxygen to prevent hypoxia) if necessary for 1 minute pre suction (10–20% above maintenance)
- Turn on vacuum pressure ensuring maximum the negative pressure does not exceed 50–100 mmHg
- Put gloves on both hands (a sterile glove on top of a non-sterile glove if you are likely to touch the catheter end to be inserted)
- Attach the end of the suction catheter to the suction tubing. Keep the rest of the catheter in the sterile pack (either held in your non-dominant hand or placed under your arm and held close to chest)
- Measure the catheter against the tape measure with identified catheter length
- Keeping the suction catheter sterile, withdraw it from the packaging

- Gently introduce the suction catheter, not yet applying suction, upwards and backwards into the child's nose or mouth, under direct visualisation. Do NOT apply suction pressure on insertion (if the child has a gag reflex they will cough)
- Apply suction as the catheter is slowly withdrawn – do NOT rotate the catheter or re-insert the catheter at any point
- Complete the suction pass as quickly as possible, taking into consideration the child's individual response, including oxygen saturations and heart rate, to a maximum of 10–15 seconds with applied negative pressure on withdrawal for a maximum of 5 seconds
- Observe the status of the child post suctioning
- Remove any secretions in the suction tubing by placing the tip of the tubing into water until the tubing is clear and secretions are trapped in the suction bottle
- Wrap the suction catheter around your hand and dispose of it in the glove to prevent cross contamination
- Repeat the procedure as necessary to clear secretions once the child's cardiorespiratory status has returned to baseline values. A recovery time of at least 30 seconds is usually required between suction episodes

Box 8.4: Possible complications of oropharyngeal and nasopharyngeal suctioning

Arrhythmias (an irregularity in normal cardiac rhythm)
Atelectasis (alveolar collapse)
Bradycardia (slow heart rate usually of under 60 beats per minute)
Coughing
Discomfort or pain
Hypoxia (inadequate oxygen available to tissues to allow normal function)
Hypotension or hypertension (low or high blood pressure)
Infection tachycardia (rapid heart rate with an age-appropriate increase)
Laryngospasm (spasm of the laryngeal nerve)
Overstimulation of secretions
Tracheal mucosal damage (damage to tissues of the trachea)
Vagal nerve stimulation (stimulation of the parasympathetic nervous system resulting in bradycardia)
Cardiac arrest

Post-procedure

- Allow the child recovery time following the procedure and re-assess the need for further suctioning
- Ensure the child is comfortable and discuss any elements of procedure with them as required

- Document the procedure and record the method of suction, tolerance, effectiveness and quantity and quality of secretions
- Clean suctioning circuit as per local policy

Sputum trap

You may be required to collect a sputum specimen for virology or microbiology purposes. The collection of a nasopharyngeal aspirate (NPA) may be performed in coryzal infants to isolate respiratory syncytial virus (RSV). The need to perform this invasive test should be led by hospital policy. Its use may no longer be routinely recommended except in at-risk groups such as premature infants and those with cardiac abnormalities.

Pre-procedure

Equipment required

- As for *Suctioning*
- Sputum trap
- Request form for required tests

Specific patient preparation

- As for *Suctioning*

During the procedure

- Attach the rigid prong of the trap to the suction tubing
- Using the same technique as directed (above) connect the suction catheter to the flexible end of the trap
- Perform suctioning as described above. Any secretions removed during suction will be collected within the pot. If insufficient secretions are collected to reach the collection pot, consider suctioning a small volume of sterile water through the catheter to wash secretions into the pot
- After suction, discard the suction catheter by wrapping it around your hand and disposing of it inside the glove to prevent cross contamination
- Unscrew the lid from the container of the sputum trap and replace with the plain lid
- Label the container with all the required details and send it to the laboratory for testing

Post-procedure

- As for *Suctioning*

Student skill laboratory activity

Familiarise yourself with the various types of suction catheters available to you.

- ✓ Familiarise yourself with local equipment.
- ✓ Practice suctioning on a mannequin.
- ✓ Consider how you would explain to a child and a parent about suctioning and why it may be necessary.

Inhaler and spacer devices

For most children, use of a metered-dose inhaler (MDI) is as effective as a nebuliser and therefore is the delivery method of choice. It is important that the correct delivery device and inhaler techniques are chosen for the child. The overall aim is to control symptoms with the minimum amount of therapy to allow the child a normal lifestyle.

Children under 5 years of age should use a pressurised metered-dose inhaler (pMDI) with a spacer device (National Institute for Clinical Excellence [NICE], 2000). A proportion of the inhaled drug is always swallowed. However, poor inhaler technique can mean that more than 80% of the inhaled drug is swallowed, and effectiveness is therefore diminished. The British Thoracic Society guidelines (1997) advise:

- MDI via a spacer and facemask for children aged 0–2 years
- MDI and spacer with or without a facemask for ages 3–5 years
- MDI and spacer for 5 years upwards using the mouthpiece.

All MDI inhalers require coordination of actuation (pressing the inhaler canister to release the drug) and inhalation and may be difficult to execute, especially for younger children. The purpose of the spacer device is to act as an intermediary chamber, so that the child can inhale the drug over several breaths.

Reasons for the procedure

- To assist breathing during an exacerbation of asthma or wheeziness

Inhaled therapy is specifically indicated for the delivery of inhaled bronchodilators and steroids in children with exacerbation of asthma or wheezy episodes. The inhaled route is preferred to the oral route because the drug is delivered directly to the small airways, and the onset of action is quicker, and there are fewer systemic (whole body) side-effects. It is important to distinguish between the local effects that can be attributed to the inhaled portion of the drug and the systemic effects that may result from the drug being ingested. This is one of the main reasons for a regular review of inhaler technique in children.

Pre-procedure

Equipment required

- Metered-dose inhaler
- Spacer device, depending on the age of the child and local hospital protocol. Current recommendations (NICE, 2000; British Thoracic Society/Scottish Intercollegiate Guidelines Network, 2003) suggest the dosage of the drug delivered may vary considerably according to the static charge on the spacer; it is therefore suggested that washing the spacer in general purpose detergent prior to use and allowing it to air dry will reduces static charge inside the spacer device
- A mask that fits well over the nose and mouth may be used with infants and younger children
- A valid prescription chart for the drug to be given
- Stickers for distraction

Specific patient preparation

- Explain the need for the inhaler and spacer to the child and the family in age-appropriate words
- Consider showing the child the use of the inhaler and spacer device on a family member, a cuddly toy or on yourself to help alleviate fears
- Consider involving a play specialist
- Choose the appropriate spacer device for the age of the infant or child. The spacer device allows the drug to be suspended in the chamber and inhaled by the child, allowing more medication to be deposited into the lungs and less to be absorbed in the oropharynx and gut (see *Box 8.5*)
- Choose an appropriate inhaler device for older children not requiring spacer use (see *Box 8.6*)

Box 8.5: Spacer devices

There are many different spacer devices available. Those listed here are the most commonly prescribed and used in clinical/community practice (NICE; 2003; NRTC, 2003; BTS 2004; Newell *et al*, 2006):

Babyhaler spacer devices – The valve requires only a low inspiratory flow to open and therefore does not require tipping. Parents may find these easier to handle than large-volume spacers, particularly when struggling to administer medication to a wriggling infant

Large-volume spacer volumatics or nebuhalers – These can be used with a facemask. The same technique can be undertaken using a facemask, but if used when a child is asleep, will require the operator to tip the device to an angle of 45° to enable the valve to remain open during use

Aerochambers – These are easily portable and available in different sizes. They are unsuitable for a technique that involves tidal breathing (as discussed in the procedure below). They can be used with a facemask over the child's nose and mouth, instead of using a mouthpiece. They can cause a whistling sound when used with the mouthpiece and if the child is breathing too quickly; however, if a *facemask* is used with the child and infant Aerochamber, the mask does not whistle

Box 8.6: Inhaler devices

There are many different inhaler devices and choice will depend on the age of the child and their ability to use the chosen device (NICE ,2003; NRTC, 2003; BTS, 2004; Newell *et al*, 2006):

Metered-dose inhalers (MDIs) – These are not normally used for children under 12 years of age as the child has to coordinate a controlled inhalation while simultaneously activating the device

Breath-actuated metered-dose inhalers – These may help with coordination. Once primed the drug is not released until inspiration occurs. However they actuate using a clicking sound, which can often stop the child breathing in, so affecting the dose administered. Have counters on to aid drug compliance and the ability to monitor doses taken

Dry-powder devices – These are not generally used in children less than 6 years old, due to insufficient inspiratory flow rates. The more recent dry-powder devices have counters on that aid compliance, but they depend on rapid inspiration, and lung deposition has been shown to vary widely. They are easier to use than MDIs but good technique is essential

During the procedure

Babyhaler

- Set up equipment as per the manufacturer's guidelines
- Remove the mouthpiece cover from the inhaler and shake the inhaler
- Insert the inhaler into the inhaler holder of the spacer device (some brands of MDIs may be difficult to insert or remove into/from the Babyhaler; it may be suggested to parents to insert the inhaler and shake the whole device)
- Place the facemask gently but securely over the baby's nose and mouth ensuring a good seal
- Hold the Babyhaler and inhaler securely and at an angle so that it is comfortable for yourself and the baby
- Consider swaddling the baby and holding firmly, or cradled in the arm of a parent or carer, comforting as needed. Children should be sitting in a supported position; this can be on the lap of a parent or carer to lessen the distress of the unfamiliar environment. Demonstrate holding positions for parents if necessary
- Press down on the canister once to release a dose of the medication into the Babyhaler/ spacer
- Keep the Babyhaler over the baby's nose and mouth until the child has taken 5 to 10 good breaths (this will usually take about 10–20 seconds to complete. You should be able to see the blue exhalation valve flutter with each breath
- Take the Babyhaler away from the baby's face
- Repeat steps above after 30 seconds, shaking the inhaler after every puff
- If the child becomes distressed at any point try to reassure and comfort him or her. Crying and/or screaming increases deposition of the drug in the upper respiratory tract and may increase loss of the drug through forced expiration. Consider discontinuing therapy until the child is more settled
- When completed, remove the MDI inhaler from the device and replace the protective cap

Large-volume spacer

- Set up equipment as per the manufacturer's guidelines
- Remove the mouthpiece cover from the inhaler and shake the inhaler
- Insert the inhaler into the inhaler holder of the spacer device
- Ensure the child is sitting in a supported position (sitting on the lap of a parent or carer can lessen the distress of an unfamiliar environment)
- Hold the spacer and inhaler securely and horizontally
- Place the mouthpiece in the mouth and close the lips, ensuring a good seal
- Start breathing in and out slowly and gently (the valve of the Volumatic may make a clicking sound as the valve opens and closes). This is called 'tidal breathing'
- When a breathing pattern is well established, press the inhaler once to administer a dose of the drug, leaving the device in the same position and ask the child to continue to breathe five more times (if you hear a whistling sound it may indicate the child is breathing too quickly)

- Remove the device from the child's mouth
- Wait about 30 seconds before repeating the steps above, shaking the inhaler after every puff
- If the child becomes distressed at any point try to reassure and comfort him or her. Crying and/or screaming increases deposition of the drug in the upper respiratory tract and may increase loss of the drug through forced expiration. Consider discontinuing therapy until the child is more settled
- When completed, remove the MDI inhaler from the device and replace the protective cap

Post-procedure

- Assess the child for effects of the inhaler. If still acutely wheezy or minimal air entry is heard when auscultating the chest, consult medical staff regarding further drug therapy. Continue to re-assess at regular intervals
- Ensure the child is comfortable and settled following therapy
- Document time and date the inhaler was given, how it was given and any effects noted, beneficial or adverse
- If the inhaler was given via a facemask, wipe the skin clean to remove traces of drug to prevent skin irritation or excoriation. This is particularly important if inhaled steroids were given (in which case they should also be given a drink or mouth care to remove any drug particles from the mouth)
- Subsequent washing of the spacer is usually recommended by the manufacturers weekly, however the Asthma Guidelines (British Thoracic Society/Scottish Intercollegiate Guidelines Network 2003) recommend washing every 4 weeks
- Provide parents with individual written information and instructions tailored to their child's needs and always allow time for them to digest the information and come back to you with any questions. Involve the child as much as possible, using language that can be easily understood
- Nurses are in a position to offer advice; parents need reassurance that, with proper care, acute symptoms can often be avoided

Peak flow measurement

A peak flow recording measures the maximum flow rate of a forced expiration. It is an effort-dependant test that is used as an assessment tool for children with respiratory conditions and it is by far the most common lung function test. Peak flow can only reliably be performed by children from about 6 years of age or older. However, it is important to assess the individual child's abilities to ensure the technique can be reproduced reliably.

Peak flow increases with height, so in order to predict a normal peak flow for a child, the child's height is plotted on one axis and predicted peak flow on the other axis of a nomogram (Godfrey, 1970) (see *Figure 8.2*).

***NOTE:** In an acute situation, a single peak flow reading is of no value and is contraindicated because the process of producing adequate breath for peak flow measurement exacerbates lower airways collapse.*

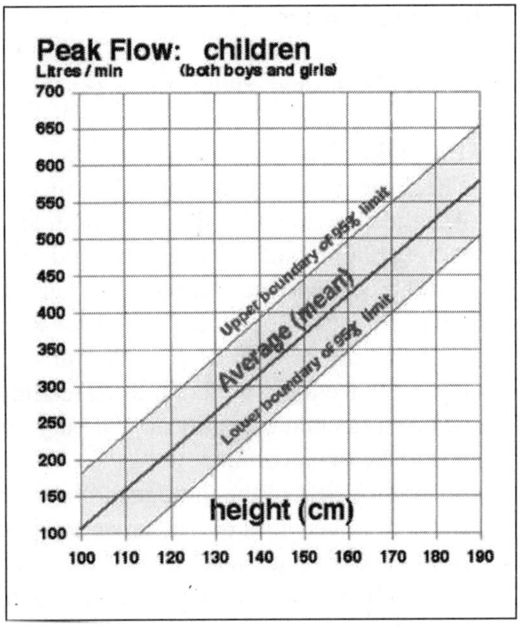

Reasons for the procedure

- To assess pulmonary function
- To aid self-management of asthma

Peak flow recordings are not indicated during acute exacerbation of asthma. They do not benefit clinical management and may lead to respiratory distress.

Figure 8.2: The normogram for peak flow in children

Pre-procedure

Equipment required

- A peak-flow meter (PFM)
- A mouthpiece
- A normogram chart with the child's height plotted to provide a predicted peak flow reading

Why use a new device? New meters are manufactured to new European Standard EN 13826 and may read differently from the traditional Wright and mini-Wright PFMs that are being phased out. The old and new devices are not interchangeable. The new standard is based on absolute flow. The new device should produce peak flow measurements that are similar to those obtained by conventional spirometry and therefore allow a more accurate assessment of peak flow across the entire measurement range (Miller, 2004).

Specific patient preparation

- Explain the need for the peak flow to the child and the family in appropriate terms for the situation and age of the child. The use of play therapy and distraction techniques should be considered to aid compliance
- Record the child's height accurately and plot the predicted peak flow on the nomogram
- Demonstrate the procedure to the child and the family. Parents can help by giving instructions using examples with which the child is familiar
- Ensure the child is standing or sitting in an upright position to assist effective lung expansion
- Explain the need for pre- and post-salbutamol peak flow recordings

During the procedure

- Set up the desired equipment as per the manufacturer's guidelines. Ensure delivery device is working correctly
- The child should stand up, if possible, or sit upright
- Check the cursor on the peak-flow meter is set to zero (0 L/min position)
- Ask the child to take a deep breath in and place the mouthpiece of the peak-flow meter in his or her mouth. It should be held horizontally with the lips sealing around the mouthpiece. Ask the child to blow hard and fast into the device, but not to block the mouthpiece with his or her tongue or by coughing
- Note the number indicated by the cursor, then return the cursor to zero
- Repeat twice more to obtain three readings – the best of these three readings should be taken (a child's peak flow will vary and is only as accurate as the technique used to undertake the recordings)
- Record the best of the three recordings on a peak flow chart (nomogram)
- If the child becomes distressed at any point try to reassure and comfort him or her
- If pre- and post-salbutamol peak flow recordings are required, the post-recordings will need to be taken 15 minutes after the administration of the salbutamol and documented as such

Post-procedure

- Ensure the child is comfortable and settled following peak flow recording
- Document the time and date and best of three recordings
- Document any adverse effects observed
- Administer medication as per the prescription chart
- Peak flow mouthpieces should be changed regularly as per the manufacturer's guidelines and local policy

Student skill laboratory activity

✓ Identify the equipment required to undertake a peak flow recording.
✓ Practice measuring and recording your own peak flow while lying, sitting and standing up.
✓ Compare your results with your predicted peak flow recording.
✓ Consider how you would instruct a child and their parents how to undertake and record peak flow recordings.

Nebuliser therapy

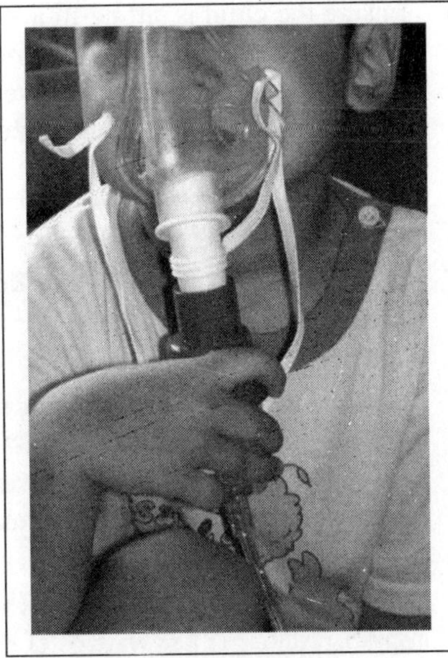

Figure 8.3: Nebuliser device

Reasons for the procedure

For most children the use of a metered-dose inhaler is as effective as a nebuliser (*Figure 8.3*) and thus the preferred delivery method of choice. Nebuliser therapy is specifically indicated in the following situations:

- To deliver inhaled steroids and bronchodilators with severe exacerbations of asthma or wheezy episodes
- To deliver inhaled steroids and bronchodilators to children who do not tolerate inhaler therapy
- To deliver certain antibiotics, predominantly those used to treat children with chronic lung conditions such as cystic fibrosis

Pre-procedure

Equipment required

- A supply of oxygen or air (delivered via pipe, cylinder, oxygen concentrator or electric portable nebuliser). Oxygen is indicated in any child requiring oxygen therapy
- A flow meter with controller
- A mask or mouthpiece (the use of a mouthpiece enhances deposition of the drug within the lower airways but is not suitable for use with infants and younger children and for individuals who are very breathless; for these a well-fitting mask should be used)
- A nebuliser device (see *Box 8.7*) – if delivering drugs that should not contaminate the atmosphere of the room ensure an appropriate nebulisation device is selected to facilitate filtration or removal of expired gases
- Oxygen tubing
- A valid drug prescription

Specific patient preparation

- Explain the need for nebuliser therapy to the child and the family in appropriate terms for the situation and age of the child. The use of play therapy and distraction techniques should be considered to aid compliance if time allows without endangering the child

- Ensure the child is sitting in a supported position or that his or her head or body is elevated to assist effective lung expansion and deposition of the drug into the lower respiratory tract. Consider sitting younger children on the lap of a parent or carer to lessen the distress of the unfamiliar treatment. Infants may be cradled in the arms of a parent or carer, or sat in an appropriate chair

Box 8.7: Nebuliser devices

There are many devices available for nebulisation, which can be achieved in two ways (Dodd, 1996)

Standard jet nebulisation – This is a continuous process which is independent of the respiratory cycle, resulting in 60–70% of the drug being wasted during expiration. The output flow rate of the device is the same as the flow rate set on the oxygen or air source. A variety of systems are available to deliver simple nebulised drugs such as salbutamol or those that require filtering such as antibiotics

Breath-assisted nebulisation – The output flow of the device is increased when the child inspires, resulting in less wastage of drug. The delivery time for the nebuliser depends on the individual child's inspiratory flow rate and depth and may be significantly quicker than standard jet nebulisation

During the procedure

- Set up desired equipment as per the manufacturer's guidelines
- Ensure the delivery device is working correctly
- Check the drug carefully against the prescription chart
- Tip the drug into the collection pot of the nebuliser. Small volumes should be diluted with normal saline to ensure greater drug delivery
- For delivery via a mask, fasten the facemask onto the child's head or hold it against their face. If the mask is held away from the mouth and the nose, much of the drug is lost, so reducing the clinical effectiveness of nebulisation
- If a mouthpiece is being used the child should place it between his or her teeth with lips sealed around it
- Turn the gas supply to a flow rate of at least 6 litres per minute (this is to ensure that the droplets of the drug are reduced to the appropriate size for inhalation and produce an adequate mist for the child to inhale)
- Encourage the patient to breathe normally through his or her mouth as an artificially increased respiratory rate or nasal breathing encourages deposition of the drug in the upper respiratory tract
- Observe for any drug specific side-effects. Inform medical staff of any observed side-effects and consider discontinuing therapy

- If the child becomes distressed at any point, try to reassure and comfort them. Crying and screaming increase the deposition of drug in the upper respiratory tract and may increase loss of the drug through forced expiration. Consider discontinuing therapy until the child is more settled. The use of an inhaler device with a facemask may be indicated if child continues to be distressed
- Nebulisation is complete when the device is not delivering any mist or is only 'spitting'

Post-procedure

- Assess the child for effects of the nebuliser. If still acutely wheezy or minimal air entry is heard consult medical staff regarding further drug therapy. Continue to re-assess the child at regular intervals
- Ensure the child is comfortable and settled following therapy
- Document the time and date the nebuliser was given, how it was given, and any effects noted, beneficial or adverse
- If the nebuliser was given via a facemask, wipe the skin clean to remove traces of drug to prevent skin irritation. This is particularly important if the child was given nebulised steroids or antibiotics (in which case they should also be given a drink or mouth care to remove any drug particles from the mouth)
- Wash the nebuliser device between uses as some solution will be left within the pot at the end of nebulisation (potential for bacterial contamination). Use warm water and a general purpose disinfectant and then dry thoroughly. Nebuliser sets should be changed regularly as per the manufacturer's guidelines and local policy

Chest drains

A chest drain is a tube that is surgically implanted within the pleural cavity. It aims to allow the lungs to expand fully and to reduce the build up of pressure on the mediastinum due to the presence of air or fluid in the pleural cavity by allowing it to drain off. It may be sited in an emergency, or in a controlled situation under local anaesthetic or general anaesthetic, as appropriate, in consideration of associated pain and distress.

How do chest drains work? They drain off the air or fluid into a bottle, whereby an 'underwater seal' prevents re-aspiration of air from the bottle into the pleural cavity. 'All-in-one' chest drainage units are supplied with the drainage tube already connected to a single multi-chambered bottle and ready to insert, simply requiring the addition of water to provide the underwater seal. The suction applied by these units is regulated by the level to which the water is filled during insertion and not by the amount of suction pressure applied at the suction source. Traditional multi-bottle systems may also be used, with or without the application of low-flow suction.

Before the surgical insertion, the nurse should explain the need for the chest drain to the child and the family. If available give them written material regarding chest drains and allow them time to absorb the information and ask any questions. A play specialist may be required to explain the procedure to the child. After insertion an X-ray of the drain is taken to ensure that it has been correctly placed. If the child has more than one chest drain placed, these should be labelled for date of insertion and location of the drain. The initial level of fluid should be marked on the bottle. The length of time that the chest drain needs to be left in place will be decided by the clinical condition of the individual patient. During this time it will need constant nursing care.

Care of chest drains

Reasons for the procedure

- To treat pneumothorax (air in the pleural cavity)
- To treat pleural effusion (fluid in the pleural cavity)
- To treat empyema (pus in the pleural cavity)
- To treat chylothorax (chyle in the pleural cavity)
- To treat haemothorax (blood in the pleural cavity)

Pre-procedure

Equipment required

- Two toothless chest drain clamps (in case of removal or breakage of the drain)
- Sterile chest drain unit (in case of removal or breakage of the drain)
- Spare sterile occlusive dressing
- Sterile gauze
- Gloves

Specific patient preparation

- Explain what is involved in caring for the chest drain to the child and the family
- Consider involving a play specialist as required
- Discuss pain management strategies with the child and family

During the procedure

Integrity of tubes

- Ensure loops of tubing do not hang from the side of the bed or chair because drainage may be impeded; they should be placed in horizontal loops next to the patient, before an appropriate length of tubing is left to travel into the bottle

- Inspect connections in the tubing for air leaks
- Observe for any bubbling of air within the chest drain unit, which may be indicative of air draining from the pleural space. Continuous bubbling may suggest an air leak at one of the connections. To check for this clamp the chest tube near the patient. The bubbling should cease if the air originates from the pleural space. If it continues check all connections. The application of suction will also create gentle bubbling; if this is too vigorous it suggests that the applied suction pressure may be too high
- For tubes located within the pleural space, examine the chest tubing for any 'swinging' of fluid (changes in pressures associated with the child's respiratory cycle); if there is no swinging it may mean the tube has become blocked. Medical staff should be informed

Fluid within the drain

- Ensure the drain is kept below the level of the chest to prevent any re-entry of fluid into the pleural cavity and that it is upright at all times with the water at the correct level to retain the water seal. If the bottle is knocked over, stand it back up and assess the child for any indications of pneumothorax. Alert medical staff
- Check the fluid level within the bottle against the initial level marked on the bottle, as the patient's condition and medical directions indicate, and record any changes. If the bottle is over two thirds full there will be increased resistance to drainage and the bottle should be changed (with the chest tube double-clamped and using a non-touch procedure)
- Check the colour and type of fluid. Record them. Any sudden changes in the rate or type of discharge should be reported to medical staff

Clamping the chest drain

- Two clamps should always be applied (double-clamping) – one close to the patient above the connection and one just below. If a chest drain is disconnected, medical staff should be alerted immediately and a new drainage bottle connected as soon as possible. The child should be assessed for any signs of pneumothorax
- Chest drains should not be routinely clamped during patient mobilisation as this can result in increased pressures within the pleural cavity. Clamps should only be used in children with a pneumothorax after radiological confirmation of chest re-expansion to allow a period of observation prior to drain removal, when changing bottles and on accidental disconnection of the drain
- Chest drain tubing should NOT be milked with clamps *or* manually as this exerts very high pressures on the pleural space or mediastinum

Care of the patient

- Regularly record observations as the patient's condition indicates, including oxygen saturations, heart rate, respiratory rate, colour, blood pressure and temperature. Auscultate the chest for equality of breath sounds. Consider the need for arterial blood gases

- Inspect the site of insertion regularly, for signs of tube displacement, infection, leakage, and bleeding or air infiltration. If the dressing over the site remains clean it should not be changed unless hospital policy or medical care dictates other
- Check the colour and type of fluid. Record them. Any sudden changes in the rate or type of discharge should be reported to medical staff
- Nurse the child in a semi-sitting position to encourage lung expansion and drainage, and consider involving a physiotherapist who can help with age-appropriate exercises to promote lung expansion (for example by blowing of bubbles)
- Monitor the use of any prescribed chest drain suction. This may be provided by a low-flow wall suction unit or a portable suction unit. Suction pressure should be prescribed by a doctor. If too high a pressure is used damage may occur to lung tissue, too low a pressure may prevent adequate lung expansion

Pain management

- Encourage the child to change position regularly to decrease pain associated with muscle spasms
- Monitor the child for any indications of pain using an appropriate pain scoring system (document the scores regularly to ensure the child's pain is being effectively controlled (always use the same scoring system to ensure validity of scores). A child who is in pain is reluctant to move in bed or to take deep breaths, lessening the effectiveness of treatment
- Encourage use of non-pharmacological (distraction therapy and positioning) and pharmacological pain-relieving methods
- Ensure the child receives adequate analgesia. Combine simple analgesics such as paracetamol with non-steroidal drugs such as diclofenac and, if indicated, opiates such as codeine or morphine
- Document time and effectiveness of any analgesia given

Post-procedure

- Ensure any changes in the patient's condition or care are documented and reported as appropriate to medical staff

Removal of the drain

The decision to remove the drain will be made by medical staff following clinical examination and/or chest X-ray. The process should performed by two people to ensure the child's safety. At least one of these two people should have performed the procedure before.

Reasons for the procedure

- To discontinue drainage as indicated by clinical condition

Pre-procedure

Equipment required

- Two toothless chest drain clamps
- Sterile occlusive dressing
- Sterile gloves
- Clinical waste bag and bin
- A paper suture may be required if not using a 'purse-string' closure

Specific patient preparation

- Explain the procedure of removing the chest drain to the child and the family
- Consider involving a play specialist and the use of distraction therapy during removal
- Discuss use of analgesia with the child and family and ensure the child is given adequate prescribed analgesia at an appropriate time prior to removal of drain
- Consider using Entonox to give child some feeling of control over the procedure (see the section on pain management in *Chapter 7*)

During the procedure

One care provider will remove the chest tube, and the other will seal the site using suture (this may be a purse-string suture).

- Wash hands. Use an aseptic manner to reduce risk of introducing infection
- Double-clamp the chest drain, one close to the patient, above the connection, and one just below
- Disconnect any suction pressure
- If the child is old enough to respond appropriately, ask him or her to take three big breaths in and out and then hold their breath until you tell them to breathe out again. The aim is to quickly but smoothly remove the tube during while the patient holds their breath (to prevent air being sucked into the pleural space)
- Your assistant should then quickly seal the entry site with the paper or purse-string sutures
- The child should then be instructed to breathe normally again while an occlusive dressing is applied

Post-procedure

- Re-assess the child's oxygen saturations, respiratory rate and depth, and heart rate
- A repeat chest X-ray may be indicated to look for a pneumothorax post drain removal
- Ensure the child is comfortable
- Observe the site of the drain for bleeding and infection
- Consider sending the tip of the chest drain for microscopy

Glossary of terms relating to respiratory care

Allergen	A foreign substance that initiates an allergic reaction
Alveolus	An air sac in the lungs
Apnoea	Cessation of breath lasting at least 10 seconds
Arrhythmia	An irregularity in normal cardiac rhythms
Asthma	A respiratory disorder characterised by recurrent episodes of difficulty in breathing, wheezing and coughing
Atelectasis	Collapse of the alveoli
Auscultation	The act of examining by listening to body sounds
Bradycardia	A slow heart rate, usually lower than 60 beats per minute
Bronchiolitis	An infection of the bronchioles, affecting mainly babies and often characterised by presence of respiratory syncytial virus (RSV)
Bronchus	One of the two large branches of the trachea that leads to the lungs
Cyanosis	A blue, grey or purple discolouration of the mucous membranes and skin caused by deficient oxygenation of the blood
Dyspnoea	Laboured, difficult breathing
Expiration	The expelling of air from the lungs (exhalation)
Hypo/hypertension	Low/high blood pressure
Hypoxia	Inadequate oxygen of tissues so that normal function is not possible
Inspiration	The drawing in of air into the lungs (inhalation)
Laryngospasm	Spasm of the laryngeal nerve
Pre-oxygenation	The giving of extra oxygen to prevent hypoxia
Pulmonary	Related to the lungs
Respiratory system	The organs and structures that carry out gas exchange, including the nose, pharynx, larynx, trachea, bronchi and lungs
Stenosis	An abnormal constriction or narrowing
Tachycardia	A rapid heart rate
Tachypnoea	A rapid respiratory rate
Tidal volume	The amount of air inhaled or exhaled during a normal breath
Vagal nerve stimulation	Stimulation of the parasympathetic nervous system resulting in bradycardia

References

Aylott M (2006a) Observing the sick child: Part 2a. Respiratory assessment. *Paed Nurs* **18**(9): 38–44

Aylott M (2006b) Tracheostomy tube change. In: Glasper EA, McEwing G, Richardson J, eds. *Oxford Handbook of Children's and Young Persons Nursing*. Oxford University Press, Oxford

Aylott M (2006c) Tracheostomy tube suctioning. In: Glasper EA, McEwing G, Richardson J, eds. *Oxford Handbook of Children's and Young Persons Nursing*. Oxford University Press, Oxford

Bateman NT, Leach RM (1998) ABC of oxygen. Acute oxygen therapy. *BMJ* **317:** 798–801

British National Formulary (2007) *British National Formulary*. BMJ/RPS Publishing , London

British Thoracic Society (1997) British Guideline on the Management of Nebulisers. *Thorax* **52**(Suppl 2): S1–S24 www.brit-thoracic.org.uk

British Thoracic Society (2004) *British Guideline on the Management of Asthma*, revised edition. www.brit-thoracic.org.uk/sign/index.htm

British Thoracic Society and Scottish Intercollegiate Guidelines Network (2003) British Guideline on the Management of Asthma. *Thorax* **58**(Suppl 1)

Dodd M (1996) Nebuliser therapy: what nurses patients need to know. *Nurs Stand* **10**(31): 39–42

Godfrey S (1970) Nomogram. *Br J Dis Chest* **64:** 15

Griggs A (1998) Tracheostomy: suctioning and humidification. *Nurs Stand* **13**(2): 49–56

Medical Devices Agency (2001) *Tissue necrosis caused by pulse oximeter probes*. Medicines and Healthcare Products Regulatory Agency, London

Miller MR (2004) Peak expiratory flow meter scale changes; implications for patients and health professionals. *Airways J* **2**(2): 80–82

National Institute for Clinical Excellence (2000) *Guidance on the Use of Inhaler Systems (Devices) in Children Under the Age of 5 Years with Chronic Asthma*. Technology Appraisal Guidance No 10. NICE, London

National Institute for Clinical Excellence (2003) *Inhaler Devices for Routine Treatment of Chronic Asthma (Aged 5–15 Years)*. Technology Appraisal Guidance No 38. NICE, London

National Respiratory Training Centre (2003) *Paediatric Asthma Diploma Module Handbook*. National Respiratory Training Centre, Warwick

Newell K, Hume S (2006) Choosing the right inhaler for patients with asthma. *Nurs Stand* **21**(5): 46–48

Pease P (2006) Oxygen administration: Is practice based on evidence? *Paed Nurs* **18**(8): 14–8

Woodrow P (2002) Managing patients with a tracheostomy in acute care. *Nurs Stand* **16**(44): 39–46

Further reading

Advanced Life Support Group (2005) *Advanced Paediatric Life Support: – The Practical Approach*, 4th edn. BMJ Publishing Group, London

Allibone L (2003) Nursing management of chest drains. *Nurs Stand* **17**(22): 45–54

Ashurst S (1995) Clinical oxygen therapy. *Brit J Nurs* **4**(9): 508–14

Asthma UK (2006) *Demo to help your patients with their inhaler technique*. www.asthma.org.uk

Avery S (2000) Insertion and management of chest drains. *NT Plus* **96**(37): 3–6

Aylott M (2006) Developing rigour in observation of the sick child: Part 1. *Paed Nurs* **18**(8): 38–44

Aylott M (2007) Observing the sick child: Part 2c. Respiratory auscultation. *Paed Nurs* **19**(2): 38–44

Aylott M (2007) Observing the sick child: Part 2b. Respiratory palpation. *Paed Nurs* **19**(1): 38–44

Barry P, O'Callaghan C (1997) Nebuliser therapy in childhood. *Thorax* **52**(Suppl 2): S78–S88

Bruce E, Howard R, Franck L (2006) Chest drain removal pain and its management: a literature review. *J Clin Nurs* **15:** 145–54

Buglas E (1999) Tracheostomy care: tracheal suctioning and humidification. *Brit J Nurs* **8**(8): 500–04

Casey G (2001) Oxygen transport and the use of pulse oximetry. *Nurs Stand* **15**(47): 46–53

Chandler T (2000) Oxygen saturation monitoring. *Paed Nurs* **12**(8): 37–42

Chandler T (2001) Oxygen administration. *Paed Nurs* **13**(8): 37–42

Dewar AL, Stewart A, Cogswell JJ, Connett GJ (1999) A randomised controlled trial to assess the relative benefits of large volume spacers and nebulisers to treat acute asthma in hospital. *Arch Dis Childhood* **80:** 421–23

Frey B, Shann F (2003) Oxygen administration in infants. *Arch Dis Childhood: Fetal Neonat* **88**(2): F84–F88

Hough A (2001) *Physiotherapy in Respiratory Care. An Evidence-Based Approach to Respiratory and Cardiac Management*, 3rd edn. Nelson Thornes, Cheltenham

Kamps AWA, Brand PLP, Roorda RJ (2002) Determinants of correct inhalation technique in children attending a hospital-based asthma clinic. *Acta Paediatrics* **91**: 159–63

Kannan S (1999) Practical issues in non-invasive positive pressure ventilation. *Care Crit Ill* **15**(3): 76–79

Levy ML (2004) *Asthma Rapid Reference*. Mosby, London

McNamara VM, Crabbe DCG (2004) Tracheomalacia. *Paediatr Resp Rev* **5**: 147–54

Moore T (2003) Suctioning techniques for the removal of respiratory secretions. *Nurs Stand* **18**(9): 47–53

O'Callaghan C, Barry PW (2000) Asthma drug delivery devices for children. *BMJ* **320:** 664

O'Callaghan C, Barry PW (2000) How to choose devices for asthma. *Arch Dis Childhood* **82:** 185–91

Pierart F, Wildhaber JH, Vrancken I, Devadason SG, LeSouef PN (1999) Washing plastic spacers in household detergent reduces electrostatic charge and greatly improves delivery. *Eur Resp J* **13:** 673–78

Place B (1998) Pulse oximetry in adults. *Nurs Times* **94**(50): 48–9

Serra A (2000) Tracheostomy care. *Nurs Stand* **14**(42): 45–55

Trachsel D Hammer J (2006) Indications for tracheostomy in children. *Paediatr Resp Rev* **7:** 162–69

Williams R, Rankin N, Smith T, Galler D, Seakins P (1996) Relationship between humidity and temperature of inspired gas and the function of the airway mucosa. *Crit Care Med* **24**(11): 1920–29

Wilson M (2005) Paediatric tracheostomy. *Paed Nurs* **17**(3): 38–44

Woodrow P (2003) Using non-invasive ventilation in acute wards: Part 1. *Nurs Stand* **18**(1): 39–44

Useful websites

Airways Extra (National Respiratory Training Centre and Asthma UK)
www.airwaysextra.com

Peak Flow
www.peakflow.com

Aaron's Tracheostomy Page
www.tracheostomy.com

Chapter 9

Fundamental aspects of cardiovascular care

Gemma Blagdon, Louise Butler, Sally Cooke, Laura Ho and Margaret Porter

This chapter covers those aspects of cardiovascular medicine that are specifically relevant to the nursing of a child or young person. The issues covered include:

- Electrocardiography
- Venepuncture
- Intravenous cannulation
- Central lines

The electrocardiograph (ECG)

ECG monitoring is one of the most valuable diagnostic tools in general medicine and is essential to recognise disorders of cardiac rhythm (Jevon, 2000). Continuous cardiac monitoring provides a visual display of a child's heart rate and rhythm. Furthermore, it enables you to analyse the electrical activity of the heart, evaluate conduction patterns, estimate heart size, assess muscle function and electrolyte imbalance in conjunction with medical colleagues.

There are two basic types of continuous ECG monitoring:

- Hard-wire monitoring
- Telemetry

In hard-wire monitoring, the child is connected via a cable from electrodes placed on their chest to a bedside monitor. However, telemetry is a more convenient method of monitoring the cardiac rhythm, whereby the child can be mobile and play away from their bed space while attached to a battery-powered transducer, which relays the heart rhythm signals to a receiver. The monitor senses any abnormal events and an alarm sounds.

Cardiac monitoring must never replace your nursing observations of the sick child. It can, however, be used as part of an overall child physical assessment, performed against background knowledge of the child's history, treatment (including drugs) and coexisting haemodynamic (circulatory) status (Mehta and Dhillon, 2004).

Glossary of terms in cardiovascular medicine

Arrhythmia	An abnormal heart rhythm
Arterial blood pressure	An invasive direct measurement of the pressure exerted by the blood on the walls of the blood vessels
Bradyarrhythmia	An abnormally slow heart rhythm
Cannulation	The insertion of a cannula or tube into a hollow body organ
Central line	A vascular infusion device that terminates at, or close to, the heart or in one of the great vessels
Central venous pressure	The pressure in the thoracic vena cava near the right atrium (therefore it is essentially the same as right atrial pressure)
Dysrhythmia	An abnormal heart rhythm
Electrocardiograph	A record of the electrical activity of the heart
Epicardial pacing	A method for temporary pacing or sensing of the atria or ventricles by attaching the pacing leads to the epicardial surface (usually used in the diagnosis and treatment of postoperative dysrhythmias)
Heart block	Interrupted electrical impulse to heart muscles. Sometimes the signal from the upper (atria) to lower (ventricles) chambers of the heart is impaired or does not transmit
Oesophageal pacing	A temporary cardiac pacing method in which leads are placed within the oesophagus to effect atrial pacing for the diagnosis and treatment of dysrhythmia
Pacing	Regulation of the rate of contraction of the heart muscle by an artificial cardiac pacemaker
Sinus node dysfunction	A disorder of impulse generation and conduction
Tachyarrhythmia	An abnormally fast heart rhythm
Transcutaneous pacing	A temporary cardiac pacing method in which large-surface, high-impedance electrodes are applied to the anterior and posterior chest walls to deliver high-current stimuli of long duration for pacing of the ventricles
Transthoracic pacing	A temporary cardiac pacing method in which a hooked pacing lead is attached to the ventricular endocardium by insertion through the chest wall or epigastric area and then the ventricular wall (used in emergency situations, usually cardiac arrest, as an alternative to transcutaneous pacing)
Transvenous (endocardial) pacing	A permanent or temporary cardiac pacing method in which the pacing leads, inserted by means of a catheter, are connected to the endocardium via the venous circulation (the pulse generator may be implanted or external)
Venepuncture	Puncturing of a vein in order to obtain blood samples

ECG monitoring

Reasons for the procedure

- To identify arrhythmias
- To detect electrolyte imbalances (particularly high and low potassium levels)
- To evaluate palpitations (fast heart beats felt in the chest, neck or ears)
- To investigate history of syncope (dizziness/fainting)
- To monitor heart failure
- To investigate chest pain (comparatively rare in children)
- To monitor patients after cardiac surgery
- To monitor the effectiveness of cardiac medication
- To assess patients during cardiopulmonary resuscitation (McChance and Heuther, 2006)

Pre-procedure

Equipment required

- Disposable chest leads (3)
- ECG leads and cable
- Cardiac monitor
- Alcohol wipes (if necessary)

Specific patient preparation

- Inform the child and/or parents where appropriate about the requirement and nature of cardiac monitoring (Jowett, 1997)
- If the child's skin feels greasy or wet due to sweat (common in children with cardiac disease) you may need to cleanse the child's skin with alcohol wipes where the electrode pads are to be sited in order facilitate a good contact and thus a good reading. Avoid using alcohol wipes indiscriminately especially with in infants who tend to have fragile/sensitive skin (Chamley *et al*, 2005)

During the procedure

- Position the red electrode on the right clavicle (right collar bone) in the mid-clavicular line (an imaginary line drawn mid-way between the suprasternal notch – the indentation or hollow over the throat – and the tip of the shoulder)
- Apple the yellow electrode to the left clavicle, again in the mid-clavicular line, as bone transmits electricity well

- Apply the green electrode to the last (bottom) rib of the lower left anterior rib cage (*Figure 9.1*)
- Attach the colour-coded cables to the electrodes and the monitor
- Switch on the cardiac monitor and set to lead II (Cooke and Metcalfe, 2000) (lead II selects the preferred electrical view across the heart)
- Endeavour to obtain the best possible trace. This depends on the waveform being large enough for you to distinguish each component of the PQRST complex (Tortora and Derrickson, 2007) (*Figure 9.2*) as a clear, well-defined tracing that travels horizontally across the screen

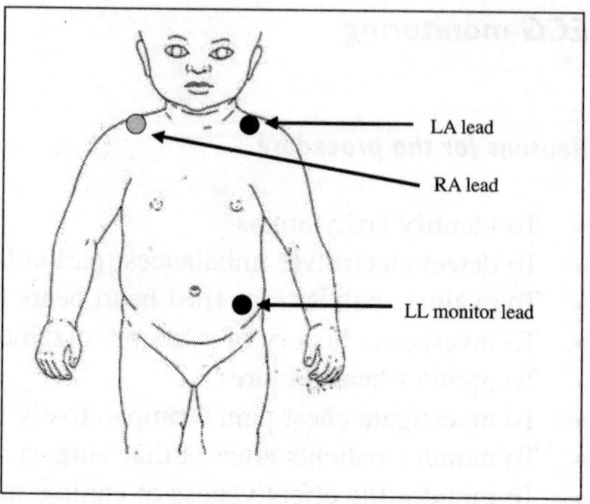

Figure 9.1: Three-lead positioning ECG system. RA, right atrial; LA, left atrial

Post-procedure

- Thank the child for their help in getting a fine picture
- Remove the electrode pads gently from the child's chest, encouraging the child to help you do this at their pace
- Wash their skin if necessary with a cloth, warm water and soap and dry thoroughly to leave the child comfortable
- Check the skin around the electrode sites for allergic reactions or sensitivity, and report any to the medical staff
- Assess the cardiac trace
- Report findings to the medical staff
- If abnormalities are present, a 12-lead ECG may be requested by medical staff

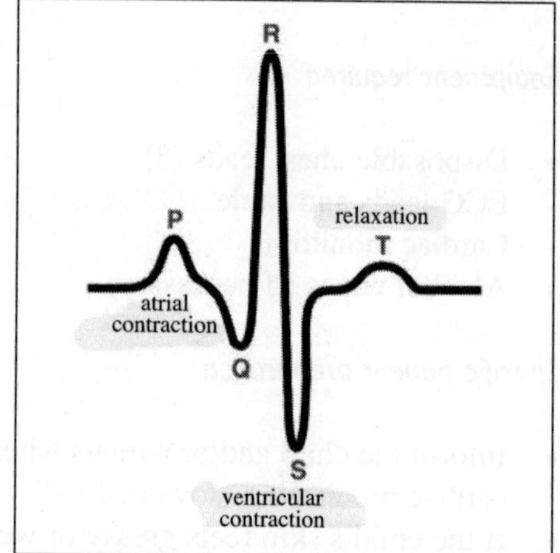

Figure 9.2: PQRST wave complex. P, atrial contraction; T, relaxation; S, ventricular contraction

Difficulties experienced with ECG monitoring

Numerous problems may be encountered with ECG monitoring. Some arise because of the limitations of the monitoring system and some because of improper technique (Jevon, 2000).

Flat-line trace

- Immediately check the child! If the child is not in distress the most likely cause is mechanical
- Check that the monitor is switched on
- Check that the electrodes are properly connected
- Check that the correct monitoring lead on the monitor is selected
- Check that the ECG gain is set properly

Poor-quality trace

- Check all the connections and the brightness display, and ensure that the electrodes are attached properly
- Check that the electrodes are in date and the gel sponge is moist
- Clean the skin with an alcohol wipe

Interference and artefacts

- Check for poor electrode contact, ensure that contact is secure and reliable
- Check for movements of the child (reassure and keep them warm)
- Consider electrical impedance (eg. an infusion pump or computer games console by the bed can cause a fuzzy appearance on the trace)
- Minimise interference by applying electrodes over bone rather than muscle (Resuscitation Council UK, 2006)

Wandering baseline

- Consider the child's chest movements and position, as the height of the QRS complexes varies in response to both
- Try changing electrodes or selecting a different monitoring lead

Recording a 12-lead ECG

A 12-lead ECG is a non-invasive procedure that records the electrical activity of the heart from many different angles or views. It is used to measure the rate and regularity of heart beats, as well as the size and position of the chambers, the presence of any damage to the heart, and the effects of drugs or devices used to regulate the heart, such as a pacemaker (Tortora and Derrickson, 2006).

Reasons for the procedure

- To assist diagnosis prior to interventions such as surgery
- To identify different types of heart disorders
- To monitor cardiac arrhythmias
- To detect electrolyte disturbances
- To monitor the effectiveness of medication

Equipment required

- ECG machine
- Disposable electrodes
- Alcohol wipes (if necessary)

Specific patient preparation

- Explain to the child and parent that an ECG is necessary and why and importantly what this involves in order to gain consent and the child and/or parent(s) help with the procedure (National Patient Safety Agency [NPSA], 2004)
- Make sure the child is undressed to the waist to expose the chest
- Ensure that the child is in a comfortable position, either sitting or lying supine

During the procedure

- Wash your hands (Department of Health, 2003)
- If the child has oily skin, cleanse the electrode sites with alcohol wipes (to enable better contact with the electrodes)
- Attach the four limb electrodes to the palmar aspect of each hand and each ankle
- Apply the six chest leads as described below (it is helpful that each lead is labelled) (see *Figure 9.3* and *Box 9.1*)
  - Place lead V1 in the 4th intercostal space to the right of the sternum
  - Place lead V2 in the 4th intercostal space to the left of the sternum
  - Place lead V3 directly between leads V2 and V4
  - Place lead V4 in the 5th intercostal space (mid-clavicular)
  - Place lead V5 directly between leads V4 and V6
  - Place lead V6 in the 5th intercostal space (mid-axillary)(Tortora, 2005)

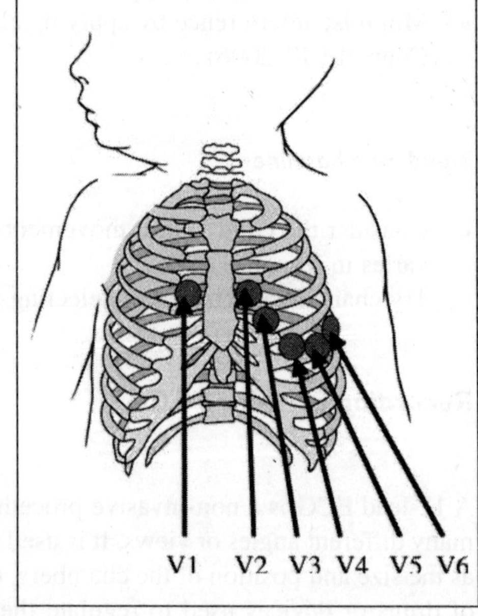

Figure 9.3: Placement of the leads of the 12-lead ECG

- Attach the ten corresponding leads from the ECG machine to the electrodes, ensuring they are connected correctly
- Encourage the child to relax and refrain from movement (where this is not possible try to distract the child to minimise movement or distress)
- Press 'Start' to commence 12-lead recording
- Label the ECG correctly with the child's name and hospital number, and the date and time

Post-procedure

- Inform the child and/or parent that the procedure is complete and thank them for their assistance
- Thank the child for their help in getting a fine picture
- Remove the electrode pads gently from the child's chest (encourage them to help you do this at their pace)
- `Wash the skin if necessary with a cloth, warm water and soap, and dry thoroughly to leave the child comfortable
- Check the skin around the electrode sites for allergic reactions or sensitivity, and report any to the medical staff
- Wash your hands (Department of Health, 2003)
- If any abnormalities are present, report and to the medical staff immediately
- Record procedure and action in the child's notes including date and time (Nursing and Midwifery Council [NMC], 2004)

Box 9.1: Tips to help locate ribs and spaces (Aylott, 2007)

The suprasternal notch is the hollow U-shaped depression just above the child's sternum, between the clavicles. The sternum (or breastbone) consists of the manubrium, the body and the xiphoid process.

1. Walk your fingers down the manubrium a few cm until you feel a distinct bony ridge – this is the manubriosternal angle, which is continuous with the second rib and is a useful place to start counting ribs
2. Palpate lightly down to the 2nd rib and slide down to the second inter-costal space. Now count down the intercostal spaces until you reach the 4th one (beneath 4th rib; ie. the intercostal space is always numbered by the rib above it) and place the V1, V2 and V3 leads
3. Then palpate down to the 5th intercostal space and place the V4, V5 and V6 leads

Non-invasive temporary pacing

Non-invasive temporary pacing may be used in emergency situations to treat heart rate and rhythm disturbances, which are compromising cardiac output. This kind of pacing is useful in cases of:

- Post-cardiac surgery (but damage may occur to the conduction system resulting in heart block)
- Bradyarrhythmia that compromises cardiac output
- Sinus node dysfunction (overdrive pacing is used to terminate refractory tachycardias such as atrial flutter)
- Failure to respond to inotropic agents, oxygen or anti-arrhythmic therapy

Types of pacing

Epicardial pacing

- Pacing wires are inserted at the time of cardiac surgery
- Two wires allow pacing of either the atria or ventricles
- Ventricular wires exit on the left side of the chest (LV). Atrial wires exit on the right side of the chest (RA)

Transvenous (endocardial) pacing

- A wire is inserted into a central vein into the right atria, usually using fluoroscopy imaging for correct placement
- Associated with increased risk of pneumothorax, air emboli, haemorrhage, infection, and arrhythmia

Oesophageal pacing

- An electrode is placed up the nose into the oesophagus and passed until it lies behind the left atrium
- Children often experience discomfort, particularly if the voltage is high and diaphragmatic pacing occurs

Transthoracic pacing

- A needle is inserted into the chest wall and an epicardial pacing wire is attached to the epicardium

Transcutaneous pacing

- Easiest method to use in an emergency because the two electrodes are easy to place on the chest wall
- The anterior electrode is placed in the right subclavicular area, lateral to the sternum
- The lateral (apex) electrode is placed on the left anterior aspect of the trunk, lateral to the left nipple, on the mid-axillary line of the 5th intercostal space

Permanent pacing

- Permanent pacemakers provide electrical stimuli to cause cardiac contraction
- The pacing systems consist of a pulse generator and pacing leads
- It is inserted subcutaneously in the chest wall or submuscularly in the abdomen of neonates (infants less than 28 days of age)

Modes of pacing

The North America Society of Pacing and Electrophysiology and the British Pacing and Electrophysiology Group (1993) have developed a code to describe the various pacing modes used. This system usually consists of three letters, but sometimes four or five are used.

The *first* letter signifies the chamber that is paced:

- A = atria
- V = ventricles
- D = dual chamber
- O = none

The *second* letter signifies the chamber that is sensed:

- A = atria
- V = ventricles
- D = dual chamber
- O = none

The *third* letter signifies the response to a sensed beat:

- T = triggered
- I = inhibited
- D = dual
- O = none

You might use a code such as VOO or DVI during a pacing procedure. The T position (triggered) is rarely used; it signifies the location of the sensed intrinsic (patient's own) events. If fixed pacing is used, the pacemaker will give a pre-set heart rate but it does not synchronise with the patient.

Common types of pacing using the coding system

In fixed pacing

- Either AOO or VOO
- This has no sensing function but delivers fixed pacing regardless of underlying rhythm

In demand pacing

- AAI for atrial demand pacing (eg. in sinus node slowing)
- VVI for ventricular demand pacing (eg. in complete heart block)
- Senses the underlying rhythm and paces in response as programmed

In AV sequential pacing

- Improves cardiac output
- DVI paces the atrium and the ventricle and senses the ventricle
- DDD paces the atrium and the ventricle and senses both the atrium and ventricle

Parameters of pacing

Rate of pacing

The rate depends on:

- The age of the child
- Indications for pacing
- The clinical response

Energy output of pacing

Energy output is usually set at a voltage that is two or three times higher than the threshold (the smallest stimulus required to excite the heart consistently). To determine the threshold, turn down the voltage slowly and note at what point there is loss of capture (ie. the pacing output fails to stimulate the heart).

Sensitivity of pacing

This refers to the level at which any sensed electrical activity is recognised by the pacemaker as a cardiac event. The sensitivity is increased in small increments until 'sensing' is achieved. However, no sensing or sensitivity setting is required on a fixed-rate setting (ie. when a minimum rate is set, in order that the heart rate does not drop below this setting irrespective of sensitivity).

Two parameters can be adjusted for sensitivity:

- **AV delay –** the delay between the ventricular spike and the atrial spike (approximately 100 msec)
- **Threshold –** useful for determining the reserve capacity of pacing energy output. The threshold voltage is prone to vary and tends to increase in the first few days after implantation of temporary pacing wire

Failure of a temporary pacemaker

The following measures must only be performed by staff competent to perform the changes. If you are NOT competent to do so, ask a senior colleague for assistance immediately.

- Start with the obvious – check whether the system is switched on!
- Check all attachments of wires, to exclude short circuit
- Try to alter the child's position (this can alter threshold)
- Increase the energy output (in case the threshold has increased)
- Set a fixed rate if the child is on demand mode (in case the pacemaker is being inhibited by inappropriate sensing)
- Change the batteries (one at a time) or try installing a new pacing box

If unable to resume pacing and the cardiac output is still compromised, phone the emergency resuscitation number 2222 and report to attending medical staff immediately, who may prescribe an intravenous infusion of isoprenaline in addition to other resuscitative measures.

Care of a child requiring temporary pacing

- Explain all procedures and care in an age/developmentally appropriate way to both the child and the family (NPSA, 2004)
- Ensure that the child's psychological well being is maintained by providing appropriate play. The child may sit out of bed or be gently mobilised to the play room for telemetric monitoring, particularly if post cardiac surgery when time is required for repair and recovery of the child's conduction system
- Nurse in an appropriate environment with an emergency resuscitation trolley, defibrillator and medications available
- Maintain venous access while the temporary pacing system in place
- Nurse the child on cardiac monitoring with an appropriate alarm set
- Record heart rate, blood pressure, and oxygen saturations at least hourly. Always assess the child's own pulse as the ECG monitor may be showing only the pacemaker's electrical stimuli. The child may be in electromechanical dissociation and so require resuscitation
- Record a 12-lead ECG daily
- Check the threshold of the temporary pacing box daily
- Check and document the pacing mode, rate, and current 4 hourly every 4 hours
- Change the position of monitoring electrodes daily to avoid skin sensitivity
- Assist the child with maintaining hygiene needs
- If the child requires a permanent pacemaker, provide education and information for the child and parents

Venepuncture

Venepuncture is defined as the procedure of entering a vein with a needle in order to obtain blood samples for laboratory analysis. Venepuncture in children is a fairly common occurrence and is often undertaken to aid diagnosis. It is a procedure only to be performed by members of staff who have received particular training and are certified as competent within specific age bands (Royal College of Nursing, 2005).

Reasons for the procedure

- To obtain blood for laboratory analysis

Pre-procedure

Equipment required

- Completed request forms
- Clean tray
- Non-sterile gloves and apron
- Disposable tourniquet (for children over 5 years of age)
- Alcohol-impregnated swabs
- Sterile gauze swabs
- Small plaster (ensuring that the patient is not allergic to the adhesive)
- Sharps container
- Appropriate specimen containers (seek local advice to ensure that the right ones are used)
- An appropriate needle to obtain the sample depending on the age/size of the child:
  - *For larger infants and young children:* a butterfly needle (the position of the needle and syringe can changed independently) (Willock *et al*, 2004)
  - *For infants:* a single-winged needle (infants' veins often collapse with the slightest suction pressure, so the single-winged needle allows blood to be dripped directly into the specimen tube) (Phillip and Beckett, 2000)

Consider pain relief for this painful procedure

- Topical local anaesthetics penetrate the nerve fibres and block sodium channels thus preventing generation of action potentials. Examples are:
  - EMLA (eutectic mixture of local anaesthetics) – for children over 1 year; apply 1 hour – before venepuncture (Lander, 1996a, 1996b)
  - Ametop (tetracaine 4%) – for infants older than 1 month; apply 30–45 minutes before venepuncture (Hewitt, 1998)
  - Ethyl chloride spray commonly described by children as 'cold spray' because it is a volatile liquid that evaporates rapidly and cools the skin to below 10°C (at this temperature nerve impulses cannot be generated but adjacent pain receptors are stimulated to produce the sensation of freezing) (BNFc, 2007) – spray onto the skin for 5–10 seconds until the skin takes on a whitish tinge (it should be stored carefully at room temperature and should never be inhaled as there have been reports of solvent abuse causing hallucinations, ataxia, short-term memory loss, cardiac arrhythmias, respiratory arrest and death; BNFc, 2007)
- Other forms of pain relief are:
  - Nitrous oxide (Entonox) (Willock *et al*, 2004); see *Chapter 7*
  - Non-nutritive sucking of sucrose for neonates (Stevens *et al*, 2003)

Specific patient preparation

- Explain all procedures and care in an age/developmentally appropriate way to both the child and the family (NPSA, 2004)
- Obtain consent prior to the procedure. The child, or their carer, may give consent so long as they are informed of the implications, potential side effects and alternatives. If competent, seek informed consent directly from the child (British Medical Association, 2001; Department of Health, 2001)
- Ensure that the child's psychological well being is maintained by providing appropriate play
- Identify a suitable vein and ensure that there are no intravenous infusions or transfusions in progress near the site. Venous access in children is also difficult because of the size of their veins and because they are covered by subcutaneous fat. The best veins are normally found in the antecubital fossa region – but take care to avoid the brachial artery (Das and Sharma, 2002). Other potential sites include the veins of the hands, wrist and feet (particularly useful for venepuncture in neonates and infants). Taking time to identify a suitable vein in advance of the procedure allows you to address the issue of pain relating to the procedure

During the procedure

- Ensure that you have adequately prepared the child and/or parent before you begin and re-affirm informed consent (NPSA, 2004)
- Enlist the assistance of a colleague or play specialist if necessary (Smalley, 1999)
- Ensure that the procedure takes place in a well lit, quiet environment (eg. a treatment room)
- Although obvious, first check that the child's identity matches that on the request forms
- Wash your hands, put on gloves and an apron and maintain an aseptic technique throughout (Department of Health, 2003; Conroy, 2004)
- Put the child's hand or foot in a bowl of warm water, if required, to aid dilation of the vein in preparation for venepuncture
- Assemble the equipment required as determined earlier
  - If using a butterfly needle, attach a syringe
  - If using a single-winged needle, open the required blood bottles in preparation
- Ensure that the child is in a comfortable position. Position a young child on the lap of a carer or nurse lap with his or her limb concealed from view. The limb should be supported firmly during the procedure in order to avoid sudden movements (Royal College of Nursing, 2003a)
- If you have not already done so, remove the occlusive dressing or cling film, and wipe off any excess anaesthetic cream applied earlier – DO NOT REPALPATE THE INSERTION SITE ONCE IT HAS BEEN CLEANED (Hindley, 2004)
- Prepare the child's skin by cleansing the site for 15–30 seconds with swabs soaked in 70% alcohol and allow to dry (at least 30 seconds) (Franklin, 1999)
- Support the child's limb on a pillow, for example pointing downwards to encourage blood flow by gravity. Ask your assistant to support and hold still the appropriate limb

- In older children, apply a disposable tourniquet tightly 8–10 cm above the intended venepuncture site (it works by obstructing venous return and dilating the veins). It can be useful to immobilise the vein by applying gentle traction to the child's skin a few cm below the proposed site using your non-dominant hand
- Holding the venepuncture device in your dominant hand and insert the needle into the vein by 0. 5–1 cm at an angle of 30°
  - If you are using a butterfly needle, gently draw back on the syringe plunger until enough blood is obtained
  - If you are using a single-winged needle, allow the blood to drip directly into the specimen containers (Phillip and Beckett, 2000)
- Once sufficient specimens have been obtained, instruct your assistant to relax pressure around the limb, or release the tourniquet
- Place gauze gently over the needle and remove the needle, applying pressure only after the needle has been removed
- If you used a syringe, decant the blood into the appropriate containers, labelled correctly at the bedside to reduce the risk of errors (British Committee for Standards in Haematology, 2003)
- Dispose of the needle and syringe directly into sharps container – do *not* re-sheathe needle
- Continue to apply pressure until haemostasis occurs (usually within 2 minutes, but longer if the child is being treated with anticoagulants). The limb should remain extended while pressure is being applied in order to prevent bruising
- Once bleeding as ceased, apply a suitably sized adhesive dressing (having first checked that the child is not allergic)
- Remove gloves and apron and discard of appropriately
- Wash your hands (Department of Health, 2003)

Post-procedure

- Gently invert blood specimen tubes that contain additives to mix the contents – do *not* shake as this might cause haemolysis (British Committee for Standards in Haematology, 2003)
- Place the pre-labelled sample tubes with the correct request forms in the appropriate plastic bags and arrange transfer to the laboratory
- Monitor the puncture site for bruising, haemorrhage, haematoma and infection
- Document the procedure as appropriate, including what investigations have been requested (NMC, 2004)

Student skill laboratory activity

- ✓ Assemble the equipment required to undertake venepuncture on an infant or child.
- ✓ Locate appropriate veins on the mannequin.
- ✓ Practice the procedure in the mannequin.
- ✓ Dispose of equipment appropriately.

Intravenous cannulation

Intravenous (IV) cannulation involves the insertion of a short flexible plastic tube into a vein using a hollow needle as an introducer. The procedure must only be performed by a member of staff who has received particular training and is certified as competent within specific age bands (Royal College of Nursing, 2005). More usually, the role of the children's nurse is to support the child and the cannulating practitioner during the procedure. Therefore, the nurse requires sufficient knowledge of IV cannulation to be able to assess a child's psychological and physical needs before the procedure is attempted.

> *REMEMBER – A cannula should not be sited where there is evidence of cellulitis, dermatitis, bruising or infection. It is preferable to avoid previous cannula sites and brachial arteriovenous fistulas (Das and Sharma, 2000) and to avoid limbs affected by conditions such as fractures, skin grafts, planned limb surgery, rheumatoid arthritis and stroke. For the child's comfort and mobility, it is preferable to use the non-dominant limb. If appropriate discuss the position of the cannula with the child. Indeed, children with long-term illnesses are invaluable in advising you where best to try for and place and IV cannula.*

Reasons for the procedure

- To administer intravenous medication
- To deliver intravenous fluids including blood or blood components

Pre-procedure

Equipment required

- Clean non-sterile tray
- Gloves

- Apron
- Alcohol-impregnated swabs
- Appropriate sized cannula
- T-piece connector (use a SmartSite if child has latex allergy)
- Bung or needleless connector
- 5 mL syringe of 0.9% NaCl to flush
- Bio-occlusive dressing, preferably moisture-permeable (see *Chapter 15*)
- Splint
- Bandage
- Disposable tourniquet for cannulation of child over 5 years of age
- Sharps container

Select IV cannula device

- Unless otherwise indicated, use the smallest gauge of cannula for the prescribed therapy (Scales, 2005) which helps protect the endothelial lining (intima) of the vessel and ensures there is sufficient blood flow past the cannula
- If the cannula is too large, blood flow is inhibited so that drugs remain in prolonged contact with the vein wall, resulting in chemical phlebitis (Crow, 1996)

Consider pain relief for this painful procedure

- Topical local anaesthetics penetrate nerve fibres and block sodium channels so preventing generation of action potential. Examples are:
  - EMLA (eutectic mixture of local anaesthetics) – for children over 1 year; apply 1 hour before venepuncture (Lander, 1996a, 1996b; Tak and van Bon, 2006)
  - Ametop (tetracaine 4%) – for infants older than 1 month; apply 30–45 minutes before venepuncture (Hewitt, 1998)
  - Ethyl chloride spray commonly described by children as 'cold spray' because it is a volatile liquid that evaporates rapidly and cools the skin to below 10°C (at this temperature nerve impulses cannot be generated but adjacent pain receptors are stimulated to produce the sensation of freezing) (BNFc, 2007) –spray onto the skin for 5–10 seconds until the skin takes on a whitish tinge (MB: the spray should be stored carefully at room temperature and should never be inhaled as there have been reports of solvent abuse causing hallucinations, ataxia, short-term memory loss, cardiac arrhythmias, respiratory arrest and death; Broussard *et al*, 2000)
- Other forms of pain relief include:
  - In neonates, consider non-nutritive sucking of sucrose or a pacifier (Stevens *et al,* 2003) or breast-feeding during the procedure (Halimaa, 2003)
  - Distraction therapy at an age-appropriate level is suitable for all ages (Willock *et al,* 2004)
  - Nitrous oxide (Entonox) (Willock *et al*, 2004) is particularly useful in children over 4 years of age. It has a rapid onset of 4 minutes (BNFc, 2007) and produces short-acting effective pain relief (see *Chapter 7*)

– A 'cough technique' is a low-cost and effective way of relieving pain (Usichenko *et al,* 2004) although the exact mechanism not known and it is only suitable in older age children
– In extreme circumstances (intense needle phobia) the child may be administered conscious sedation with midazolam or chloral hydrate (BNFc, 2007)

Specific patient preparation

- Explain all procedures and care in an age/developmentally appropriate way to both the child and the family (NPSA, 2004)
- Obtain consent prior to the procedure (Lavery, 2003). The child, or their carer, may give consent so long as they are informed of the implications, potential side effects and alternatives. If competent, seek informed consent directly from the child (British Medical Association, 2001; Department of Health, 2001). For IV cannulation, assumed or verbal consent is adequate (Scales, 2005)
- Ensure that the child's psychological well being is maintained by providing appropriate play
- Identify a suitable vein before commencing and ensure that there are no intravenous infusions or transfusions in progress near the site. Optimal cannula sites vary according to the age and the condition of the child – see *Figure 9.4* for suitable sites in the arm and *Figure 9.5* for suitable sites in infants. The dorsal aspect of the hand is usually the first choice in children as the metacarpal veins and the dorsal venous arch is usually easy to visualise and palpate; however, younger children and infants may have superficial fat which makes these veins less accessible. The radial end of the dorsal venous arch continues to form the cephalic vein, while the ulnar end of the dorsal venous arch forms the basilic

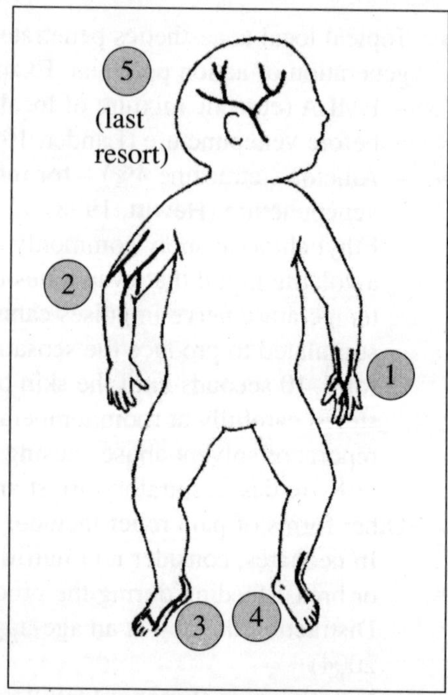

Figure 9.5: Five sites for cannulation in an infant

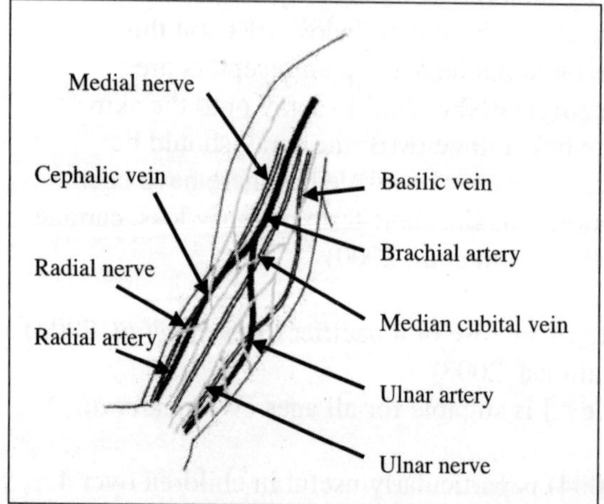

Figure 9.4: Selecting a vein for cannulation in the arm

vein (Moore and Dalley, 1999). The cephalic and basilic veins extent up to the forearm and make good veins to cannulate; they are connected at the ante cubital fossa by the median cubital vein, which runs diagonally between the two. There is great variation in the patterns of veins in this area. However, these veins are frequently accessed as they are easily visualised and palpated. Cannula sites in this area are particularly prone to mechanical phlebitis as the cannula is easily dislodged or kinked following flexion of the elbow (Scales, 2005). Taking your time to identify a suitable vein in advance of the procedure allows you to address the issue of pain relating to the procedure

During the procedure

- Ensure that you have adequately prepared the child and/or parent before you begin and re-affirm informed consent (NPSA, 2004)
- Enlist the assistance of a colleague or play specialist if necessary
- Ensure that the procedure takes place in a well-lit, quiet environment (eg. a treatment room)
- Wash your hands, put on gloves and apron and maintain an aseptic technique throughout (Department of Health, 2003)
- Assemble the equipment required for the procedure as determined by your pre-procedure assessment
- Draw up 5*mL of 0.9% NaCl into a syringe and prime the T-piece (or Smart-Site connector)
- Ensure that the child is in a comfortable position. Position young children on a carer's or nurse's lap with the limb concealed from their view, and supported firmly to avoid sudden movement (Royal College of Nursing, 2003a)
- If you have not already done so, remove the occlusive dressing or cling film, and wipe off any excess anaesthetic cream applied earlier to your selected the site for cannulation
- Prepare the child's skin by cleansing the site, for 15–30 seconds with swabs soaked in 70% alcohol and allow it to dry (at least 30 seconds) – DO NOT REPALPATE THE INSERTION SITE ONCE IT HAS BEEN CLEANED (Hindley, 2004)
- Support the child's limb on a pillow, for example, pointing downwards to encourage blood flow by gravity. Ask your assistant to support and hold still the appropriate limb
- In older children, apply a disposable tourniquet tightly 8–10 cm above the intended cannulation site (it works by obstructing venous return and dilating the veins)
- Apply anaesthetic spray, if using, immediately prior to insertion of the cannula, to ensure maximum analgesic effect
- It can be useful to immobilise the vein by applying gentle traction to the child's skin a few cm below the proposed venepuncture site using your non-dominant hand (Royal College of Nursing, 2003b)
- Hold the cannulation device in your dominant hand, checking that the bevel of the needle is facing upwards at the selected angle and insert the needle into the vein. With a steady smooth action, keeping the skin taut, continue to insert the needle until there is 'flashback' (blood in the syringe as a result of backflow) or until puncture of the wall is felt. When flashback is seen, gently advance the cannula off the needle until it is inserted up to the hub. A secondary

flashback of blood will be seen along the length of the cannula. Keep traction on the vein with the other hand – DO NOT re-introduce the needle into the cannula as this can cause damage to the cannula and predispose to catheter embolus
- Instruct your assistant to relax pressure around the limb, or to release the tourniquet
- Apply digital pressure to the vein above the cannula while removing the needle (to avoid spillage of blood) and dispose of the needle directly in the sharps container
- Attach the T-piece and flush the cannula
- Apply a sterile Luer lock cap
- Secure the cannula with a suitably sized moisture-permeable sterile adhesive dressing, ensuring that the insertion site is visible (Royal College of Nursing, 2003b) (see *Figure 9.6*)
- Immobilise the limb using a suitable splint; scalp cannulas need to be protected with a sterile pot padded with gauze
- Ensure the patient is comfortable and safe, explaining any restrictions of movement and bathing to the child and parent
- Remove gloves and apron and discard of appropriately
- Wash your hands (Department of Health, 2003)

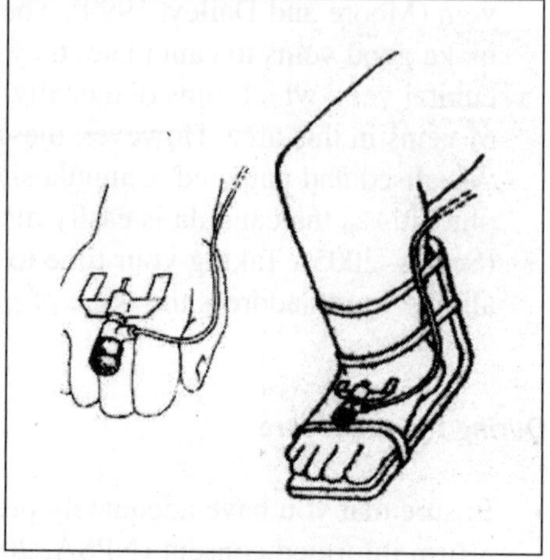

Figure 9.6: Taping and splinting of cannulae on the hand and foot

Post-procedure

- Document the procedure as appropriate (NMC, 2004), recording:
  - Date and time of insertion
  - Name of who inserted the cannula
  - Site of cannula
  - Size of the cannula
- See *Chapter 15* for more information about monitoring the IV cannula site and VIP (visual infusion phlebitis) scoring. A phlebitis score should be used to assess the cannula site (Royal College of Nursing, 2003a). Studies have shown that implementation of care plans and guidelines for cannula care have decreased the incidence of thrombophlebitis (Ahlqvist *et al*, 2006)
- Flush the cannula with normal saline at least every 12 hours, or after each drug administration, to maintain patency and reduce catheter-related complications. A pulsatile (push–pause technique) is advocated as this action creates turbulence inside the lumen and flushes any adherent substances (Ingram and Lavery, 2005); there are no significant advantages in using heparinised saline for this purpose as Fujita *et al* (2006) maintained that it is the flushing action itself that is responsible for patency rate rather than the heparin

Student skill laboratory activity

- ✓ Assemble the equipment required to cannulate a child.
- ✓ Identify veins on the forearm, hand and foot on another student and the mannequin.
- ✓ Practice cannulation on the mannequin.

Central lines

A central line, sometimes referred as a central venous access device, is inserted into a vein via either a central vessel or a peripheral vessel (Galway *et al*, 2003). A central line is placed:

- To aid in diagnostic procedures, such as blood sampling or central venous pressure (CVP) monitoring which is used to guide fluid volume administration
- To administer medications, parenteral nutrition, fluids and blood products

A short-term (non-tunnelled) percutaneous central venous catheter is inserted into a vein less than 2.5 cm from the skin exit site (Galway *et al*, 2003). It should enable days to weeks of intravenous access. Central venous catheters have between one and five lumens. Multi-lumen catheters are particularly useful because they allow the administration of several medications or fluids at once.

Common veins for placement

- Jugular vein
- Subclavian vein
- Femoral vein

Principles of caring for a child with a central line

Asepsis

The principles of asepsis are essential, most importantly:

- Hand washing
- Minimal line handling
- Cleansing of access points prior to use (Department of Health, 2003)

Inspection

The insertion site should be inspected hourly and assessed for signs of:

- Phlebitis (erythema, pain and swelling)
- Infection

Appropriate, and swift, action should be undertaken if any such signs are noted, and these findings should be reported to the medical staff immediately (RCN, 2003b).

Administration sets

Change the administration sets at the designated times:

- Blood products – at least every 12 hours
- Solution sets – at least every 72 hours
- Parenteral nutrition – at least every 24 hours

Appropriate cannulation-site dressing

Dressings are applied to minimise contamination and maximise stability of the insertion site. According to Treston-Aurend *et al* (1997) an ideal dressing should provide:

- An effective barrier to bacteria
- Secure fixation of the central line
- Sterility
- Easy application and removal
- Comfort

Transparent dressings provide all the characteristics of an ideal dressing and also allow easy inspection of the line insertion site (Royal College of Nursing, 1999). Moreover, Keenlyside (1993) found such dressings to be highly desirable as they have reduced moisture accumulation and they contribute to an improved condition of the child's skin surrounding the insertion site. However, when there is an accumulation of debris beneath the dressing, the dressing must be removed, the site cleansed and dressing re-applied using an aseptic technique. See procedure below.

Maintaining a closed system

In order to prevent complications such as air embolus it is important to maintain a closed system. This can be maintained by:

- Using Luer lock connections only to provide a secure link between the central line and the administration set
- Firmly clamping the central line when bungs or lines are changed

Maintaining patency of the catheter

Catheter occlusion is a common complication due to clot formation. Partial occlusion or total occlusion can occur. Partial occlusion refers to the inability to withdraw blood from the line, whereas total occlusion is when fluid or medication is unable to be infused into the line (McIntosh, 2003). Several factors can influence catheter occlusion. These include:

- Catheter type
- Location of the distal tip
- Flushing technique
- What is being infused into the catheter
- A normal physiological response taking place

It is therefore important to appreciate how central line patency can be maintained. Intermittent flushing with 0.9% NaCl followed by a heparin–saline solution (10 units/mL) is usually sufficient to maintain patency. 0.9% NaCl is used first to clean the internal lumen of the catheter. Heparin–saline (10 units/mL) is used as it prevents the build up of fibrin, and therefore clot formation. Use the push–pause method to flush the catheter as this creates turbulent flow that is effective in cleansing the internal diameter of the catheter. Intermittent flushing should be completed using a positive-pressure technique which is often achieved by clamping the central line while completing the flush (Royal College of Nursing, 2005).

Changing the dressing on a central-line insertion site

Reasons for the procedure

- To prevent infection
- Maintain secure fixation of line

Pre-procedure

Equipment required

- Sterile dressing pack
- Line clamp if necessary
- Alcohol gel

- Alcohol-based cleansing preparation (eg. chlorhexidine in 70% alcohol or a pre-impregnated swab; but aqueous chlorhexidine for neonates)
- Sterile occlusive dressing
- Bacteriological swab
- Sterile gloves
- Disposable apron

Specific patient preparation

- Explain all procedures and care in an age/developmentally appropriate way to both the child and the family (NPSA, 2004)
- Obtain consent prior to the procedure. The child, or their carer, may give consent so long as they are informed of the implications, potential side effects and alternatives. If competent, seek informed consent directly from the child (British Medical Association, 2001; Department of Health, 2001)
- Ensure that the child's psychological well being is maintained by providing appropriate play

During the procedure

- An aseptic technique should be used in order to prevent cross-infection
- The child should be placed in a supine position in order to prevent air embolus
- The individual undertaking the procedure should undertake effective hand-washing. Alcohol gel should be applied to the hands
- Open a sterile field and any other additional equipment required
- Apply sterile gloves and loosen the dressing. Adhesive removal wipes should be used to allow easy removal
- If the central line site is red and discharging, a bacteriological swab should be taken. This is in order to identify any causative organism and allow effective treatment of any infection
- The site should be cleaned with 70% chlorhexidine in alcohol or pre-impregnated swab (in neonates use aqueous chlorhexidine). It should be allowed to dry completely to ensure the disinfection process is complete
- An occlusive dressing should be applied ensuring that there are no folds or creases in order to minimise skin irritation
- Remove gloves and dispose of all equipment in the clinical waste bag

Post-procedure

- Praise the child and thank parents for their assistance with the procedure
- Document the procedure as appropriate, including what investigations have been requested (NMC, 2004)

Removal of a short-term (non-tunnelled) percutaneous central line

Reasons for the procedure

- To remove a line that is no-longer required
- To remove a line that is septic and/or malfunctioning

Pre-procedure

Equipment required

- Sterile dressing pack
- Gauze
- Occlusive dressing
- Alcohol gel
- Sterile gloves
- Apron
- Stitch cutter
- Sterile specimen container
- Sterile scissors
- Clinical waste bag and sharps container
- Skin cleansing solution (eg. chlorhexidine in 70% alcohol or pre-impregnated swab; but aqueous chlorhexidine for neonates)
- Bacteriological swab for site

Specific patient preparation

- Explain and discuss the procedure with the child and their family. Preparation prior to the procedure is important and a play specialist should be utilised as appropriate. Ensure that consent is gained to enable the procedure to take place

During the procedure

- Place the child in the Trendelenberg position, whereby the head is slightly lower than the feet, which helps to prevent air embolus (Smith *et al*, 2005)
- Wash your hands effectively and apply alcohol gel to reduce the risk of cross-infection (Department of Health, 2003)
- Open the sterile field and any other additional equipment required
- Loosen the dressing covering the central line. Skin adhesive remover wipes should be used to allow ease of removal
- Apply sterile gloves and clean the insertion site with an alcohol-impregnated swab

- Ensure that the central venous catheter is clamped or the 'On–Off' switch is set at the off position
- Use a stitch cutter to cut the skin suture as close to the skin as possible and remove that is securing the central venous catheter
- If possible ask older children or teenagers to perform the Valsalva manoeuvre (bear down as if staining to have a bowel movement)
- Cover the insertion site with several sterile topical gauze swabs to reduce spay or aerosols
- Hold the catheter with one hand near the point of insertion and pull firmly and gently. As the catheter starts to move press the site firmly. This pressure should be maintained for at least 5 minutes (to allow the puncture in the vein to close)
- When the bleeding has ceased the site should be covered with a gauze pad and sterile dressing
- If the central venous catheter is removed due to infection, the tip should be examined in the laboratory. Approximately 5 cm of the tip of the catheter should be cut off with sterile scissors and placed in a sterile container. This will be sent to microbiology for MC&S in order to detect the causative organism and guide effective treatment
- Any equipment should be disposed of in the appropriate container (eg. sharps bin or yellow clinical waste bag)
- It should be ensured that the child is comfortable. The child should be closely observed for any complications of the procedure

Student skill laboratory activity

- ✓ Assemble the equipment necessary to change the dressing covering a short-term (non-tunnelled) percutaneous central line.
- ✓ Assemble the equipment to safely remove a short term (non-tunnelled) percutaneous central line.
- ✓ Practice changing the dressing on the central line using a mannequin.
- ✓ Practice removing a central line on the mannequin.
- ✓ Practise accessing the central line and aseptically attaching an infusion using a mannequin.
- ✓ Dispose of all equipment appropriately.

Management of arterial lines and catheters

Intra-arterial access is used in paediatric critical care to provide continuous accurate monitoring of systemic blood pressure and allow access to easily sample arterial blood (McGhee and Bridges, 2002). The placement of the arterial catheter, a small plastic tube, can be technically challenging due to the small diameter of the arteries of infants and children, and the invasive nature of the catheter can lead to complications of haemorrhage, thrombosis and infection (Clarke and Kruse,

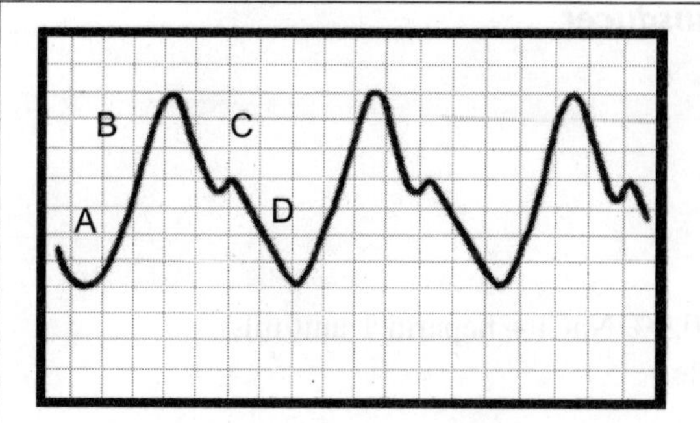

Figure 9.7: Normal arterial pressure waveform. A, the anacrotic limb (correlates with ventricular systole and the QRS) (McGhee and Bridges, 2002; Smith et al, 2004); B, systolic pressure measured at the peak of the arterial waveform (McGhee and Bridges, 2002); C, the dicrotic notch (correlates with the closing valve) (Smith et al, 2004); D, diastole

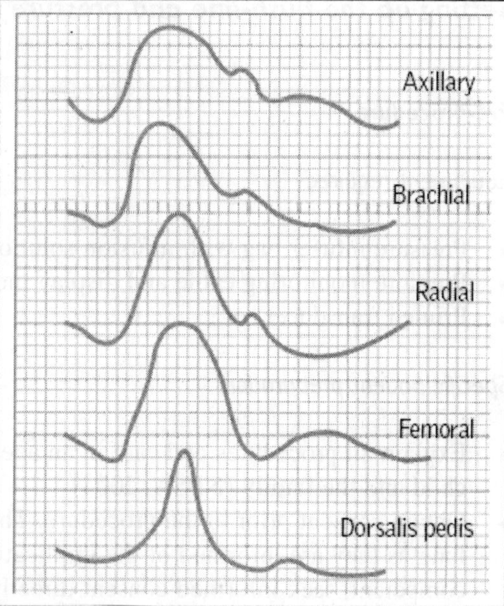

Figure 9.8: Arterial pressure waveforms in the axillary, brachial, radial, femoral and dorsalis pedis arteries

1992). Although the risks and complications are low, the potential for devastating injury exists and therefore deserves the greatest respect whenever the placement of an arterial catheter is considered (Schindler, 2005). A variety of sites can be used most commonly the radial, brachial, axillary, femoral or dorsalis pedis artery (Clark and Kruse, 1992). Due to the nature of the necessity of arterial monitoring, the child is usually sedated while the arterial catheter is inserted by an experienced medical practitioner. Nurses are required to set up the flush-line and pressure transducer once the arterial line has been placed, and to maintain its functioning.

Features of a properly functioning arterial line

- Blood can be drawn from the catheter
- The system can be zeroed (a procedure that will vary according to the monitors in use but which should be performed at the level of the 4th intercostal space or mid-axillary line; Imperial-Perez and McRae, 2002)
- A mechanism is present that ensures the catheter remains clear
- A dependable waveform is present on the monitoring screen

A normal arterial pressure waveform is shown *Figure 9.7*. Arterial pressure waveforms in different arteries can be seen in *Figure 9.8*.

Setting up the flush-line and pressure transducer

Pre-procedure

Equipment required

- Pressure infuser bag with infusion solution (0.9% NaCl + heparin 1 unit/mL)
- Pressure monitoring cable and display module
- Primed transducer set

Specific patient preparation

- Explain all procedures and care in an age/developmentally appropriate way to both the child and the family (NPSA, 2004)
- Obtain consent prior to the procedure. The child, or their carer, may give consent so long as they are informed of the implications, potential side effects and alternatives. If competent, seek informed consent directly from the child (British Medical Association, 2001; Department of Health, 2001)
- Ensure that the child's psychological well being is maintained by providing appropriate play

During the procedure

- The catheter is zeroed and the monitoring equipment calibrated
- The arterial line site must be observed regularly for signs of discolouration and poor perfusion. The potential disconnection and subsequent haemorrhage should be detected quickly and therefore the site should never be covered up (Garretson, 2005)
- Ensure there are no bubbles within the system
- Ensure that the arterial line is clearly marked so to prevent any drugs being injected via this route

Post-procedure

Monitor the arterial lines for the occurrence of the following problems (Imperial-Perez and McRae, 2002; McGhee and Bridges, 2002).

- If there is no arterial waveform trace on the bedside monitor:
  - check stopcocks are in the 'on' position
  - check all connections are tight
  - check the transducer cable is connected

- check the arterial catheter is connected
- check the monitor is set up correctly
- check for kinks in the catheter
- check for clots in the catheter by trying to withdraw blood (do not flush as clot may be flushed into the patient)
- check the pressure bag is sufficiently inflated to 300 mmHg

- If there is a sudden increase in blood pressure:
  - check the patient first – it may be real
  - check if there has been a sudden bolus of vasoactive drugs
  - check all drug infusions for errors
  - check the pump is functioning properly
  - check the level of the transducer (if it is below the phlebostatic axis it may give a higher reading)
  - check whether the patient is awake and/or anxious, assess them and re–assure or sedate them
- If there is a sudden decrease in blood pressure:
  - check the patient first – it may be real
  - check whether the catheter has become disconnected during infusion of a vasoactive drug
  - check all drug infusions for errors
  - check whether the iv pump has stopped or is malfunctioning
  - check the level of the transducer (if it is above the phlebostatic axis it may give lower reading)
  - consider any side-effects of recently administered analgesics or sedatives
- If there is a dampened waveform (*Figure 9.9*):
  - check the pressure of the bag is 300 mmHg
  - check for kinks in the arterial catheter
  - check the level of fluid in the pressure bag
  - check for loose connections
  - check the stopcocks are in the correct positions

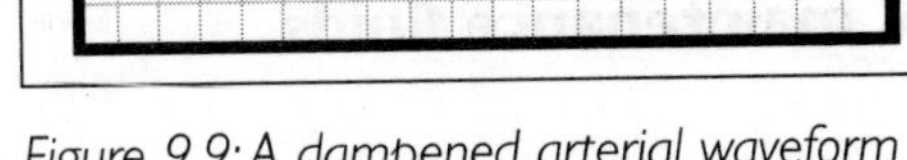

Figure 9.9: A dampened arterial waveform

- If you are unable to draw blood:
  - check the stopcocks are in the correct positions
  - check all connections
  - check for kinks in the catheter
  - check for clots in the catheter (do *not* flush as clot may be flushed into the patient)
- If there is any bleeding from the site:
  - check the transducer is properly connected to the arterial catheter
  - check for arterial 'oozing' from the insertion site; if so, apply a small absorbent dressing and an occlusive dressing and continue to monitor
  - consult medical staff if problem is the bleeding is significant
- If the arterial catheter is dislodged (eg. if someone has tripped over the transducer tubing, the patient is moving around in bed, or the transducer catheter is caught on equipment):
  - immediately apply pressure to the site for 5 minutes

- get a colleague to check blood pressure manually (especially if there is heavy blood loss)
- inform medical staff and prepare to assist with re-insertion
- remember always to prepare a new transducer tubing set-up – never re-use the 'old' set up

In all cases, consult the medical staff if the problem is not resolved.

Complications of arterial lines (Garretson, 2005)

- Haemorrhage
- Infection
- Thrombosis

Removal of arterial lines

- The patient should have a normal INR (international normalised ratio) – blood clotting time
- Clamp the T-piece and remove monitoring equipment
- While wearing gloves, remove the occlusive dressing and cannula and apply pressure to the site with sterile gauze
- Apply pressure for about 5–10 minutes until haemostasis has been achieved
- Apply a clean dressing

IV maintenance fluids

Maintenance fluid is the amount of fluid the body needs to replace usual daily losses from the respiratory tract, skin, urinary and gastrointestinal tracts. A well child usually drinks more than maintenance requirements. If a child takes in significantly less than maintenance requirements, he or she will gradually become dehydrated. The requirement for maintenance fluid varies with the weight of the child, thus infants need more fluid per kilogram of body weight than older children and adults do. Various medical conditions also affect these requirements (see *Box 9.2*). Fluid requirements are dynamic, with many conditions increasing or decreasing daily fluid requirements (for example, daily fluid requirements increase by 12% for every degree Celsius rise in body temperature over 37.5°C (Marieb, 2004). Therefore, careful input and output records must be kept. However, body weight loss or gain is the most reliable and accurate measurement of fluid loss and gain.

Box 9.2: Factors that decrease and increase daily fluid requirements

Decreased fluid requirements
Meningitis
Heart failure
Renal failure
Increased fluid requirements
Fever
Sweating
Vomiting
Diarrhoea
Burns

Practitioners administering intravenous medication must have undertaken suitable education and training in the theory and practice of the skill and be deemed competent in all aspects of intravenous therapy (Royal College of Nursing, 2005).

Infusion of IV maintenance fluids

IV maintenance fluids are needed in the following clinical situations (Ingram and Lavery, 2005):

- To replace fluid loss
- For fluid resuscitation
- For fluid challenge
- Therapeutic use
- To administer medication
- To maintain hydration

Risks associated with infusion of fluids

There are a number of risks associated with infusion of IV fluids (Quinn, 2000). Please refer to *Chapter 15* for more on wounds and care of intravenous cannula sites.

- Extravasation commonly referred to as 'tissuing'
- Phlebitis
- Thrombophlebitis
- Embolism

- Bacterial contamination
- Particulate contamination
- Incompatibility
- Allergic reactions
- Fluid overload

Types of therapeutic fluids

Therapeutic fluids that are prescribed for intravenous administration can be divided into two basic types (see *Box 9.3*):

- Crystalloids (simple solutions of small solutes)
- Colloids (suspensions of macromolecules, or in the case of blood, cells)

The most commonly used crystalloids are saline and dextrose, where the dissolved solutes are sodium chloride and glucose respectively. The standard saline solution is 0.9% saline (NaCl), often referred to as 'normal saline, which contains 150 mmol/L of NaCl, and is therefore not normal at all, being slightly hypertonic, and hypernatraemic. Dextrose is usually given as 5% dextrose, which means that it contains 5 g of glucose per 100 mL of water. This solution is roughly isotonic to serum, but the glucose is rapidly utilised, leaving behind pure water. A host of other crystalloids exist but they are beyond the scope of this chapter. Multiple colloid preparations are available, but the essential ones are either natural (blood, human albumin or plasma) or synthetic (where the macromolecule is manufactured). In common synthetic colloids, hydrolysed gelatine is suspended in saline.

Box 9.3: Examples of crystalloids and colloids

Crystalloids
Sodium chloride
Sodium lactate (Hartmann's solution)
Glucose
Dextrose saline
Ringer's solution

Colloids
Albumin
Gelatin-based solutions
Blood

Choice of therapeutic fluid

The choice of IV fluid depends on some basic rules. A child with serious intravascular volume depletion, hypotension and reduced cardiac output is shocked, from haemorrhage, plasma loss (eg. with burns injury), or water loss. The aim here is to restore intravascular volume with a fluid that remains in the vascular compartment, and may even draw water from the intracellular space, into the blood system. A fluid with a high oncotic pressure would do this job. Blood remains the fluid of choice to treat someone with blood loss. Colloid is the fluid of choice in resuscitation when blood loss is not pronounced, or while waiting for blood. Any crystalloid will enter the vascular space, then distribute around the other compartments (Marieb, 2004). By containing sodium (the main extracellular cation), saline will expand the interstitial and intravascular compartments more than dextrose, most of which will enter the intracellular space. 5% dextrose is isotonic to plasma. A bolus of 5% dextrose will cause immediate expansion of the vascular compartment but, as its glucose content is rapidly metabolised, the remaining water will distribute itself between all compartments and very little will remain within the blood space. For this simple reason, dextrose is not a fluid of resuscitation.

Maintenance fluid requirements

Well children with normal hydration but no oral intake require an amount of fluid that is termed 'maintenance'. Maintenance fluid is the volume of daily fluid intake that replaces the insensible losses from breathing, through the skin and in the stools, and at the same time allows excretion of the daily production of excess solute load (eg. urea, creatinine, electrolytes) in a volume of urine (Tortora, 2005). A child's maintenance fluid requirement decreases proportionately with increasing age and weight (Methany, 2000). Fluid requirements are better estimated by weight than age, to take into account the possibility of an underweight or overweight child. Fluid requirements in children are based on body weight according to the Holliday–Segar method (Willock and Jewkes, 2000). *Box 9.4* shows the baseline requirements for a normal healthy child according to weight (kg). You will see that 100 mL per hour (2500 mL/day) is the normal maximum amount. Many remember these as the '100, 50, 20' and '4, 2, 1' rules of thumb. It is important to note fluid requirements are higher with increased losses such as fever, diarrhoea, vomiting, sweating. Fluid restrictions may be required in some medical cases such as heart failure and those children should be carefully monitored. It is important, however, to maximise fluid intake within this restriction.

For example:

- A 5 kg infant would require 500 mL per day
- A 14 kg child would require 1000 + 200 = 1200 mL per day
- A 25 kg child would require 1000 + 500 + 100 =1600 mL per day

The requirement for both sodium (Na) and potassium (K) in the healthy child is 1 mmol/kg per 24 hours. The recommended fluid to be infused as maintenance for well children with normal hydration is:

0. 45% NaCl with 5% glucose + 20 mmol KCl per litre (Stewart, 2007)

Box 9.4: Normal fluid requirements for children according to body weight

Body weight (kg)	Fluid requirement per 24 hours	Fluid requirement per hour
First 10 kg	100 mL/kg	4 mL/kg
Second 10 kg	50 mL/kg	2 mL/kg
Each subsequent kg	20 mL/kg	1 mL/kg

But remember, this represents basal requirements and not sick children.

It is important to note that this usual maintenance fluid should NOT be given if:

- Serum potassium is low
- Serum sodium is low
- For volume resuscitation
- For replacement of fluid deficit in dehydrated children
- For initial management of children with acute neurological conditions such as meningitis

Daily decisions about intravenous fluid intake are made by medical staff based on serum sodium, clinical signs of hydration and weight change. Fluid therapy is intended to maintain the normal volume and composition of body fluids and, if needed, to correct any existing abnormalities. In children, the most common abnormality is hypovolaemia, primarily due to vomiting and diarrhoea from gastroenteritis. Thus, it is useful clinically to divide fluid therapy into maintenance (maintenance therapy) and deficit requirements (repletion therapy).

- *Maintenance therapy* replaces the ongoing losses of water and electrolytes under normal physiologic conditions
- *Repletion therapy* replaces the existing water and electrolytes deficits that are needed to return the patient to a normal volume and electrolyte status

Thus, in a patient who is hypovolaemic, fluid therapy will include both repletion and maintenance therapy.

Unwell children (with or without abnormal hydration) require maintenance fluids. They may also need extra to replace fluid deficits due to dehydration, and possibly more fluid to replace abnormal ongoing losses for example from drain sites.

Maintenance requirements for young infants

Maintenance fluids are calculated differently for neonates and young infants up to 2 months of age (as shown in *Box 9.5*). However, these fluids must be adjusted in the following conditions:

- In infants requiring phototherapy or under a radiant warmer – fluid requirements increase by 150%
- In infants with neurological illnesses like meningitis – fluid requirement decrease by 70%

Daily decisions about intravenous fluid intake are made by medical staff based on serum sodium, clinical signs of hydration and weight change.

- Sodium and potassium requirements in healthy neonates (up to 28 days of age) is 2–3 mmol/kg per 24 hours
- For most infants the appropriate starting maintenance intravenous fluid is 0. 45% NaCl + 10% glucose

Box 9.5: Maintenance fluid requirements for newborns and infants up to 2*months of age

Day 1	2–3 mL/kg/hour
Day 2	3 mL/kg/hour
Day 3 to 2 months	4 mL/kg/hour

All neonates on intravenous fluids should have daily sodium, potassium and acid–base measurements, and regular assessment of weight and clinical signs of hydration, to guide medical decisions on fluid volume and electrolyte content.

Administering IV maintenance fluids

Pre-procedure

Equipment required

- Plastic tray (freshly cleaned with detergent and water and dried thoroughly)
- Prescription of the fluid to be infused
- 5–10 mL syringe contain sterile normal saline to flush the cannula
- Drip/infusion stand

- Appropriate giving set (for infusion device to be used)
- Gloves
- Alcohol-impregnated swab
- Splint to immobilise the limb
- Bandage
- Tape to secure bandage

Specific patient preparation

- Check that the cannula to be used has not exceeded its recommended insertion time of 72 hours (Royal College of Nursing, 2005). If the cannula has exceeded its insertion time; report to the medical staff that the cannula required replacement
- Explain all procedures and care in an age/developmentally appropriate way to both the child and the family (NPSA, 2004)
- Obtain consent prior to the procedure. The child, or their carer, may give consent so long as they are informed of the implications, potential side effects and alternatives. If competent, seek informed consent directly from the child (British Medical Association, 2001; Department of Health, 2001)

During the procedure

- Assemble equipment in the tray
- Check (Watt, 2003a; 2003b):
  - Correct child
  - Correct medicine
  - Correct dose
  - Correct time
  - Correct route
- Check the intravenous fluid:
  - Is the packaging is intact?
  - What is the expiry date? Is the fluid in date?
  - Is the fluid clear with no evidence of particulate contamination?
  - Record the batch number of the bag on the prescription sheet
- Wash your hands and put on non-sterile gloves (Department of Health, 2003)
- Remove the outer packaging and hang the infusion bag on the drip stand. Remove packing from the giving set and ensure the roller clamp is closed
- Remove the protective cover from around the infusion port using a twisting action, taking care not to touch the inside of the port which must be kept sterile (Hindley, 2004)
- Twist the protective cover from the sterile spike of the giving set and fully insert the spike into the infusion port, being careful to maintain sterility of both (Dougherty, 2002)
- Priming the infusion set is an aseptic procedure so care must be taken not to contaminate the system. To prime the line, squeeze the drip chamber until it is half full, then hold the end that will be connecting to the patient and release the roller clamp, usually half way, and

allow the fluid to flow slowly into the line. If the giving set has a sensor disc this should be grasped between the thumb and forefinger while the fluid is passing through (to prevent any air bubbles in the disc) (Infusion Nurses Society, 2006)

- Once the fluid has reached the end of the administration set, ensure all air bubbles have been expelled and close the clamp
- If you have been trained to do so, place the infusion set into the pump according to the manufacturer's instructions (Quinn, 2000; NPSA, 2004)
- Put on a fresh pair of gloves
- Take the equipment to the child. Check (Watt, 2003a; 2003b):
  - Correct child
  - Correct medicine
  - Correct dose
  - Correct time
  - Correct route
- Uncover the cannula site, check site using VIP score (see *Chapter 15*)
- If the cannula site is satisfactory, clean the bung for 30 seconds with an alcohol-impregnated swab; allow to dry for at least 30 seconds
- Using a non-touch aseptic technique throughout to keep the injection free from microbial contamination (Clinical Resource and Audit Group, 2002), insert the hub of the syringe into the bung with a push and twisting action until it is locked in place
- Slowly and smoothly flush the IV cannula with 0.5–2 mL 0.9% NaCl to ascertain patency. Patency is evidenced by the following (Ingram and Lavery, 2005):
  - The child experiences no pain or discomfort
  - There is very little resistance of the cannula to a slow flush
  - No blanching of tissue is seen around the cannula site
  - No redness of tissue is seen around the cannula site
  - No leakage of fluid is seen from around the cannula site
- If any of these occur, or you are in doubt, do not use the cannula and inform medical staff
- While instilling the flush continuously, observe the insertion site and, if able, and in terms they understand, ask the child to tell you if they feel any discomfort or pain
- If the cannula is patent, remove the protective cap from the connector part of the giving set without contaminating it
- Lock the end of the connector part of the giving set to the cannula, ensuring that it is screwed in firmly
- To prevent any complications such as kinking and pulling, the tubing can be taped in an upwards direction using appropriate dressings, and the limb can be splinted. The actual site where the cannula enters the vein should be left visible so it can be inspected regularly
- Set rate of the infusion as prescribed, open all clamps, and commence the infusion
- Dispose of needles and syringes directly after use into a sharps bin. NEVER re-sheathe the needle (MDA, 2001)
- Check the cannula is secure, comfortable and re-apply any bandage as needed

Post-procedure

- Document on the prescription chart accordingly (NMC, 2004)
- Document all the information on the infusion chart
- Enter the type of solution, the date the line was put up, and the registration number of the pump on the fluid chart
- Change the infusion set according to local policy
- Explain to the child and/or career how positioning could affect the infusion rate
- Ask the child and/or career to report any discomfort or adverse reactions to the staff
- Observe for potential complications. Inspect the cannula site and record volume of fluid infused at least hourly. Potential intravenous cannula complications are discussed in *Chapter 15*

Student skill laboratory activity

- ✓ Assemble all the equipment required for setting up an infusion.
- ✓ Set up an infusion.
- ✓ Practice calculating fluid requirements according to a child's weight.
- ✓ Practice calculating flow rates for given volumes and giving times.

Administration of blood or blood products

A transfusion consists of the administration of whole blood or any of its components to correct a clinical abnormality. Blood components include red blood cells and blood components (plasma, fresh frozen plasma, cryoprecipitate and platelets). Before commencing the transfusion, a sample of the patient's blood is taken for ABO/rhesus D testing and cross-matching. This sample should be taken less than 1 week prior to the transfusion, or according to local policy. The British Committee for Standards in Haematology (2003) claims that 39% of all 'wrong blood' incidents occurred at this stage. Careful cross-checking of patient's details and labelling the sample with these details at the bedside should be performed when collecting blood samples for cross-matching purposes.

The procedure described below is based on the British Blood Transfusion Service (UK) (British Transfusion Service, 2005) *Guidance for Best Practice*.

Reasons for the procedure

- To treat severe blood loss
- To manage specific deficiency disorders or disease processes

Pre-procedure

Equipment required

- Appropriate giving set (see below)
- Gloves
- Apron
- Suitable clean and stable surface (dressing trolley or tray)
- Blood warmer if the child is receiving more than 15 mL/kg/h and for all exchange transfusions
- Electronic infusion pump suitable for blood transfusion (NPSA, 2004)
- IV drip stand
- Observation chart
- Fluid balance chart
- Patients medical notes (check that the decision to transfuse has been recorded here)

Specific patient preparation

- When blood or blood products are required for neonates and infants up to 4 months of age, medical staff will need to obtain a maternal sample for cross-matching in addition to the patient sample (British Transfusion Services, 2005). Any antibody present in the young infant's circulation will be of maternal origin and will be of greater concentration in a maternal sample, and therefore a safer cross-match will result. Also it may be impossible to obtain sufficient sample from a small infant to perform a full compatibility test (British Committee for Standards in Haematology, 2004)
- If a maternal sample is unavailable OR the baby is transfused previously, blood or blood products which are ABO homologous with the baby will be cross-matched against the baby's own blood sample to assure compatibility (Contreras, 2001)
- Check that the child has suitable intravenous access, sited less than 48 hours previously. A small-child cannula (23 G) can be used. Check that the cannula is adequately secured with a clear sterile dressing to allow the site to be observed. Use a needleless bung on the cannula for patient safety (Watterson, 2004)
- Prior to transfusion, record baseline observations of temperature, pulse, respirations and blood pressure (checking oxygen saturations is optional)
- Check the prescription chart as to whether any medication is to be administered while the child is receiving the transfusion (such as diuretics or antihistamines)
- Finally, but most importantly, check that medical colleagues have obtained written or signed parental consent, and consent from the child if appropriate
- Ascertain whether the child has had any previous transfusions or allergies by questioning the family and checking the patient's notes
- Check that the details on the blood collection form match the details on the child's wristband and notes before going to collect the blood. Check that the blood group and rhesus factor are compatible with the child's (see *Table 9.1*) The minimum identification criteria are: name, surname, address, date of birth and hospital number (British Committee for Standards in Haematology, 2004)

- Check the child's identification details on the blood collection form against the label on the blood component
- Record the collection of blood as per local procedures
- Transport to patient in a box or tray, preferable with a lid
- The transfusion should be commenced within 30 minutes of removal from storage to prevent bacterial growth in the blood (British Committee for Standards in Haematology, 2004)

Table 9.1: Donor/recipient blood group compatibility chart

Recipient/patient ABO blood group	Donor red cells compatible with:	Donor fresh frozen plasma compatible with:	Donor platelets compatible with:
A	A or O	A or AB	A or B or O
B	B or O	B or AB	B or A or O
AB	AB, A, B, O	AB	A or B or O
O	O	O, A, B, AB	O or A or B

During the procedure

- Apply standard precautions – wash hands and put on gloves and apron (Department of Health, 2003)
- Check the child's name, date of birth, hospital reference number, expiry of product, irradiation and CMV status (see below) with the cross-match form and prescription chart with child's blood group to ensure that the child is given the correct product and in the prescribed quantity. Re-check that child/parental signed consent has been given as appropriate (Conteras, 2001)
- Inspect the blood component for signs of leaks, clumping and discolouration
- Blood and blood products to be administered to infants aged less than 1 year or immunocompromised must be from CMV(cytomegalovirus)-negative donors as CMV pneumonitis causes significant mortality (85%) and morbidity in vulnerable groups (McClelland, 2001)
- Blood and blood products must be delivered using the correct giving set with the appropriate filter to remove microaggregates and white cells present in the fluid to be transfused (Contreras, 2001)
  - Blood and fresh frozen plasma (FFP) – blood administration set has a microaggregate or filter
  - Platelets – a platelet administration set has a microparticle
  - Albumin 4. 5% – standard solution administration set
  - Salt-poor human albumin 20% – blood administration set
  - Factor VIII (cryoprecipitate) – directly via syringe or blood administration set

- Prepare the fluid for infusion and prime the appropriate administration/giving set using an aseptic, non-touch technique and observing standard precautions (Royal College of Nursing, 2003b)
- Close the roller clamp on the giving set, and using a sterile non-touch technique connect the giving set into the component bag
- Fill the drip chamber with blood component by gently squeezing the drip chamber until it is half full. This will help to prevent air entering the tubing of the giving set during transfusion
- Turn the flow regulator on slightly (usually about half-way) to slowly prime the line with the blood component. Observe the line for any air bubbles. Once primed switch the flow regulator to off
- Prepare a syringe containing at least 2 mL 0.9% NaCl for injection to use as a 'flush' using one of the two appropriate procedures described in *Chapter 7* (pp. 00–00):
  - *Withdrawing liquid medication from an ampoule into a syringe*
  - *Withdrawing medication from a vial into a syringe*
- Place the flush, the transfusion and connected giving set in the disposable tray and proceed to the child
- Re-check and confirm child's identity and transfusion to be given
- Expose and inspect the insertion site of the cannula. Ensure that the cannula is secured correctly. Check the IV cannula site for signs of infection, infiltration, phlebitis and if present *do not use* (Royal College of Nursing, 2005) and report to the medical staff
- Remove the cap from the cannula while at the same time applying digital pressure above the cannula tip to prevent fluid/blood leakage
- Inject gently 0. 5–2 mL 0.9% NaCl flush into the cannula to ensure patency. Patency is evidenced by the cannula (Ingram and Lavery, 2005):
  - The child experiences no pain or discomfort
  - There is very little resistance of the cannula to a slow flush
  - No swelling is evident
  - No blanching of tissue is seen around the cannula site
  - No redness of tissue is seen around the cannula site
  - No leakage of fluid is seen from around the cannula site
- If any of these occur, or you are in doubt, do not use the cannula and inform medical staff
- Remove the plastic guard on the giving set and screw the giving set onto the bung of the cannula
- Connect the giving set using a sterile non-touch technique
- Load into infusion device as appropriate and if are trained to do so (Medical Devices Agency [MDA], 2006) and set the transfusion to run at a rate as prescribed. The transfusion must be completed within 4 hours of commencement and within 4.5 hours of removal from storage (British Transfusion Services, 2005)
- Switch the flow regulator on, unclamp the cannula, and start the infusion at the rate prescribed, ensuring that this is appropriate to the infusion being administered (see *Box 9.6*)
- Dispose of needles and syringes directly after use into a sharps bin. NEVER re-sheathe the needle (MHRA, 2001)
- Dispose of all equipment appropriately and wash hands

- Once the infusion is completed, wash hands as before and put on gloves
- Disconnect the transfusion set and flush the cannula with 0.9% NaCl 0. 5–2 mL and check its patency as before
- Dispose of needles and syringes directly after use into a sharps bin. NEVER re-sheathe needle (MHRA, 2001; Watterson, 2004) and dispose of transfusion bag and giving set according to local policy
- Check cannula is secure, comfortable and re-apply any bandage as needed

Box 9.6: Recommended rates of transfusion (Wright, 2004)

Red cells	2–3 hours
Fresh frozen plasma	10–15 mins
Platelets	30 mins
Plasma	30 mins
Cryo	STAT bolus

Post-procedure

- Record baseline vital signs prior to commencing the infusion (Todd, 2002). Check pulse and temperature 15 minutes after starting each unit (Department of Health, 2002)
- Observe the child throughout the transfusion for:
  - Behavioural changes
  - Skin rashes
  - Oedema around the eyes
  - Breathlessness
  - Chest or abdominal pain
  - Facial flushing
- Repeat and record full vital signs on completion of transfusion. This facilitates prompt recognition of problems such as:
  - Pyrogenic reaction
  - White-cell antibody reaction
  - Allergic reaction to protein in plasma
  - Infection
  - Incorrect cross-match

If there is ANY cause for concern, stop the infusion, maintain patency of the IV cannula with 0.9% NaCl, and report to the medical staff IMMEDIATELY.

- To facilitate early detection of IV cannula complications observe the cannula site at least hourly and report to the medical staff signs of:
  - Inflammation
  - Phlebitis
  - Extravasation
- Document to maintain accurate records, provide a point of reference in the event of any queries, and prevent any duplication of treatment. If there is a transfusion reaction, follow the SHOT protocol (Serious Hazards of Transfusion) as stipulated by the British Transfusion Services (2005)
- Blood giving sets should be changed every 12 hours or between each unit if a different blood product or blood group is being transfused
- Record the volume of blood component given on a fluid balance chart
- In the event of an adverse reaction, stop the transfusion immediately and inform the medical staff. Implement the local procedure for adverse reactions. The transfusion may need to be abandoned or the flow rate reduced
- The transfusion must be completed within 4 hours of commencement and within 4.5 hours of removal from storage (British Transfusion Services, 2005)
- Dispose of waste according to waste management policy

Adverse reactions of blood and blood products

These may be acute or delayed, so early recognition and management are essential as adverse reactions can be fatal (British Transfusion Services, 2005). Delayed reactions to transfusions occur 24 hours or more following transfusion. Early signs and symptoms are shown in *Box 9.7*. Late signs and symptoms include jaundice, an unexplained drop in haemoglobin, flushing, purpura, a feeling of tiredness and shivering.

Types of reaction

- Fluid overload
- Acute haemolytic reaction
- Allergic reaction
- Infective shock
- Transfusion-related acute lung injury (TRALI)
- Mild reaction (urticarial rash and/or pyrexia of less than 1. 5°C above baseline)

Box 9.7: Early signs and symptoms of adverse reactions to blood and blood products

Signs	Symptoms
Pyrexia	Chills
Urticarial rash	Unease
Wheezing	Pruritis
Rigors	Muscular pain in chest or abdomen
Oedema	Pain at infusion site
Facial flushing	Nausea
Hypertension or hypotension	Shortness of breath
Tachycardia	
Tachypnoea	
Oliguria	
Breathlessness	

Inotrope therapy

Cardiovascular physiology

Cardiac output

In order to appreciate the clinical benefits of inotropes, it is important to have an understanding of the physiology of cardiac output. Cardiac output is the amount of blood ejected from the ventricle each minute (Marieb, 2004). It is calculated by:

$$\textit{Cardiac output} = \textit{heart rate} \times \textit{stroke volume}$$

Stroke volume is the volume of blood ejected with each ventricular contraction. Cardiac output can re regulated by altering either the heart rate or the stroke volume (Tortora, 2005). For example, during exertion both heart rate and stroke volume increase, therefore cardiac output is increased to meet the body's increased metabolic needs. Cardiac output is influenced by four contributing factors (Marieb, 2004). These are:

- Heart rate
- Stroke volume
- Preload
- Afterload and contractility

Heart rate

Heart rate is affected by:

- The autonomic nervous system (it increases with sympathetic stimulation and decreases with parasympathetic stimulation)
- Circulating catecholamines (adrenaline/epinephrine and noradrenaline/norepinephrine) which are secreted by the adrenal medulla in response to stress, and have a similar effect to the sympathetic nervous system
- Exercise
- Temperature
- Age

Increasing the cardiac output by increasing the heart rate causes:

- Increase oxygen demand
- Decreased diastolic filling time (and, therefore, decreased stroke volume)
- Decreased time for coronary artery blood flow (most coronary artery filling occurs during ventricular diastole, and some during ventricular systole)

Stroke volume

This is the amount of blood ejected by the heart with each heart beat, and it is affected by:

- Preload
- Contractility
- Afterload

Preload

Preload is often referred to as 'ventricular filling pressure' or 'left ventricular end-diastolic pressure'. It relates to the degree to which the myocardium is stretched at the end of diastole. The heart is stretched by the amount of blood that returns to it, and the more blood that returns to the heart the greater the stretching of the myocardium.

- If stretched to an optimal degree, the muscle fibres shorten maximally, and the heart contracts more forcefully (Frank Starling's Law), thereby increasing the stroke volume (British and Knowles, 2004)
- If overstretched, the myocardial fibres lose their ability to completely shorten, and therefore contractility and stroke volume are reduced

In summary, the degree of stretch in the myocardial fibres at the end of diastole (just before it contracts) is determined by the volume of blood in the ventricles at that time. Therefore, preload = left ventricular-end diastolic volume.

Preload is affected by:

- Length of diastole
- Venous return
- Atrial systole
- Myocardial compliance

Contractility

This is the intrinsic ability of the myocardial muscle fibres to shorten (contract). It is affected by:

- Sympathetic nervous system
- Metabolic abnormalities
- Electrolyte imbalance
- Inotropic drugs
- Intrinsic myocardial dysfunction

Afterload

Afterload is the resistance that the ventricle must overcome in order to eject its blood. When afterload is increased, the amount of muscle-fibre shortening is decreased and, therefore, stroke volume is decreased. Afterload is affected by:

- Aortic resistance
- Peripheral vascular resistance
- Blood viscosity
- Drugs such as vasodilators

Summary of the relationship between preload, afterload, stroke volume and cardiac output

Preload
Increased preload or increased contractility leads to increased stroke volume and increased cardiac output
Decreased preload or decreased contractility leads to decreased stroke volume and decreased cardiac output
Afterload
Increased afterload leads to decreased stroke volume and decreased cardiac output
Decreased afterload leads to increased stroke volume and increased cardiac output

What is an inotrope?

Inotropes are normally secreted by the body during times of stress, but need augmentation when the stressor has exhausted the body's supplies (British and Knowles, 2004). Inotropes (also known as vasoactive drugs) are agents that affect myocardial contractility (BNFc, 2007).

Two types of inotropes exist:

- Positive inotropes – they increase the strength of myocardial contraction and are used to increase heart contractility
- Negative inotropes – they decrease the force of myocardial contraction and are commonly used to reduce cardiac afterload

Inotropes (vasoactive) agents are short-acting and are therefore given via a continuous intravenous infusion (Cooper, 2004). Furthermore a central venous site is preferred because of their local effects on the vein and the risks of severe tissue damage if there is extravasation (leakage of agent into the tissues) (BNFc, 2007).

Positive inotropes include:

- Dopamine
- Dobutamine
- Epinephrine (adrenaline)
- Norepinephrine (noradrenaline)
- Isoprenaline

Negative inotropes include:

- Beta-blockers
- Diltiazam
- Verapamil

The ultimate aim of using inotropes is to increase, or improve, cardiac output using their specific actions on the different receptor sites (Grebenik and Sinclair, 2003).

Inotropes work by acting on different adrenoreceptors (see *Boxes 9.8* and *9.9*). Thus, stimulation of:

- **Alpha-1 and alpha-2 adrenoreceptors** causes arterial and venous vasoconstriction in order to increase systemic vascular resistance and improve venous return to the heart
- **Beta-1 adrenoreceptors** increases heart rate and improves myocardial contractility
- **Beta-2 adrenoreceptors** increases heart rate and can cause arterial vasodilation and bronchodilation. Inotropes that act on beta-2 receptors are used in order to reduce systemic vascular resistance, bronchospasm and/or acute allergic response

- **Dopamine receptors** causes renal and mesenteric vasodilation, which increases renal and mesenteric blood flow (Williams and Asquith, 2004); inotropes acting on dopamine receptors also aid coronary perfusion

Box 9.8: Inotrope effects of different receptor types

Alpha-adrenergic receptors	Found in peripheral vessels Cause vasoconstriction
Beta-1-adrenergic receptors	Found in myocardium Increase rate and force of heart contraction
Beta-2-adrenergic receptors	Found in bronchi, airways, and peripheral vessels Cause bronchodilation and vasodilation
Dopamine receptors	Found in renal and splanchnic vessels Causes renal and splanchnic vasodilation

Box 9.9: Inotropic actions of drugs on adrenoreceptors and dopamine receptors

	Alpha-1	Beta-1	Beta-2	Dopamine
Epinephrine/adrenaline	++	+++	++	0
Dobutamine	+	+++	++	0
Dopamine	+++	++	+	+++
Isoprenaline	0	+++	+++	0
Norepinephrine/noradrenaline	+++.	+	0	0

Reasons for using inotropes

Inotropes are useful (Horrox, 2002):

- When cardiac surgical repair has caused interruption of the myocardial tissue, resulting in impaired ventricular dysfunction (Williams and Asquith, 2004)
- In acute renal failure (may require low-dose inotropic support)
- In cardiogenic shock or septic shock with hypotension
- In low cardiac-output states
- When there is myocardial failure due to cardiomyopathy

Nursing considerations of a child receiving inotrope therapy

Any underlying hypovolaemia must be corrected first

The degree of stretch in the myocardial fibres at the end of diastole (just before it contracts) is determined by the volume of blood in the ventricles at that time, therefore, the heart must be adequately filled before starting inotropes for them to have any positive effect on cardiac output.

Inotropic agents have a short half-life

They have a short half-life due to re-uptake into the tissues and degradation by catechol-*O*-methyl-transferase in the liver and lungs (which is why they are prescribed at μg/kg per min as shown in *Box 9.10*). Therefore, these agents are delivered by a continuous intravenous infusion and are never bolused. A steady state is achieved within 5–10 minutes of starting continuous infusion. Catecholamines are administered by continuous infusion, preferably into a large vein (via a catheter used solely for the purpose).

Box 9.10: Doses of inotropes (BNFc, 2007)

Epinephrine/adrenaline	0. 05–1. 0 μg/kg/min
Norepinephrine/noradrenaline	0. 05–1. 0 μg/kg/min
Dopamine	1–20 μg/kg/min
Dobutamine	0.05–1. 0 μg/kg/min
Isoprenaline	0.05–0. 5 μg/kg/min

Note: The abbreviation mcg is often used for the unit μ.

Extravasation may lead to sloughing and necrosis

Always administer inotropic agents by a central venous line!

Inotropes have adverse effects

Nurse the child in a high dependency or intensive care environment. Continuously monitor the child and his or her heart rate, blood pressure, saturation monitoring, and any other haemodynamic parameters required. Be aware of, and be able to identify, all potential side-effects. These include (Horrox, 2002):

- Tachyarrhythmias
- Hypotension
- Nausea and vomiting
- Headache

Be aware of possible adverse drug interactions (eg. dobutamine is inactivated by alkaline solutions such as sodium bicarbonate and furosemide).

*Titrate – **never** bolus!*

Infusion rates are titrated against end-points such as mean arterial blood pressure, cardiac output, systemic vascular resistance, oxygen consumption and oxygen delivery. Their haemodynamic effects are predictable from knowledge of the receptor activity. Doses are prescribed by doctors using body weight with ranges to predict the relative predominance of beta- and alpha-adrenoreceptor effects.

Continuous cardiac monitoring is required

Heart rate, arterial blood pressure, central venous pressure, and fluid balance (urine output) must be monitored accurately and frequently. Prolonged use of inotropes may lead to a loss of efficacy due to down-regulation of beta-adrenoreceptors.

Double-pump to change syringe?

Inotrope infusions are run continuously and fresh infusions are required on a regular basis. Two methods of changeover are commonly used:

- Quick change method
- Double-pump method

Research has shown that haemodynamic compromise can occur to some degree with both methods and there is no statistically significant difference between them (Arino *et al*, 2004).

Glossary of terms

Agonist	A substance promoting receptor activity
Afterload	Resistance that the left or right ventricle has to overcome during systolic ejection
Antagonist	A substance inhibiting receptor activity
Cardiac output	The amount of blood ejected from the ventricle each minute
Chronotrope	An agent that affects heart rate
Half-life	The time required for the plasma concentration of a medication to be decreased by 50% after discontinuation/stopping the medication

Inotrope	An agent that affects myocardial contractility
Negative chronotrope	An agent that causes a decrease in the heart rate (eg. beta-blocker)
Negative inotrope	An agent that causes decreased contractility (eg. the beta-blocker metoprolol)
Pharmacokinetics	The factors that determine the blood concentration of medicine
Positive chronotrope	An agent that causes an increase in heart rate (eg. epinephrine/ adrenaline)
Positive inotrope	An agent that causes increased contractility
Preload	The volume of blood remaining in the ventricles at the end of diastole (or ventricular end-diastolic volume)
Steady state	The point when medication elimination is equal to medication administration (takes four to five half-lives to reach)

References

Ahlqvist M, Bogren A, Hagman S, *et al* (2006) Handling of peripheral intravenous cannulae: effects of evidence based clinical guidelines. *J Clin Nurs* **15**(11): 1354–61

Arino M, Barrington JP, Morrison AL, Gillies D (2004) Management of the changeover of inotrope infusions in children. *Intens Crit Care Nurs* **20:** 275–80

Aylott M (2007) Observing the sick child: Part 2b Respiratory palpation. *Paediatr Nurs* **19**(1): 38–44

British Committee for Standards in Haematology (2003) *Guidelines for Near Patient Testing.* BCSH www.bcshguidelines.com/guidelinesMENU.asp

British Committee for Standards in Haematology (2004) Transfusion Guidelines For Neonates and Older Children. *Br J Haematol* **124:** 433–53

British Medical Association (2001) *Consent, Rights and Choices in Health Care for Children and Young People. BMJ Books, London*

British National Formulary for Children (2007) British National Formulary. BNF/BMJ *London*

British S, Knowles H (2004) The Biology of Child Health: A Reader in Development and Assessment. Palgrave Macmillan, Basingstoke

British Transfusion Service (2005) *Guidelines for the Blood Transfusion Services in the UK.* www.transfusionguidelines.org.uk/index.asp?Publication=RB&Section=25

Chamley CA, Carson P, Randall D, Sandwell M (2005) *Developmental Anatomy and Physiology of Children: A Practical Approach.* Churchill Livingstone, Edinburgh

Clark VL, Kruse JA (1992) Arterial catheterisation. *Crit Care Clin* **8**(4): 687–97

Clinical Resource and Audit Group (2002) *Good Practice Statement for the Preparation of Injections in Near-Patient Areas including Clinical and Home Environments*. Scottish Executive, Edinburgh

Conroy F (2004) Preventing the spread of MRSA from practices such as phlebotomy is worth considering. *BMJ* **329:** 978

Contreras M (ed.) (2001) *ABC of Transfusion*, 3rd edn. BMJ Books, London

Cooke F, Metcalfe H (2000) Cardiac monitoring – 1. *Nurs Times* **96**(23): 45–46

Cooper N (2004) Acute care: Circulatory failure and the use of inotropes. *Student BMJ* **12:** 177–220

Crow S (1996) Prevention of intravascular infections ways and means. *J Intraven Nurs* **19**(4): 175–220

Das B, Sharma A (2000) Acquired brachial arteriovenous fistula in an ex-premature infant. *Clin Paediatr* **41**(2): 131–32

Department of Health (2001) *Seeking Consent: Working with Children*. The Stationary Office, London

Department of Health (2002) *Better Blood Transfusion: Appropriate Use of Blood*. HSC 2002/009. www.transfusionguidelines.org.uk

Department of Health (2003) *Winning Ways: Working Together to Reduce Healthcare Associated Infection in England*. Department of Health, London

Dougherty L (2002) Delivery of intravenous therapy. *Nurs Stand* **16**(16): 45–52

Franklin L (1999) Skin cleansing and infection control in peripheral venepuncture and cannulation. *Nurs Stand* **14**(4): 49–50

Fujita T, Namiki T, Suzuki T, Yamamoto E (2006) Normal saline flushing for maintenance of peripheral intravenous sites. *J Clin Nurs* **15:** 103–04

Galway R, Harrod ME, Crisp J, *et al* (2003) Central venous access and handwashing: variability in policies and practices *Paediatr Nurs* **15**(10): 14–17

Garretson S (2005) Haemodynamic monitoring: arterial catheters. *Nurs Stand* **19**(31): 55–64

Grebenik CR, Sinclair ME (2003) Which inotrope? *Curr Paediatr* **13:** 6–11

Halimaa SL (2003) Pain management in nursing procedures on preterm babies. *J Adv Nurs* **42**(6): 587–97

Hewitt T (1998) Prolonged exposure to topical anaesthetic cream: a case report. *Paediatr Nurs* **10**(2): 22–23

Hindley G (2004) Infection control in peripheral venous cannulae. *Nurs Stand* **18**(2): 37–40

Horrox F (2002) *Manual of Neonatal and Paediatric Heart Disease*. John Wiley & Sons Ltd, Chichester:

Imperial-Perez F, McRae M (2002) Arterial pressure monitoring. *Crit Care Nurs* **19**(2): 105–07

Infusion Nurses Society (2006) Infusion Nursing Standards of Practice. *J Infus Nurs* **29**(1) (Suppl)

Ingram P, Lavery I (2005) Peripheral intravenous therapy: key risks and implications for practice. *Nurs Stand* **19**(46): 55–64

Jevon P (2000) Cardiac monitoring. *Nurs Times* **96**(23): 43–44

Jowett N (1997) *Cardiovascular Monitoring*. Whurr Publishers, London

Keenlyside D (1993) Avoiding and unnecessary outcome. A comparative trial between IV3000 and a conventional film dressing to assess catheter related sepsis. *Prof Nurs* **8**(5): 288–91

Lander J, Hodkins M, Najarali S, McTavish J, Oollette J, Frieson E (1996a) Determinants of success and failure of EMLA. *Pain* **64:** 89–97

Lander J, Hodkins M, Najarali S, McTavish J, Oollette J, Frieson E (1996b) Evaluation of a new topical anaesthetic agent: a case report. *NT Research* **45**(1): 50–53

Lavery I (2003) Peripheral intravenous cannulation and patient consent. *Nurs Stand* **17**(28): 40–42

Marieb EN (2004) *Human Anatomy and Physiology*, 6th edn. Addison-Wesley, San Francisco

McChance KL, Huether SE (2006) *Pathophysiology: The Biologic Basis for Disease in Adults and Children*, 5th edn. Elsevier Mosby, St Louis

McClelland DBL (ed.) (2001) *Handbook of Transfusion Medicine*, 3rd edn. HMSO, London

McGhee BH, Bridges MEJ (2002) Monitoring arterial blood pressure: what you may not know. *Crit Care Nurs* **22**(2): 60–79

McIntosh ND (2003) Central venous catheters: reasons for insertion and removal *Paediatr Nurs* **15**(1): 14–16

Medical Devices Agency (MDA) (2006) *Sterilisation Disinfection and Cleaning Medical Equipment: Guidance on Decontamination from the Microbiology Committee to Department of Health Medical Devices Agency*. MDA, London

Mehta C, Dhillon R (2004). Understanding paediatric ECGs. *Curr Paediatr* **14:** 229–236

Methany NM (2000) *Fluid and Electrolyte Balance*, 4th ed. Lippincott, London

Moore KL, Dalley AF (1999) *Clinically Orientated Anatomy*. Lippincott Williams and Wilkins, Philadelphia

National Patient Safety Agency (2004) *Right Patient- Right Care. NPSA, London*

North America Society of Pacing and Electrophysiology and the British Pacing and Electrophysiology Group (1993) The NASPE/BPEG defibrillator code. Pacing Clin Electrophysiol **16**(9): 1776–80

Nursing and Midwifery Council (2004) *Guidelines for Records and Record Keeping*. NMC, London

Phillip R, Beckett M (2000) Step-by-step guide. Neonatal blood sampling time for safe devices *J Neonat Nurs* **6**(3) (four-page insert)

Quinn C (2000) Infusion devices: risks functions and management. *Nurs Stand* **14**(26): 35–41, 43

Resuscitation Council UK (2004) *Advanced Life Support Manual*. Resuscitation Council UK, London

Royal College of Nursing (1999) *Guidance for Nurses giving Intravenous Therapy*. Royal College of Nursing, London

Royal College of Nursing (2003a) *Restraining, Holding Still And Containing Children and Young People: Guidance Nursing Staff*. Royal College of Nursing, London

Royal College of Nursing (2003b) *Standards for Infusion Therapy.* Royal College of Nursing, London

Royal College of Nursing (2004) *Right Blood – Right Patient– right Time. Guidance for Improving Transfusion Practice*. Royal College of Nursing, London

Royal College of Nursing (2005) *Competencies: An Education and Training Framework for Peripheral Venous Cannulation in Children and Young People*. Royal College of Nursing, London

Scales K (2005) Vascular access: a guide to peripheral venous cannulation. *Nurs Stand* **19**(49): 48–52

Schindler PW (2005) Catheterisation of the radial or brachial artery in neonates and infants. *Paediatr Anaesth* **15**(8): 677–82

Smalley A (1999) Needle phobia. *Paediatr Nurs* **11**(2): 17–20

Smith SF, Duell DJ, Martin BC (2005) *Clinical Nursing Skills: Basic to Advanced*, 6th edn. Pearson Prentice Hall, New Jersey

Stevens B, Yamada J, Ohlsson A (2003) Sucrose in newborn infants undergoing painful procedures. *Cochrane Review Issue 3*. Update Software, Oxford

Stewart P (2007) New maintenance fluid guidelines for children: is 0.9% sodium chloride with 5% glucose a good choice? *Anaesthesia* **62**(4): 322–24

Tak JH, van Bon WHJ (2006) Pain and distress reducing interventions for venepuncture in children. *Child Care Develop* **32**(3): 257–68

Todd AAM (2002) Evidence-based use of blood products. *Curr Paediatr* **12:** 304–09

Tortora GJ (2005) *Principles of Human Anatomy*, 10th edn. Wiley, Danvers

Tortora GJ, Derrickson B (2006) *Principles of Anatomy and Physiology*, 11th edn. Wiley, Danvers

Tortora GJ, Derrickson B (2007) *Introduction to the Human Body: The Essentials of Anatomy and Physiology*, 7th edn. Wiley, Danvers

Treston-Aurend J, Olmsted RN, Allen-Bridson K, Craig CP (1997) Impact of dressing materials on central venous catheter infection rates. *J Intraven Nurs* **20**(4): 201–06

Usichenko TI, Pavlovic D, Foellner S, Wendt M (2004) Reducing venepuncture pain by a cough trick; a randomised cross over volunteer study. *Anaesthes Analges* **98**(2): 343–45

Watt S (2003a) Safe administration of medicines to children: Part 1. *Paediatr Nurs* **15**(5): 4

Watt S (2003b) Safe administration of medicines to children: Part 2. *Paediatr Nurs* **15**(5): 40–44

Watterson L (2004) Monitoring sharps injuries. *Nurs Stand* **19**(3): 33–38

Williams C, Asquith J (2004) *Paediatric Intensive Care Nursing*. Churchill Livingstone, London

Willock J, Jewkes F (2000) Making sense of fluid balance in children *Paediatr Nurs* **12**(7): 37–43

Willock J, Richardson J, Brazier A, Powell C, Mitchell E (2004) Peripheral venepuncture in infants and children. *Nurs Stand* **18**(27): 43–50

Wright E (2004) Therapeutic plasma exchange in children. *Paediatric Nursing*, **16**(9): 39-42

Chapter 10

Fundamental aspects of gastrointestinal care

Dawn Ashbee and Karen Dick

Enteral feeding

Feeding via the enteral route remains the most effective method to deliver nutrients into the body and should be encouraged if at all possible. For children unable to maintain optimum nutrition orally, enteral feeds can be administered many ways, including:

- Nasogastric tube
- Gastrostomy
- Jejunal tube (rare)

Enteral feeding at a rate of 1–2 mL/kg/h helps to maintain gastrointestinal integrity and immunological function, prevents biliary cholestasis, and reduces bacterial translocation (Brogden, 2004). Enteral nutrition (feed) is provided in pre-packed liquid or powder to be reconstituted. Pre-packed feeds are sterile until handled; some require decanting into giving sets for administration, while others come ready to hang as part of a closed sterile system. This closed system minimises the potential for bacterial contamination. Powdered feed that requires reconstitution should be made in a clean environment designated for that task (National Institute for Clinical Excellence [NICE], 2003a).

Nasogastric tube feeding

A nasogastric tube is a tube that is passed through the nostril and down the oesophagus into the stomach. Orogastric tubes can be used instead in neonates as neonates are obligatory nose breathers. A nasogastric tube is the most commonly used route for supplemental enteral feeding in the nutritionally compromised child (Dougherty and Lister, 2006). The use of a polyvinyl chloride (PVC) tube is indicated only for short-term use, approximately 7–10 days. For long-term use a polyurethane tube (silk) should be used (NHS Quality Improvement Scotland, 2003).

Passing a nasogastric tube

Reasons for the procedure

- To administer medication
- To supplement oral feeding often during acute illness, eg. a child with acute respiratory distress or heart failure
- To provide complete long-term nutrition, eg. poor or no swallow reflex
- To decompress the gut, eg. bowel obstruction
- To decompress air from the stomach, eg. following bag-valve mask ventilation

Pre-procedure

Equipment required

- Nasogastric tube: use a PVC tube if for less than 10 days or a silk tube if for longer than 10 days; consider the child's age, nasal cavity size and other relevant anatomical issues
- Syringe with minimum capacity of 30–50 mL, to ensure pressure does not exceed the bursting pressure of the tube (*Figure 10.1*)
- Water for lubrication if required (*not* KY Jelly)
- pH indicator strips (*Figure 10.1*)
- Plastic apron and gloves – mouth and eye protection should be available
- Water and straw for child to drink if appropriate
- Hydrocolloid dressing
- Adhesive tape to secure tube to hydrocolloid dressing on cheek
- Vomit bowl and tissues
- Oxygen and suction

Specific patient preparation

- Prepare the child and his or her family by giving the reasons for the carrying out the procedure and explaining the risks and benefits
- Ensure that there are no known contraindications, eg. obstruction, trauma, or recent surgery to the nasal or upper gastrointestinal tract
- Ensure oxygen and suction are available, with appropriately sized mask and suction tubing attached
- Check patient identification
- Wash hands to prevent cross infection
- If possible, position child in a semi-upright

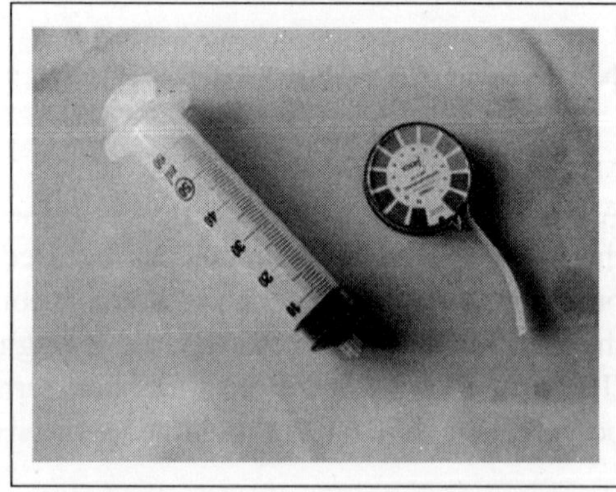

Figure 10.1: 50 mL syringe and pH paper

position, with head tilted slightly forward to reduce cervical flexure; swaddle babies and very young children so that arms are kept tucked away and cannot pull out tube during procedure

- Wash hands again
- Measure length of nasogastric tube required (measure from tip of nose, to the ear lobe and down to xyphoid process; in infants, measure nose to ear, to the mid-point between the tip of the sternum and the umbilicus). Make a mental note of distance using numbers on the tube (if no numbers present, mark the tube with tape or a permanent marker)
- Select a nostril using child's preference and skin integrity as a guide; often the nasogastric tube is inserted in nostrils alternately as required
- Place hydrocolloid dressing such as Granuflex or DuoDerm on the child's cheek to form a protective barrier (Watson and Hodgkin, 2005)
- *If using a silk tube* flush it through with 10 mL of water to lubricate the tube internally immediately before passing the nasogastric tube (Dougherty and Lister, 2006)

During the procedure

- Wash hands and put on gloves and apron
- Lubricate end of tube with water (not KY Jelly as this affects the pH value)
- Encourage the child to take a sip of water and to swallow to help the tube pass down (Tortora, 2005). Swallowing covers the trachea with the epiglottis, minimising the risk of passing the tube into the trachea. Allowing a baby to suck on a dummy also stimulates the above action
- Insert tube into nostril and advance it to the nasopharynx, allowing the tip to seek its own passage until the measured length is reached
- If the tube is difficult to pass, check for coiling and withdraw and rotate it slightly before re-advancing, to help the tube to pass any obstruction (NHS Quality Improvement Scotland, 2003)
- *If using a silk tube* (with guide wire) pass it with a guide wire in place. In order to confirm tube placement the guide wire must be removed
- Aspirate the tube with a 30 mL or 50 mL syringe
- Once aspirate is obtained place a sample on pH paper. Gastric placement is confirmed with pH of 5 or less (Heiselman *et al*, 1993) (see *Box 10.1* for measures to take if no aspirate is obtained)

Box 10.1: What to do if no aspirate is obtained

Instil 3–5 mL of air to push the lumen away from wall and then check for aspirate
Try oral fluids, if not contraindicated
Lie the child on his or her left side
Try advancing or retracting the tube slightly
Wait 5–10 minutes and try again (Methany *et al*, 1993)
A pH of 6 means there is doubt about the tube's position, and a pH of 7 or more means the tube is incorrectly positioned and needs to be re-passed (Tait, 2001)
Do not use the tube to feed or give medication without first confirming correct placement
If at any time during the procedure the patient becomes distressed, cyanosed, vomits, coughs or complains of pain, stop and withdraw tube immediately
Once placement is confirmed, tape the tube in place

Litmus paper is no longer recommended for testing pH because the pink colour change suggestive of acid can also be obtained from bronchial secretions, which have a pH of between 5.5 and 7 (see *Box 10.1*), and therefore does not provide confirmation of correct placement (NHS Quality Improvement Scotland, 2003).

Auscultation involves passing air down the nasogastric tube into the stomach – known as the whoosh test. It is an unreliable method of confirming tube placement (National Patient Safety Awareness [NPSA], 2005). Do not assume that lack of coughing, distress or respiratory compromise is an indicator of correct placement (NPSA, 2005).

Post-procedure

- If location is unconfirmed despite using some of the techniques listed, an X-ray may be recommended
- Secure the tube comfortably to the cheek and allow the child to calm down and relax; discourage them from pulling out tube by using distraction techniques
- Remove gloves and apron and wash hands
- Dispose of equipment as per hospital policy
- If a silicone tube was used, the guide wire should be wiped down using an alcohol wipe and stored in a clean re-sealable bag labelled with patient details. Do not discard
- Document in the child's nursing notes, including the size and length of tube, what distance was passed and which nostril was used (Nursing and Midwifery Council [NMC], 2004)

Complications

Complications of passing a nasogastric tube include:

- Nausea and vomiting
- Nose bleeding
- Aspiration
- Pressure sores to nasal flange and nasal stenosis when tube is in long-term use
- Mucosal damage/gastric erosion to gastrointestinal tract
- Nose–intracranial penetration

Removing a nasogastric tube

Reasons for the procedure

- To change the feeding device (change to gastrostomy)
- To stop nasogastric feeding in children:
  - who no longer need feeding via a nasogastric tube
  - who are achieving appropriate oral intakes
  - in whom the stomach no longer needs emptying of air or gastric contents

Pre-procedure

Equipment required

- Apron and gloves
- Tissues and vomit bowl
- Adhesive remover

Specific patient preparation

- Inform child of procedure
- Ensure they are comfortable
- Discuss child and family involvement

During the procedure

- Wash hands and put on gloves and apron
- Remove tape, if child is anxious an adhesive remover can be used
- Encourage child to take a deep breath, as the child exhales pull the nasogastric tube out

Post-procedure

- Dispose of waste as per hospital protocol
- Remove gloves and apron and wash hands to prevent cross infection
- Ensure the child is comfortable
- Document removal in the child's notes

Complications

Complications of removing a nasogastric tube include:

- Nausea and vomiting
- Trauma to nasal passage
- Discomfort

Gastrostomy

A gastrostomy is a surgical opening (stoma) through the abdomen into the stomach, in which a feeding device is inserted that allows the child to be fed directly into his or her stomach, as defined by Great Ormond Street Hospital for Children NHS Trust and UCL Institute of Child Health (GOSH/ICH, 2007). A gastrostomy tube is shown in *Figure 10.2*.

Reasons for the procedure

- To assist with feeding difficulties
- Neurological disorders such as:
  - cerebral palsy
  - acquired brain injury
  - spina bifida
- Gastrointestinal disorders such as:
  - malabsorption
  - foregut dysmotility
  - inborn errors of metabolism, eg. mitochondrial disorders
- Difficulty swallowing (and/or risk of aspiration)
- Long-segment tracho-oesophageal atresia and/or fistula (Sullivan and McIntyre, 2005)

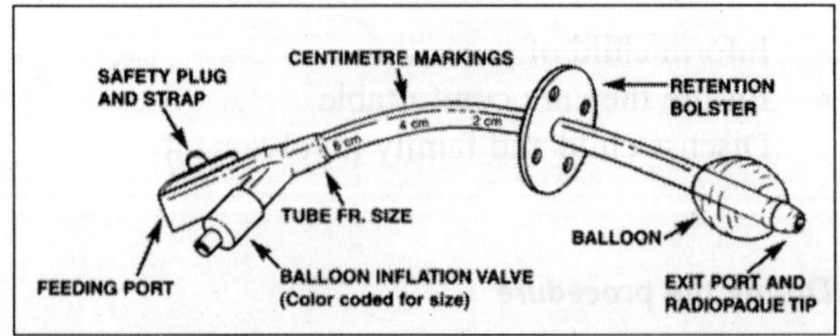

Figure 10.2: Gastrostomy tube

The types of gastrostomy tube

- PEG tube (ie. percutaneous endoscopic gastrostomy) – a tube inserted into the stomach through a small incision in the abdominal wall using an endoscope; it can last up to 2 years (see *Figures 10.3 and 10.4*)
- Balloon device – a transparent silicone tube with an internal balloon and external ring flange, placed initially via surgical laparotomy or laparoscopically; it can last up to 6 months (*Figure 10.5*)
- Mini balloon button – a low-profile silicone device with an internal balloon device, replaced in an existing stoma tract or laparoscopically; it can last up to 6 months (*Figure 10.6*)

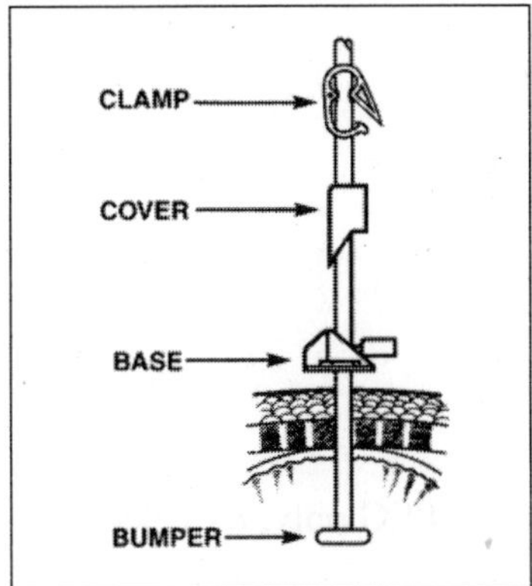

Figure 10.3: PEG tube

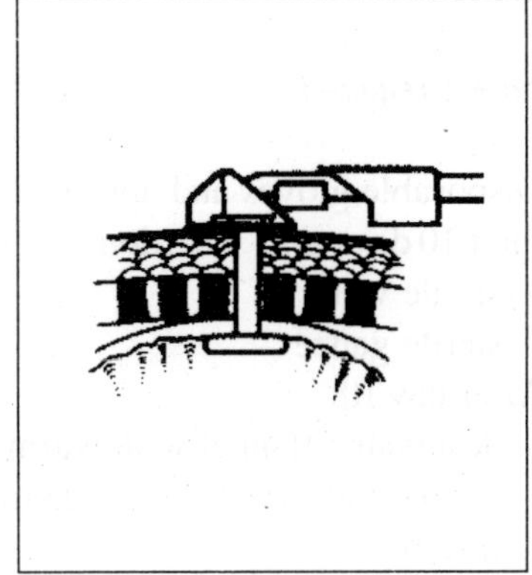

Figure 10.4: PEG tube fixation device

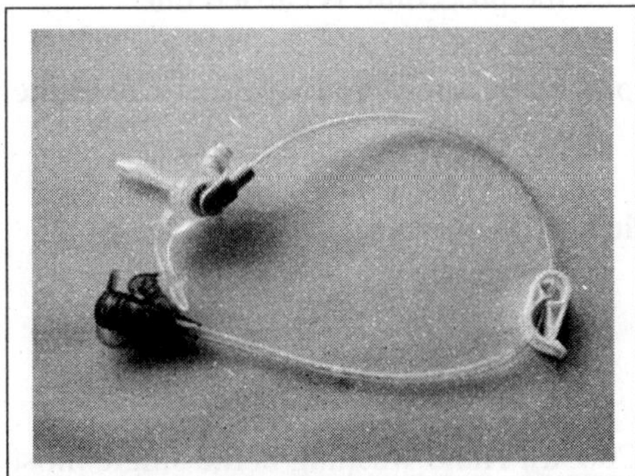

Figure 10.5: Silicon balloon device

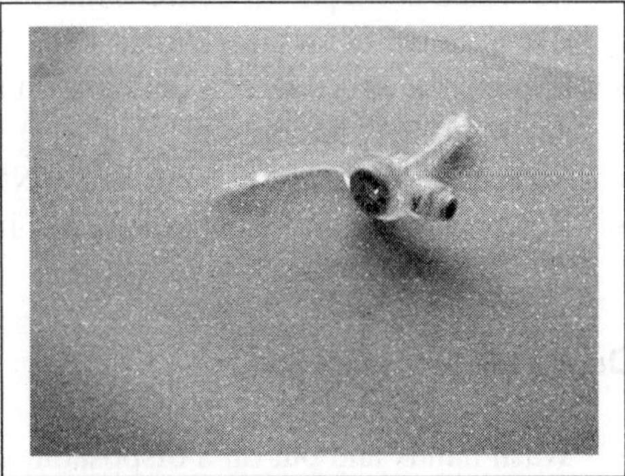

Figure 10.6: Mini button

Care of the gastrostomy

Reasons for the procedure

Daily skin care should be performed:

- To prevent infection
- To prevent skin breakdown (NICE, 2003a,b)

Pre-procedure

Equipment required

- Disposable gloves and apron
- First 10 days post insertion:
  - sterile water
  - sterile gauze
- After day 10:
  - designated flannel with warm, mildly soapy water
  - cotton buds (useful for cleaning right-angled connector of PEG only; 8 weeks after insertion)

Specific patient preparation

- Informed child/parent consent must be obtained before the procedure is carried out (Department of Health, 2004)
- Explain the procedure to the child in an age/developmentally appropriate manner and to the parents if they are present
- Screen the bed to provide privacy (NMC, 2004)
- Read and follow the manufacturer's instructions (Medical Devices Agency [MDA], 2000)

During the procedure

- Wash hands and put on a disposable apron (NICE, 2003a). Hand washing is the single most important step in preventing the spread of infection
- Cleanse around the stoma and device daily using appropriate equipment. Use this opportunity to check the stoma site for:
  - leakage
  - infection
  - irritated skin
  - granulation

- Report any of the above to medical staff immediately
- During cleansing, using the gauze or flannel as appropriate, clean the skin underneath the device ensuring that the button/PEG can rotate freely, stopping at a different point each time to allow for air circulation. This helps to prevent adhesions to the tract and soreness due to granulation under the base
- *Button only* – usually able to do from 8 weeks after insertion (allows stoma tract to form) – deflate and re-inflate the balloon with the prescribed amount of water/saline water every week, as recommended by manufacturers, in order to check that the gastrostomy balloon is intact
- Ensure that the child is redressed and comfortable

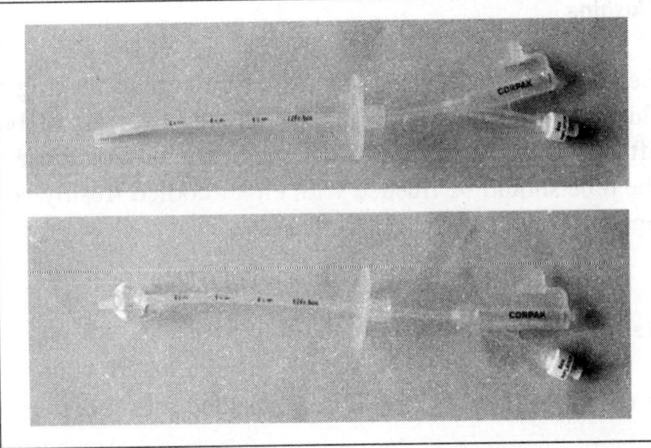

Figure 10.7: PEG (percutaneous endoscopic gastrostomy) tube showing the balloon not inflated (top) and the balloon inflated (bottom)

Post-procedure

- Discard clinical waste including gloves and apron according to trust policy
- Wash hands (NICE, 2003a)
- Record the procedure in the child's nursing records (NMC, 2004)
- Maintain good oral hygiene in order to prevent infection and maintain the child's mouth in a healthy condition

Administering feed and/or medication via an enteral tube

The principles of feeding using a nasogastric tube or a gastrostomy are the same. In both cases, feed can be administered as a set number of boluses throughout the day, as a continuous feed, or as a combination of both. The gastrostomy and nasogastric tube can be used to provide a child's full nutritional requirement, or to 'top up' what a child is able to take orally.

Flushing

Before, after and during the use of an enteral feeding tube, it is recommended that the tube is flushed to prevent blockage. The feeding tube should be flushed with fresh tap water before and after feeding or administering medications. For those patients who are immunocompromised, the tube should be flushed with either cooled freshly boiled water or sterile water from a freshly opened container (NICE, 2003a).

Reasons for the procedure

A child can have an enteral feeding tube for numerous reasons, such as:

- To provide adequate oral intake to maintain optimal fluid and nutritional status
- To provide nutrition for children with long-term disability and inability to feed (eg. no swallow reflex)
- To feed child during acute illness, such as bronchiolitis (nasogastric tube only)

Pre-procedure

Storage of feed

Pre-packed feeds should be stored as per manufacturer's instructions. Once opened, a pre-packed feed can be stored in the fridge for 24 hours. This also applies to feeds reconstituted from powder. Ensure feed is always given at room temperature to reduce the risk of diarrhoea or shock due to bacterial contamination.

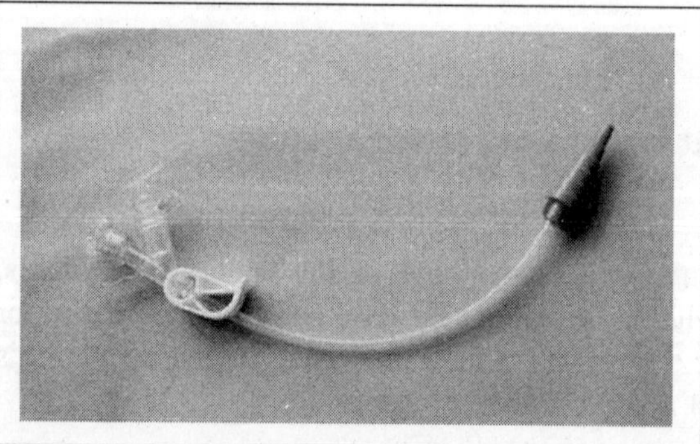

Figure 10.8: Feeding extension tube

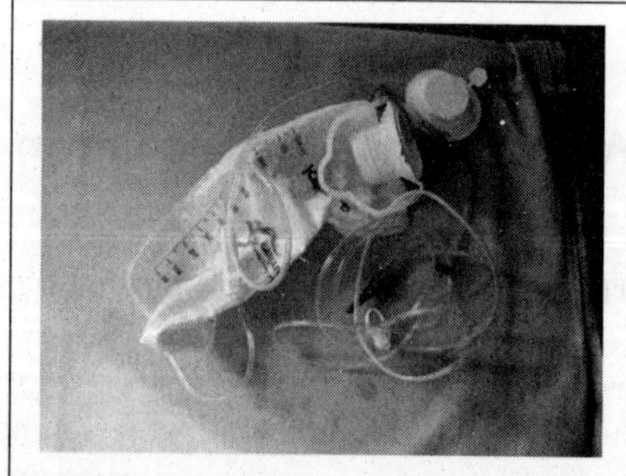

Figure 10.9: Feed bag and feeding extension set

Equipment required

Nasogastric feeding

- Gloves and apron
- 30 mL or 50 mL syringe to aspirate
- pH paper
- Feed as directed by dietician
- Feed pump
- Giving set and container, for continuous feeding
- 50 mL syringe with plunger removed, for bolus feeds
- Water to flush

Gastrostomy feeding

- Gloves and apron
- Extension set for mini balloon button
- 10 mL syringe to flush
- Feed as directed by dietician
- Feed pump
- Giving set and container, for continuous feeding
- 50 mL syringe with plunger removed, for bolus feeds
- Water to flush

Specific patient preparation

- Inform child of procedure
- Ensure they are comfortable
- Discuss child and family involvement

During the procedure

- Wash hands as per hospital policy, and put on gloves and apron
- *Nasogastric tube only* – attach a 30/50 mL syringe and aspirate per recommendations, to ascertain correct positioning (Wilkes-Holmes, 2006)
- *Button only* – prior to connecting the clean extension set to the button, release the clamp and flush the tube with water so that the child is not given a bolus of air. Then re-clamp the tube. Connect the extension set to the button as per manufacturer's instructions
- With all devices, flush the tube with the prescribed amount of water using a gentle 'push', usually 10–20 mL. With a gastrostomy this checks for leakage around the site and with a nasogastric tube it makes sure the tube is not blocked

Continuous feeding

- Sterile feeds (pre-packed) can be hung for a maximum of 24 hours, provided they are handled using a clean technique. Non-sterile feeds, modified feeds or feeds that are decanted into a container are at greater risk of bacterial contamination and should have a hanging time of no longer than 4 hours. (NICE, 2003a; NHS Quality Improvement Scotland, 2006)

- Feed containers and giving sets should be discarded after 24 hours
- Run feed through the giving set to prime the line then re-apply the roller clamp until ready to administer the feed. Avoid touching any internal part of the giving set (non-touch technique). Keep the end connection sterile by leaving the cover in place
- Hang feed on pump stand and load the giving set into the appropriate pump
- Ensure the drip chamber (if present) in the giving set is only half full, so that the pump can read the drips accurately
- When ready, securely attach the connector to the feeding port
- Turn the pump on, set rate and volume to be infused, open clamps and commence feed
- Re-check frequently to ensure feed is running correctly and child is comfortable

Bolus feeding

- Connect 50 mL syringe with the plunger removed to the feeding port
- Pour in the prescribed amount of feed (this may not fit in the syringe all in one go, so do in stages)
- If the tube has a clamp, release it in order to allow feed to flow
- Gravity will cause the feed to be administered
- Holding the syringe higher will cause the feed to flow faster
- Give bolus feeds over approximately 20 minutes to prevent dumping syndrome (see *Complications*)

Giving medications

- Depending on their quantity and consistency, medicines can be given as a slow push or as a bolus
- Flush the tube with water before administering medications, between each medication and after all medications have been given (NICE, 2003a)
- Use liquid medications whenever possible
- If medication is only available in tablet form, check this can be crushed because the efficacy of some formulations can be impaired or lost by crushing (Estoup, 1994)
- If unsure of any potential problems about administering medication, contact a pharmacist for advice

In all cases

- Place baby or child at a 30° angle to minimise the risk of reflux, vomiting and potential aspiration (NHS Quality Improvement Scotland, 2003)
- Once the feed/medication is complete, apply clamp as appropriate
- Flush the tube again with water usually 10–20 mL to prevent the tube from blocking

- Remove the giving set/syringe and replace the spigot into the end of the tube
- *PEG only* – with the clamp closed, curl the tube up and fasten to the skin to prevent air entering the stomach and to make the gastrostomy less visible
- *Button only* – disconnect the extension set and close the button port to prevent air entering the stomach and to make the gastrostomy less visible

Post-procedure

- Dispose of waste as per hospital policy
- *Button only* – the extension set must be washed with warm soapy water and stored in a specific container
- Remove gloves and apron
- Wash hands to prevent cross infection
- Document on the fluid chart and in the child's nursing notes (NMC, 2004)
- If giving medication, sign the prescription chart to state that medication has been given

Complications

Complications of enteral tube feeding include:

- Nausea
- Vomiting
- Diarrhoea
- Reflux
- Aspiration
- Abdominal distension (Dougherty and Lister, 2006)
- Blocked feeding tube (warm water, carbonated soft drinks and pineapple juice are all recommended for unblocking tubes)
- Dumping syndrome (this condition causes bloating, nausea, diarrhoea, pallor and weakness. It is caused by feed exiting the stomach and entering the small intestines too quickly) (Borkowski, 1998)
- Difficulty in testing correct placement of a nasogastric tube as per recommendations
- Patients suffering from gastro-oesophageal reflux may be on antacids to reduce the acidity of their gastric contents; be aware that this makes it difficult to obtain an acidic aspirate for confirmation of tube placement (Colagiovanni, 2000)
- Gastric pH rises with continuous feeding, again making it difficult to obtain an appropriate pH reading. Stopping the feed returns the pH to normal, so enabling an acidic aspirate to be obtained (Colagiovanni, 2000)

Stoma care

A stoma is a surgically created opening along the gastrointestinal tract, through the abdominal wall, that allows a passage for stool. It is formed when part of the bowel becomes non-functioning, causing an obstruction. The stoma is sited above the malfunctioning section of bowel (Kean, 2002). Often, the formation of a stoma is a temporary measure while surgical correction of the malfunction is performed. However, some children have permanent stomas if their abnormal bowel cannot be corrected.

There are two types of gastrointestinal stoma – an *ileostomy* which involves the formation of a stoma using a portion of the small intestine (ileum), and a *colostomy* which uses part of the large intestine (colon) (Kean, 2002).

Many conditions can cause children to require formation of a stoma. These are just a few of the causes:

- Imperforated anus
- Hirschsprung's disease
- Inflammatory bowel disease
  - Crohn's disease
  - Ulcerative colitis
- Neonatal necrotising enterocolitis

As the stoma is not a normal passage for stool, the child has no control. Therefore, a bag is placed over the stoma to collect the stool as it is passed. These bags or pouches come in all shapes and sizes, as one-piece or two-piece, drainable or non-drainable, to name just some. When the child's stoma is first formed a discussion takes place between the parents, the child, and their caregivers, to decide which pouch is best for that child's own lifestyle. Because of the variety of pouches, each has its own method of emptying.

Changing a stoma bag and cleaning the stoma

Reasons for the procedure

- To replace a leaking bag
- To clean and check the stoma site
- To empty the stoma bag

Although there are many types of pouches, the principles of changing them remains the same. Drainable pouches can be emptied several times before they need changing and can stay in place for several days. Closed (non-drainable) pouches have to be changed each time they need to be emptied.

Pre-procedure

Equipment required

- Gloves and apron
- Incontinence pads or sheets to prevent soiling of surrounding area
- Sterile gauze wipes
- Warm water
- Clinical waste bag
- Adhesive remover
- Container to drain bag contents (if possible)
- Scissors
- Template for stoma size
- New bag and clip

Specific patient preparation

- Explain the procedure to the child and parents as appropriate (negotiate about how much the they wish to do themselves)
- Reassure the child and/or parents, as appropriate, that a stoma has no nerve endings and therefore will not be sensitive to touch
- Ensure privacy
- Read the manufacturer's instructions (MDA, 2000)
- Prepare a new bag before removing the old one so that the procedure is not rushed. Using a template with the same size and shape of the stoma, cut a hole in the flange of the new bag
- It is sometimes useful to stretch the opening with a finger to ensure a snug fit (Merenstein and Gardner, 2006)
- Discuss with the child and family the best position for the child throughout the procedure (in babies and younger children this will generally be lying down)

During the procedure

- Wash hands, put on gloves and apron, and place an incontinence sheet under the child to protect from drips and spillages of the bag's contents
- It is advisable to drain the bag of contents (if the bag is drainable) before removing it, to prevent unnecessary spillages
- Remove the old bag by carefully peeling it off with one hand, starting at the top, while gently pressing down on the skin with the other. This helps to minimise trauma to the skin. If the child is particularly anxious, an adhesive removal agent can aid the removal of the old bag
- Discard the old bag into a clinical waste bag (never flush them down the toilet)
- Cleanse the skin using warm water and gauze:
  – if using soap, rinse well

  - do not use cotton wool (can leave fluff in the stoma)
  - do not use baby wipes (can inhibit adhesion of the new bag and therefore can cause leakage)
- Ensure the skin is dried thoroughly before sticking on the new bag. Take care not to rub or accidentally poke the stoma as this can cause surface bleeding
- Take this opportunity to monitor the health of the stoma and surrounding skin
  - the stoma should look similar to the inside of your cheek – a healthy pink colour – so if it appears dusky or dark in colour, inform the child's doctor immediately
  - bleeding from inside the stoma or any signs of inflammation to the stoma or surrounding skin should be reported
- If prescribed, apply skin barrier cream to the skin immediately around the stoma, sparingly so as to not interfere with the adhesive properties of the appliance
- Double-check that the new flange has been cut to ensure a close fit around the stoma (to prevent effluent coming into contact with child's skin)
- Apply the new appliance, directing the opening of the bag towards the side of the abdomen for ease of draining, and so it does not lie in the young child's nappy (causing discomfort or a potential risk of infection and urinary tract infection)

Post-procedure

- Ensure child and family are comfortable
- Dispose of soiled items in clinical waste
- Remove gloves and apron
- Wash hands as per hospital policy
- Document in the child's nursing records, noting the amount and consistency of the bag contents and the health of the stoma (NMC, 2004)

Complications

Complications of changing/cleaning the stoma include:

- Leakage from under the flange causing discomfort and soiling of clothing
- Infection to stoma site or surrounding skin
- Effluent dermatitis
- Discomfort
- Contact dermatitis

References

Borkowski S (1998) The Mic-ky experience with the pediatric patient. *Wound, Ostomy Cont Nurs* **21**(5): 195–98

Bott L, Usson MO, Guimber D, *et al* (2001) Contamination of gastrostomy feeding systems in children in a home-based enteral nutrition program. *J Pediatr Gastroenterol Nutr* **33:** 266–70

Brogden B (2004) Current practice in administration of parenteral nutrition: venous access. *Br J Nurs* **13**(18): 1068–73

Clinical Resource Efficiency Support Team (1994) *Guidelines for the Management of Enteral Tube Feeding in Adults*. CREST www.library.nhs.uk/guidelinesfinder/ViewResource.aspx?resID=36156

Colagiovanni L (2000) Preventing and clearing blocked feeding tubes. *Nurs Times Plus* **96**(17): 3–4

Department of Health (2004) *National Service Framework for Children, Young People and Maternity Services*. DH, London

Dougherty L, Lister S (2006) *The Royal Marsden Hospital Manual of Clinical Nursing Procedures, 6th edn. Blackwell Publishing, London*

Estoup M (1994) Approaches and limitations of medicine delivery in patients with enteral feeding tubes. Crit Care Nurs **14**(1): 68–81

Great Ormond Street Hospital for Children NHS Trust and UCL Institute of Child Health (2007) *Enteral Feeding*. GOSH&ICH www.ich.ucl.ac.uk/gosh/clinicalservices/Dietetics_and_nutrition/InformationforFamilies

Gussull MA, Cabre E (2001) Home enteral nutrition in gastrointestinal diseases. *Clin Nutr* **20**(Suppl 2): 63–67

Heiselman DE, Robin R, Milkovich G, Black LD (1993) Naso-intestinal tube placement with a pH sensor feeding tube. *J Parental Enteral Nutr* **17**(6): 562–65

Kean Y (2002) Paediatric stomas and why they are formed. *Nurse 2 Nurse* **3**(1): 24–26

McConnell E (2001) Clinical do's & don'ts; administering total parenteral nutrition. *Nursing* **31**(11): 17

McGrath JM (2006) Family presence during procedures: Breathing life into policy and everyday practices. *Newborn Infant Nurs Rev* **6**(4): 242– 45

Medical Devices Agency (2000) *Single Use Medical Devices: Implications and Consequences of Re-Use*. DB2000 (04). MDA, London

Merenstein GB, Gardner SL (2006) *Handbook of Neonatal Intensive Care*, 6th edn. Elsevier, London

Methany N A, Titler MG (2001) Important facts about intestinal feeding tube placement. *Gastroenterol Nurs* **29**(2): 112–25

Methany N, Reed L, Wiersema M, McSweeney M, Wehrle MA, Clark J (1993) Effectiveness of pH measurements in predicting feeding tube placement: An update. *Nurs Res* **42**(6): 324–31

National Advisory Service for Parents of Children with a Stoma (2002) Our Special Children: A Practical Guide to Stoma Care in Babies and Young Children. www.ccs.org.nz/catalog/toileting2005.doc

National Institute for Clinical Excellence (2003a) *Infection Control: Prevention of Healthcare-Associated Infection in Primary and Community Care*. www.guidance.nice.org.uk/page.aspx?o=CG002NICEguideline/

National Institute for Clinical Excellence (2003b) *Essential Steps to Safe Clean Care: Enteral Feeding*. www.dh.gov.uk/prod_consum_dh/groups/dh_digitalassets/@dh/@en/documents/digitalasset/dh_4136276.pdf/

National Patient Safety Awareness (2005) *Reducing the Harm Caused by Misplaced Nasogastric Feeding tubes*. NPSA, London

NHS Quality Improvement Scotland (2003) *Nasogastric and Gastrostomy Tube Feeding*. NHSQIS, Edinburgh

Nursing and Midwifery Council (2004) *Code of Professional Conduct*. NMC, London

Sullivan PB, McIntyre E (2005) Gastrointestinal problems in disabled children. *Curr Paediatr* **15:** 347–53

Tait J (2001) Going nasogastric. Current thinking in nasogastric tube techniques. *Compl Nutr* **1**(2): 27–28

Tortora GJ (2005) *Principles of Human Anatomy*, 10th edn. Wiley, Danvers

Watson NFS, Hodgkin W (2005) Wound dressings. *Surgery* **23**(2): 52–55

Wilkes-Holmes C (2006) Safe placement of nasogastric tubes in children. *Paed Nurs* **18**(9): 14–17

Workman BA, Bennett CL (2003) *Key Nursing Skills*. Whurr Publishers, London

Useful websites

National Advisory Service for Parents of Children with a Stoma
www.naspcs.co.uk

NHS Quality Improvement Scotland
www.nhs.healthquality.org

Chapter 11

Fundamental aspects of musculoskeletal and integumentary care

Alan Glasper, Jane McConochie and Sue Twells

Orthopaedic nursing skills

The term 'orthopaedics' is derived from two Greek words, *ortho* meaning straight and *paedia* relating to children, literally 'the rearing of straight children'. The term was utilized in the nineteenth century because many children were malformed by diseases of bone and associated muscles, joints and ligaments. In addition to poorly treated fractures, diseases such as rickets and osteomyelitis impacted negatively on a child's gait and mobility. To this day the prevention of infection and the preservation of function remain the mantra of the children's orthopaedic nurse. Dame Agnes Hunt is widely regarded as the pioneer of orthopaedic nursing for sick children (Carter, 2001). She suffered herself from osteomyelitis as a child and went on to found one of the best known orthopaedic hospitals in the world in Oswestry in Shropshire.

Children who require orthopaedic nursing care are often immobilised and require treatment at home or in hospital that may last for many weeks.

Applying a plaster cast and cast management

A plaster cast is made up of plaster of Paris bandages or synthetic materials. Plaster of Paris is less frequently used now, increasingly replaced by fibreglass or lighter and sturdier materials. This procedure will focus on the application of plaster of Paris and fibreglass casting.

Reasons for the procedure

- To prevent and correct deformities
- To provide support
- To provide pain relief
- To protect injury

- To immobilise fractures
- To improve function by stabilizing the joint
- To permit early ambulation and weight bearing

Pre-procedure

Equipment required

- Equipment trolley
- Plaster of Paris
- Softband padding and stockinette
- Plaster of Paris slabs if required and plaster strips to finish
- Plastic sheeting and aprons and plastic-covered pillows
- Plaster scissors
- Bucket or bowl of water at 20–25°C, and a wash bowl and towel for the child
- Rubbish bag
- Elbow or knee rest
- Instruction leaflets
- Felt padding

Specific patient preparation

- Remove any jewellery and clothing on the affected limb (to stored safely by the child's family or according to local policy)
- Check the prescription for correct details
- Prepare an equipment trolley in readiness for undertaking the procedure for the casting
- Ensure the child is appropriately positioned for the limb or body in the case of spicas to be casted. For upper limb casting, the child is nursed in a supine position, with the shoulder abducted at 90°, elbow flexed at 90° and the digits held towards the ceiling. In lower-limb casting, the child is positioned sitting up for a below-knee plaster of Paris, and supine for a full-length or cylinder plaster; a footrest may be used to maintain the ankle in a neutral position during application

As this procedure is likely to be performed in a plaster room, the environment of care should be suitably child orientated. Such rooms are normally bleak places, so mobile equipment such as Starlight's distraction boxes (www.starlight.org) should be used. Parents should be offered suitable protective clothing and plastic overshoes. Plaster of Paris and expensive modern shoes are not compatible!

During the procedure

Application of plaster of Paris

- Apply a stockinette for comfort, and to protect the skin of the child from the sharp edges of the plaster. It needs to be measured and cut a little longer than the plaster and then rolled up and applied to the limb. It is important to note that the application of stockinette is contraindicated if there is likelihood of swelling, as it may create a tourniquet effect and cause constriction
- Protect bony prominences with a layer of Softband. Apply a layer of Softband smoothly and evenly over the stockinette. The width of padding is usually 10–15 cm for legs and 5–10 cm for arms but depends on the age of the child. Apply the padding by rolling distally to proximally, tearing it off to go around joints
- Select an appropriate-sized plaster for casting: 8–10 cm for upper limbs and 10–15 cm for lower limbs (also age- dependent). Prepare the plaster roll by unrolling the first 5–8 cm then, keeping hold of the end, immerse it into the container of lukewarm water (20–25°C) until the bubbles stop. Cold water retards the setting process while warm water quickens it. With one end of the role in each hand, gently squeeze to get rid of excess water
- Begin bandaging at one end of the cast, rolling away from its applicator. Applied it evenly, covering about one-third of the previous turn
- During application, use the palms of the hands and palmar eminences, rather than the fingertips, to constantly smooth and mould, in order to fuse the bandages into one. It is important to maintain the limb position throughout the application, to which end an additional nurse may be required to assist
- After application, rest the limb on a pillow to prevent the cast from denting (plastic or rubber pillows should not be used as they trap heat under the cast, preventing heat dissipation and prolonging drying). Where necessary, trim the edges of the cast and turn back the proximal and distal ends of the stockinette over the cast edges, making a neat finish to prevent discomfort or injury

Application of fibreglass cast

- Fibreglass casts are becoming increasingly popular because they are durable, lightweight and waterproof. However, fibreglass is difficult to mould and significantly more expensive than plaster of Paris, and is less used for acute injury, because frequent cast changes are required
- The patient preparation and the procedure are as for the application of plaster of Paris, except that wearing gloves is mandatory for handling the fibreglass material (a nylon stockinette and padding should be used), and the roll of casting should be opened immediately before using
- Fibreglass material must be applied with a little more pressure than plaster of Paris, and it conforms more easily if applied spirally, squaring the upper and lower ends by making horizontal turns
- Apply the cast so as to decrease the amount of trimming needed because fibreglass casts cannot be cut by a cast knife or scissors

- After application, the cast takes approximately 7 minutes to dry by the open-air drying method, and weight bearing is only allowed after 20 minutes

Post-procedure

- Elevate as appropriate, especially if swelling is anticipated. Elevating the limb will help prevent excessive swelling and may prevent the need for bi-valving
- Allow to dry naturally at room temperature and leave uncovered for 48 hours. Be careful not to put excessive pressure on the cast with your fingers at the drying stage as indentations can result in development of unnecessary plaster sores. This is especially so for hip spicas where the child's position has to be changed every 2 hours to prevent pressure sores. When nursing children in hip spicas prone to supine you will need to adjust the pillows and foam blocks to accommodate the shape of the spica, especially if the knee in plaster is flexed. Drying times will vary and depend on the thickness of the plaster cast. As a rule, for regular, non-weight-bearing plaster casts the drying time is 24 hours (note that for weight-bearing plaster casts the drying time is at least 48 hours). The child is allowed to bear weight after an X-ray shows reduction and immobilisation of the fracture but normally tibial fractures will require a minimum of 2 weeks of non-weight bearing
- Exercise joints that are not encased in plaster
- In consultation with medical staff, clarify whether the child is allowed to bear weight on the cast. If cast edges become rough, cover the rough ends with tape. Wash the skin area around the cast but taking care not to wet it
- Hip spicas and other body casts, especially in very young children, will need to be protected from urine and excrement. Waterproof sleek tape can be used around all the edges. The smell of these plasters can become very unpleasant and therefore the area around the groin requires strict hygiene
- Monitor for cracking, denting or softening of the cast, swelling, discoloration, soreness, unpleasant smells, discharges and undue or increasing pain, and report to medical staff. Note that when a child is discharged in a cast, full care instructions must be given to the family, as well as a telephone number of someone to contact for advice. Some units adhere the instructions to the cast itself
- If the cast has been applied over a wound – for example after an open reduction or surgery – the cast should be monitored for blood loss. This can be achieved by drawing a felt-tip line around the discoloration to determine further and excessive blood loss

It is vital to undertake neurovascular observations as part of a neurovascular assessment and you should monitor for numbness or pins and needles, cyanosis or discoloration of the toes or fingers. Feel the extremities with your own fingers and check for warmth or coldness. Ascertain that the child can wiggle his or her fingers or toes and in the case, for example, of supracondylar fractures of the humerus, check the integrity of the radial pulse. Compartment syndrome is still a worrying complication of limb fractures. Always carry out neurovascular assessment to prevent a child from developing a potential life-long disability. The five P's of neurovascular assessment are shown below.

The five P's of neurovascular assessment (Andrews, 1990)

Pain
Pallor
Paraesthesia
Pulselessness
Paralysis

Pain and pallor are *early* indicators of damage
Paraesthesia, pulselessness and paralysis are *late* signs of damage.

Always carry out neurovascular assessment to prevent a child from developing a potential life-long disability.

General cast rules

- Fingers and toes need to be exercised
- Limbs must be kept elevated when resting
- The plaster must not get wet
- No pencils or knitting needles are to be used for scratching ('nothing smaller than an elbow' should be put down a cast!)
- A child in plaster should not be placed next to any heating element such as an electric fire or radiator – the risk of burns is high

Removing a plaster cast

Although plaster casts can be removed with plaster shears it is customary to use an oscillating saw which emits fluctuating levels of high frequency noise and can cause a vibration sensation in the bone. Some children find this very uncomfortable. In fact, children can find the whole process frightening, so the nurse should take steps to prepare the family for the procedure. Anxiety reactions can be partially mitigated by the use of ear protectors (Katz *et al*, 2001).

Student skill laboratory activity

✓ Identify the equipment required for the application of a plaster cast
✓ Practice applying a plaster cast on a suitable mannequin

Skin closure

Skin closure is the alignment and bringing together of skin edges to facilitate optimal healing. Skin closure comprises a number of methods: suturing, stapling, glueing, hair tying and the use of adhesive closure strips. The method of skin closure depends on the nature of the wound.

Sutures

Suture material is either absorbable or non-absorbable. Absorbable sutures such as surgical gut (catgut) or vicryl take around 4 weeks to dissolve, thus are most useful for internal and deeper wounds (Cole, 2003). Non-absorbable sutures such as nylon, polypropylene or silk are most suitable for wounds of the dermis and epidermis. Suture thickness is measured by gauge, with 6.0 being the smallest and 3.0 the thickest. When used for skin closure, non-absorbables must be removed or they will lead to infection.

Glueing

Glue is often used as an alternative to suturing for simple, dry lacerations. It works through polymerisation and achieves a good cosmetic result (Farion, 2003). Charters (2000) identified glue as most successful on scalp lacerations.

Adhesive closure strips

These are available in a wide variety of lengths and widths. They can be used in conjunction with staples and sutures to provide additional support. Used on their own, adhesive closure strips do not require local anaesthetic for application. They are most commonly used for simple, superficial lacerations. Adhesive closure strips cannot be used for deep wounds or be applied to hairy, oily skin surfaces (Gottrup, 1999).

Hair-tying

This closure method is only suitable for simple scalp lacerations that are not actively bleeding. Hair ties or the hair apposition technique (HAT) has been described by Hock *et al*, (2002) who conclude that the technique can be used in simple lacerations of the scalp, where hair on both sides of the laceration are apposed with a single twist and secured with tissue adhesive, and is an acceptable alternative to other methods of skin closure. Clearly hair is important and children with hair length of less than 3 cm will not make suitable candidates for this procedure.

Reasons for the procedure

- To support the damaged tissues while healing occurs
- To minimise the risk of developing a localised infection and reduce the risk of future bleeding
- To provide a visually aesthetic result

Pre-procedure

Equipment required

- Appropriate closure equipment
- 0.9% normal saline (warmed)
- 50 mL syringe
- 19 G needle
- Dressing pack
- Additional dressings to cover wound as required
- Gloves
- Goggles (or other protective eye equipment)
- Lidocaine hydrochloride
- Sterile forceps
- Sharps bin

Specific patient preparation

- Undertake a comprehensive wound assessment (*Box 11.1*) to identify the skin closure method to be used and the material required
- The wound should be appropriately cleansed and debrided if required. To remove the debris from the wound, high-pressure irrigation using a 50-mL syringe and a 19-G needle is most effective (Richardson, 2004). This provides 4–15 p.s.i. (pounds per square inch) and safely removes contamination from the wound without causing further damage (Bergstrom, 1994). The wound should be infiltrated with a prescribed local anaesthetic, such as lidocaine hydrochloride (British Medical Association and Royal Pharmaceutical Society of Great Britain, 2003)

Box 11.1: Factors to be considered in a wound assessment

Establishing cause of the injury/wound
Duration of the wound
Depth of the wound
Site of the wound
Tissue type involved
Presence of infection
Pain
Measuring the wound
The wound edge
Condition of the surrounding skin

During the procedure

Adhesive closure strips

- The correctly sized closure strips are selected for the wound – the strip must cover the diameter of the wound and have a clean and dry area at either side for it to securely adhere to. Strips are available in 3 mm, 6 mm and 12 mm sizes
- Starting at the middle of the wound, the first closure strip is applied by apposing the wound edges together. This can either be achieved by using forceps or a sterile, gloved finger, depending on where the wound is located
- Starting in the middle and applying other strips towards the outward edge of the wound will maintain skin position and prevent the wound healing in a displaced manner. Careful wound-edge alignment will ensure a good cosmetic result
- The strips should ideally be 3 mm apart (Richardson, 2003) to allow draining of any exudates or bleeding

Suturing

- Nurses should not attempt to suture unless they are competent to do so
- Facial wounds in children require particular consideration and should be carefully assessed before being managed by a highly competent nurse or doctor
- The suture needle is held in a pair Spencer Wells forceps and is inserted about 5 mm from one skin edge, which is itself held and supported with more forceps. The suture is pulled through into the open wound
- The needle is next inserted separately through the open wound and should exit through the skin on the opposite side of the wound, about 5 mm from the edge
- Skin edges should be slightly elevated during this procedure to aid wound healing. The suture is knotted on one side of the wound line. If sutures are tied too tightly, tissues can become damaged; sutures that are tied too loosely fail to hold tissues in adequate apposition and may result in delayed healing and in scar lines that are cosmetically unacceptable

Hair-tying

- This involves taking hair from both sides of a scalp wound and tying it across the wound to achieve tissue apposition. It can be achieved through a series of evenly spaced hair knots for a secure closure line. The knots can be further fixed with tissue adhesive. Aoki (1996) reinforces the value of this technique which preserves the hair by avoiding shaving (particularly useful where children may have concerns about their body image)
  - After cleaning, select 10–20 hairs on each side of the wound tie them to their opposite number using the suture technique. Although the hair suture knots can be reinforced with glue this is not always necessary
  - After 5–7 days the knots can be untied after wetting the hair with an antiseptic lotion (but if left will grow out)

Glueing

- After cleaning the wound (making sure in the case of the scalp that the child's own hair is not embedded in the wound) appose the wound edges
- The glue vial is squeezed gently either to spread a thin line of adhesive along the length of both sides of the wound or to 'spot weld' the wound closed by applying a series of dots along its length. Be careful not to squeeze glue into the wound itself and avoid the embarrassment of glueing yourself to the child (Charters, 2006)
- The wound needs to be held together for 30 seconds to allow polymerisation

Post-procedure

- Dispose of equipment as per local policy
- Correct documentation of the closure procedure
- Ascertain the patient's tetanus status in accordance with the Department of Health (2002) recommendations for immunisations
- Apply additional dressing if required

Student skill laboratory activity

✓ Assemble the equipment needed for skin closure and practice skin closure on appropriate mannequin

Removal of skin closure material

The main principle behind suture removal is to ensure that no part of the suture that is visible above the skin should be drawn underneath the skin. This prevents infection developing in the healing wound tissue (Workman and Bennett, 2003). The principle behind all wound closure material is to hold the wound edges in apposition to promote effective and timely wound healing, to produce minimal scar tissue, and to prevent wound infection. Sutures are removed after 3–10 days depending on the site and type of the wound (Wyatt, 2003). Adhesive closure strips can remain in place for 5–7 days for simple lacerations (Cole, 2003). If strips lose their adhesiveness before the wound-healing process is complete, more strips can be applied over the top of the existing strips to secure the wound for a longer period of time. When ready, they are simply removed by peeling off alternate strips from the wound – warmed 0.9% sodium chloride solution may reduce their adhesiveness. Hair ties do not need to be removed unless they cause irritation; otherwise they will grow out as the surrounding hair grows.

Reasons for the procedure

- To remove dressings because the wound has healed
- To prevent further complications (delayed removal causes the body to respond as though a foreign object remains within the scar tissue, which may result in further scarring)

Pre-procedure

Equipment required

- As for aseptic technique including sterile dressing pack with forceps and gloves
- Sterile stitch cutter, or sterile scissors, according to the wound closure material
- Normal saline
- Suitable dressing if necessary
- Sharps container

Specific patient preparation

- Establish whether all or interrupted sutures are to be removed
- Discuss with the child and parents what is going to happen
- Show the child on a doll what you are going to do (involve the play specialist when necessary to provide distraction)
- Position the child to expose the wound site If dressings are present, loosen and remove following standard precautions
- Examine the wound and skin integrity before removing the sutures. The wound should show signs of healing. Excessive wound inflammation or discharge should be reported to the nurse in charge before proceeding, as a wound swab may be required and only alternative sutures removed on this occasion
- Establish the number of sutures to be removed
- When removing any type of wound-closure device, inform the child that they may feel slight discomfort, such as a pulling or stinging sensation
- Moisten dried crusts with warmed 0.9% sodium chloride solution, wearing clean gloves

During the procedure

Individual or interrupted sutures

- Hold the knot with sterile forceps and slightly lift it away from the surface of the skin
- Slide the stitch cutter or scissor tips under the suture opposite to the knot, as close to the skin surface as possible, and cut the suture here (*Figure 11.1*)
- Using the forceps pull the suture upwards from the knot end

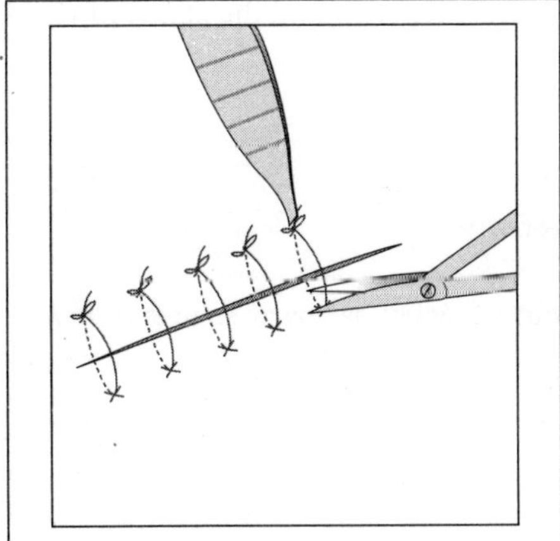

Figure 11.1: Individual or interrupted suture removal

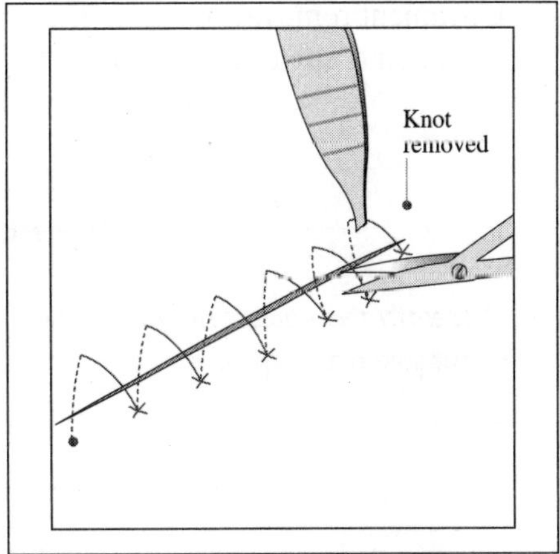

Figure 11.2: Continuous suture line removal

- Use the tips of the scissors held slightly apart or the edge of the blade cutter to gently press on the skin when the suture is drawn out, to ease its withdrawal and lessen the resistance from the skin
- Place removed sutures on some gauze - if the wound is longer than 15 cm, remove alternate sutures first to determine wound integrity. If healing has taken place sufficiently then all the sutures can be removed (Nicol *et al,* 2003; Workman and Bennett, 2003)
- Count and discard the sutures
- If necessary, clean the wound site with normal saline and place a suitable dressing over the suture line if the patient wishes, for his or her comfort (Workman and Bennett, 2003).

Continuous suture line

- Cut the first suture at the end furthest from the knot
- Use the forceps to lift the next suture and loosen it from the skin. It is imperative that only one end of the suture is cut to ensure complete removal of the entire suture (*Figure 11.2*)
- The exposed part of the suture should not be pulled through the tissues
- Repeat this process along the suture line, until all portions have been removed
- If any part of the wound edge appears to be gaping, skin-closure strips can be applied to assist the healing process
- A suitable dressing may be applied and the wound site cleaned as necessary

Post-procedure

- Dispose of equipment as appropriate, ensuring that sharp objects such as stitch cutters are disposed of in the sharps bin

- Document removal of suture material in the nursing records, reporting on the status of the wound and any changes to the planned intervention

Student skill laboratory activity

✓ Identify the equipment you would require to remove sutures. Practice removing sutures form a suitable mannequin.

Traction

Traction means the drawing of an injured or diseased part of the body along a plane. In order to pull an object in one direction and therefore efficiently treat the disease or fracture, there must be an equal force or counterthrust in the opposite direction. This is known as counter traction. There are two main ways to apply traction – fixed and sliding.

Methods of traction

Fixed traction

Fixed traction is illustrated in *Figure 11.3*. This is the traction between two fixed points, as in a traditional Thomas' splint. The two fixed points in this case are the force applied to the pull of the extension cords tied to the end of the splint, and the force that is transmitted along the parallel bars pushing against the ischial tuberosity.

Sliding traction

This is also known as balanced traction and is shown in *Figure 11.4*. In sliding traction there must be two opposing forces, this time balanced and each of comparable weight. In sliding traction, the bed is tilted so that the child tends to slide or move in the opposite direction to that of the traction force. The balance is the traction from the limb by the weights, and the counter traction is the patient's own weight sliding in the opposite direction.

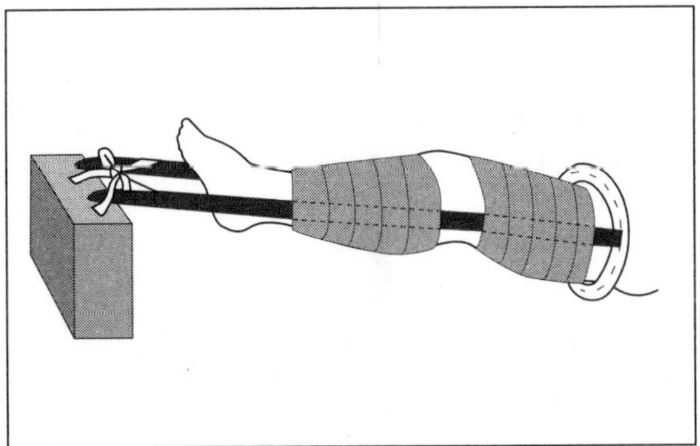

Figure 11.3: :A fixed traction

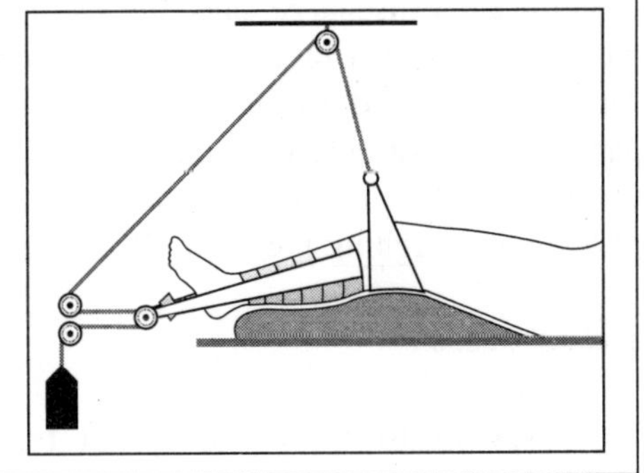

Figure 11.4: :A sliding traction

Types of traction used in childhood disorders

Four types of traction are used in childhood disorders (Silverwood, 2006).

Simple skin traction (Pugh's traction)

Pugh's traction is frequently used to reduce pain or muscle spasm in children with leg or hip problems prior to surgery or more permanent fixation. Weights are attached to the extension tapes of either the adhesive or non-adhesive foam extension strips via a swan-neck traction pulley at the end of the bed. Care must be taken to keep the securing bandages loose enough to prevent swelling and allow good circulation to the part of the limb beyond the spot where the traction is applied. Only a moderate amount of pull can be exerted using skin traction because excessive weight applied to the skin surface can cause serious skin irritation, thus rendering the treatment useless. (Doman, 2006)

Thomas splint traction

This splint was invented by Hugh Owen Thomas, a bone setter in Liverpool in the late nineteenth century. Originally used to treat hip disorders, it is now universally used in the initial treatment of fractures of the femoral shaft. In children, the Thomas splint can utilise either a fixed traction method or a sliding traction method as a temporary measure prior to the use of internal or external fixation (which allows earlier discharge).

Gallows traction

This special type of fixed traction is appropriate for very young children with fractured femurs (*Figure 11.5*). It uses the child's own body weight to maintain traction, with the legs suspended and attached by skin traction to a Balkan beam fixed to the child's cot. It is important to stress that the child's bottom should be raised off the bed surface to allow maximum traction. To promote early discharge, once the swelling has subsided, the child is placed in a hip spica (broomstick variety). This will depend on home circumstances as some parents may not able to manage a child in a hip spica. Gallows traction is only used in children under 2 years of age and weighing not more than 16 kg.

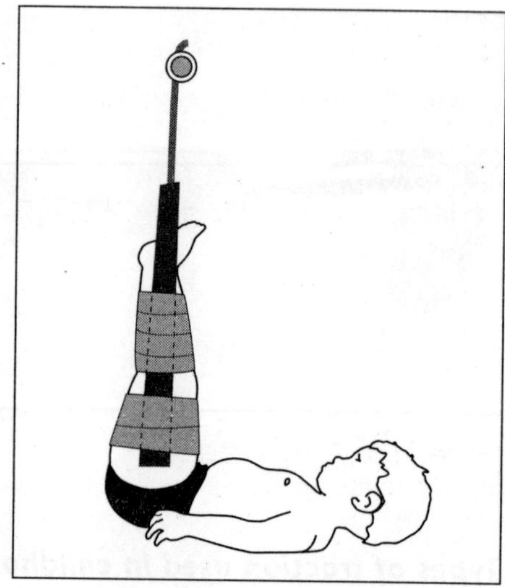

Figure 11.5: A gallows traction

Skeletal traction

This type of traction is now not regularly used in children because surgical interventions have improved greatly, allowing internal fixation of fractures and thus early discharge. Skeletal traction is sometimes used to treat fractures of the femur that are difficult to align, for example, or where there has been skin damage. It may be used in conjunction with a Thomas splint and Pearson's flexion knee piece. Although rare, when this is advocated a sterile metal pin is inserted through an area of strong bone such as the tibial tuberosity. Traction by means of weights is then applied to the pin via a stirrup which is clamped to the ends of the pin. The traction cords are then allowed to run through a pulley at the foot of the elevated Balkan beam bed-end where the weights hang free.

Applying simple skin traction (Pugh's traction)

Reasons for the procedure

- To reduce dislocation or fracture
- To prevent movement of the injured part, thus facilitating bone healing
- To reduce and overcome muscle spasm
- To prevent and correct deformity
- To rest joints (eg. irritable hip)
- To allow healing in the optimum position

Pre-procedure

Equipment required

- Non-adhesive traction kit
- Bandages
- Swan-neck

Specific patient preparation

- Ascertain the need for either an adhesive or non-adhesive traction kit or appropriate bandages
- Prepare the bed with appropriate Balkan beam bed frame and pulleys, swan-neck and weights as prescribed. Some hospitals have special beds and cots with orthopaedic frames already attached
- Provide appropriate information to the child and family members using a variety of methods
- Involve a play specialist to provide distraction/pre-procedural play when required

During the procedure

- Ascertain the integrity of the child's skin
- Check allergy status of the child with the parent/guardian
- Administer prescribed analgesia where necessary
- Measure the traction extensions against the unaffected limb to avoid causing pain making sure that you have left enough space to allow the child to plantar flex the foot without restriction when the spreader bar is inserted. Cut off the excess material with scissors
- Starting at the malleolus of the foot apply the extensions to the medial and lateral aspects of the leg. Keep the extensions straight to prevent medial or lateral rotation of the limb and to ensure that the malleoli are covered by the foam padding. If you are using adhesive extensions, peel back the adhesive covering slowly to enable you to apply the material to the skin without causing wrinkles, which in turn could damage the child's skin integrity
- Apply bandage (not too tightly) starting just above the malleoli. Leave the knee free
- Take the traction cords at the spreader and pass through the pulley over the swan neck and attach securely to the prescribed weights
- Elevate the foot of the bed to provide the counter traction ensuring that the child does not slide down the bed too much
- Ensure neurovascular observations are recorded

Post-procedure

- Bandages should be checked and only renewed as appropriate, but 4-hourly observations of neurovascular function should be recorded
- Nutrition may find be difficult as the child is in bed. The nurse in consultation with the family should devise a suitable diet of small frequent, easily digested meals with plenty of fibre and fluids. A fluid balance chart should be kept until the child has resumed a normal pattern of eating and drinking
- The child will find it difficult to adapt to their new position and confinement to bed so nurses have developed a number of strategies to help, and will involve parents in the management of elimination (because some children may be discharged home in a hip spica

(Holmes *et al*, 1983; Clayton, 1997). Eaton (2000) stresses the importance of involving children's community nurses when sick children are transferred between healthcare boundaries and nurses must assess the ability of parents to manage a child in traction or plaster at home

Applying a Thomas splint

Reasons for the procedure

- *As for simple traction (Pugh's) above*

Pre-procedure

Equipment required

- Suitable bed with Balkan beam to use with various types of traction and a Thomas splint (modern splints can be used on either leg and are fully adjustable with half rings secured with Velcro (*Box 11.2*)
- Skin preparation material as required
- Skin extension (or rarely pin holder for skeletal traction)
- Ready-made foam slings which come in different sizes and are disposable and have Velcro fastenings
- Crepe bandages and adhesive strapping
- Scissors
- Possible Pearson knee flexion piece (rare)
- Traction cord
- Pulleys as required
- Prescribed weights
- Suspension system

Specific patient preparation

- Shaving as necessary (in older children)
- Position and alignment
- Pain relief
- Clean the skin around the ring of the Thomas' splint
- Expose the affected limb and remove clothing

During the procedure

- Prepare the splint by using the foam slings to create a cradle along the length of the Thomas' splint for supporting the limb
- Depending on the fracture, the splint may be positioned to create 5° of knee flexion by placing additional padding in the knee region. If more than 5° of knee flexion is required, a Pearson knee flexion piece may be attached to the parallel bars of the splint.
- Apply the skin (or skeletal) traction and pass the prepared splint over the limb
- Push the splint up to the groin and adjust the tension of the slings to maintain normal bowing of the femur
- When used with as a fixed traction method at the w-shaped distal end of the splint, the skin extension cords are tied to the end of the splint with sufficient force to prevent the ring from embedding in the groin (Stewart and Hallett, 1983). When the splint, as is customary, is used with sliding traction the cords are passed over a pulley on the bed frame. In this way the traction is achieved by the pull on the extension, and the foot of the bed is elevated for counter traction. After application of the traction, the suspension system is set up to facilitate the mobility of the patient while being maintained on the Thomas' splint
- Apply crepe bandages above and below the knee to keep the extensions in place over the limb and secure them with adhesive strapping

Post-procedure

- Prevent undue pressure in the popliteal space by ensuring that the slings art and remain crease-free and if used as fixed traction ensure the pillow on which the splint rests is not hard
- Although in contemporary UK practice the use of a Thomas' splint is usually a temporary measure, children will still need to be taught to lift their buttocks off the bed frequently by using the overhead trapeze and their unaffected leg, so as to reduce risk of sacral tissue damage. Foot exercises must be encouraged regularly to the affected foot to maintain strength and prevent foot drop
- The knee should be left exposed
- Ensure good skin care, nutrition and manage elimination (as above)
- Liaise with the physiotherapist regarding exercise education

Applying gallows traction

Reasons for the procedure

- *As for simple traction (Pugh's) above*

Pre-procedure

Equipment required

- Normally gallows traction is used with adhesive extensions, but a non-adhesive traction kit may be prescribed if there are skin problems (Note: All children under a year of age presenting with a femoral fracture are screened under hospital safeguarding policies)
- Prepare the bed with an appropriate Balkan beam bed frame and pulleys where necessary

Specific patient preparation

- Provide appropriate information to the child and family members using a variety of methods
- Involve a play specialist to provide distraction/pre-procedural play when required
- Ascertain the integrity of the skin. Check allergy status of the child with the parent or guardian
- Administer prescribed analgesia where necessary

During the procedure

- Measure the traction extensions against the unaffected limb to avoid causing pain, making sure that you have left enough space to allow the child to plantar flex the foot without restriction when the spreader bar is inserted. Cut off the excess material with scissors
- Starting at the malleoli of the foot, apply the extensions to the medial and lateral aspects of the leg. Keep the extensions straight to prevent medial or lateral rotation of the limb and to ensure that the malleoli are covered by the foam padding. If you are using adhesive extensions peel back the adhesive covering slowly to enable you to apply the material to the skin without causing wrinkles, which in turn could damage the child's skin integrity
- Apply bandage (not too tightly) starting just above the malleoli. Leave the knee free
- Take the traction cords at the spreader and tie them to the beam above or thread the cords through the pulleys on the Balkan beam bed frame and attach to the prescribed weights
- To provide counter traction ensure that the child's buttocks are one flat handbreadth off the surface of the mattress
- Ensure that the counter traction is only maintained by the 'flat of the hand' principle as too little counter traction can cause pain from muscle spasm and may result in mal-union of the bone. Too much counter traction, as with tight bandages, may cause neurovascular impairment
- Ensure neurovascular observations are recorded

Post-procedure

> *Please note that although children adapt very well to being suspended in mid-air they do initially find the experience strange and frightening. The use of the play specialist in providing distraction at the outset is crucial, as is the partnership with the parents during and after the procedure. Children in gallows traction may become quite disruptive and fractious if not occupied and may become entangled in their traction cords if they try to spin around. The play specialist can proactively prevent or modify such behaviour by providing high-quality play materials and visual distractions with, for example, a film on DVD. These children also need considerable help in undertaking the activities of daily living (Silverwood, 2006).*

In particular skin care, elimination and nutrition are all important when nursing a child in gallows traction:

- Bandages should be checked and only renewed as appropriate, but 4-hourly observations of neurovascular function should be recorded
- Nutrition is problematic as children in Gallows traction are flat with their legs in the air. The nurse in consultation with the family should devise a suitable diet comprising small, frequent, easily digested meals with plenty of fibre and fluids. Young children in Gallows should be supervised during meal times as the danger of inhalation and choking is always present. Given the emphasis on fluids and nutrition, a fluid balance chart should be kept until the child has resumed a normal pattern of eating and drinking
- Elimination causes problems because the child in gallows traction may find it difficult to adapt to their new position and confinement to bed. Children's nurses have developed a number of strategies to help. They also need to involve parents in the management of elimination because some children may be discharged home in Gallows traction, although a hip spica is usually applied (Holmes *et al,* 1983; Clayton, 1997). Eaton (2000) stresses the importance of involving children's community nurses when sick children are transferred between healthcare boundaries and nurses must assess the ability of parents to manage a child in traction at home

External fixation and pin-site care

The use of external fixation in children is well established but the management of the skeletal pin-site skin care is subject to continuing debate (Williams and Griffiths, 2004). The presence of a pin through a bone and skin is always a potential source of infection and as the skin cannot heal around the pin-site exit it is necessary to ensure that the infection risk is minimised. Davies *et al* (2005) have described a prospective study in which patients were monitored for infection rates using two pin-site care methods. They used open and closed methods of covering the exit wounds. Although not a randomised controlled trial the study showed no significant differences in infection rates between the two groups. A sample pin-site protocol adapted from the Bristol Children's Hospital protocol is shown in *Box 11.2*.

> *Always refer to you own hospital procedure guidelines for instructions on how to undertake pin-site care.*

Box 11.2: Sample pin-site protocol

The primary aim of pin-site care is to prevent infection of the bone. Osteomyelitis is greatly feared by healthcare professionals and all steps should be taken to prevent this bone infection.

What you will need

One dressing pack

Extra packets of sterile sponge sticks

A sheet of soft-hold foam dressing

Pink chlorhexidene 0.5% or normal saline

Sterile scissors

Alcohol hand-rub

Method of pin-site dressing

Wash your hands as normal and use hospital alcohol hand-rub afterwards

Open dressing pack and set out equipment using forceps

Pour cleaning solution into the plastic receptacle

Cut foam sheets into squares about 3 cm by 3 cm.

Make keyhole dressings out of the squares by using the sterile scissors to make a 1.5 cm cut as if making a pair of shorts

Push the plastic clips up the wire or pin. These can be removed and cleaned and replaced over the new dressings

Remove the old dressings and discard in the bag provided

Wash your hands again with the alcohol rub

Clean the pin sites individually using the sponge sticks dipped into the cleaning solution, remembering to clean in one direction only but using all sides of the stick

Make sure that the skin can move freely around the pin and where necessary remove crusts with the forceps

Ensure all sites are dry – where necessary use dry gauze

Wash your hands again with alcohol rub

Cover the pin sites with at least two layers of foam dressing – with some pin sites you may need to use three or four layers. Remember to ensure that the keyhole slits in the dressings are all opposed

Push down the plastic clips and again make sure that the slit of the clip is in a different direction to the slit in the top layer dressing. Do not press the clips down too hard – they are to hold the dressing in place, not to cause a pressure sore

Dispose of the dressing pack in the normal way

Changing pin-site dressings

Dressings should be changed every 7 days unless there is:

– pain or purulent discharge from around the pin site

– any other sign of infection

References

Andrews LW (1990) Neurovascular assessment. *Adv Clin Care* **6**(6): 5–7

Aoki N (1996) Hair braiding for superficial wounds. *Surg Neurol* **46**(2): 150–51

Bergstrom N (1994) *Treatment of Pressure Ulcers*. Department of Health Care Policy Research, Nebraska

British Medical Association and Royal Pharmaceutical Society of Great Britain (2003) *British National Formulary 5*. BMA/RPSGB, London

Callam MJ, Harper DR, Dale JJ, Ruckley CV (1987) Arterial disease in chronic leg ulceration: an underestimated hazard. Lothian and Firth Valley Leg Ulcer Study. *BMJ* **294:** 929–31

Carter M (2001) From open air to high tech care: orthopaedic nursing at Oswestry 1921–2000. *Orthopaed Nurs* **20**(5): 13–16

Charters A (2000) Wound glue: a comparative study of tissue adhesives. *Accid Emerg Nurs* **8:** 223–27

Charters A (2006) Glueing wounds. In: Glasper EA, McEwing G, Richardson J, eds. *Oxford Handbook of Children's and Young Peoples Nursing*. Oxford University Press, Oxford

Clayton M (1997) Traction at home. The Doncaster approach. *Paediatr Nurs* **9**(2): 21–23

Cole E (2003) Wound management in A&E department. *Nurs Stand* **17**(46): 45–52

Davies R, Holt N, Nayagam S (2005) The care of pin sites with external fixation. *J Bone Joint Surg* **87-B**(5): 716–19

Department of Health (2002) *The Green Book: Immunisation Against Infectious Disease*. Department of Health, London

Doman M (2006) Skin traction: application and care (principles). In: Glasper EA, McEwing G, Richardson J, eds. *Oxford Handbook of Children's and Young Peoples Nursing*. Oxford University Press, Oxford

Eaton N (2000) Children's community nursing services: models of care delivery. A review of the United Kingdom literature. *J Adv Nurs* **3291:** 49–56

Farion K (2003) Tissue adhesives for traumatic lacerations: a systematic review of randomised controlled trials. *Acad Emerg Med* **10**(2): 110–18

Gottrup F (1999) Wound closure technique. *J Wound Care* **8:** 397–400

Hock MO, Ooi SB, Saw SM, Lim SH (2002) A randomised controlled trial comparing the hair apposition technique with tissue glue to standard suturing in scalp lacerations (HAT study). *Annals Emerg Med* **40**(1): 19–26

Holmes SJK, Sedgewick DM, Scobie WG (1983) Domiciliary gallows traction for femoral shaft fractures in young children. Feasibility safety and advantages. *J Bone Joint Surg* **65**(3): 288–290

Katz K, Fogeleman R, Attias J, Baron E, Soudry M (2001) Anxiety reaction in children during removal of their plaster cast with a saw. *J Bone Joint Surg* **83:** 388–90

Nicol M, Bavin C, Bedford-Turner S, Cronin P, Rawlings-Workman BA, Bennett CL (2003) *Key Nursing Skills*. Whurr Publishers, London

Richardson M (2003) Wound closure. *Emerg Nurse* **11**(3): 25–32

Richardson M (2004) Procedures for cleansing, closing and covering acute wounds. *Nurs Times* **100**(4): 54–59

Silverwood B (2006) Caring for children with orthopeadic disorders. In: L Glasper A, J Richardson, eds. *A Textbook of Children's and Young Peoples' Nursing*. Churchill Livingstone, Edinburgh

Stewart JDM, Hallett JP (1983) *Traction and Orthopaedic Appliances,* 2nd edn. Churchill Livingstone, London

Williams H, Griffiths P (2004) The effectiveness of pin-site care for patients with external fixators. *Br J Commun Nurs* **9**(4): 206–10

Workman BA, Bennett CL (2003) *Key Nursing Skills.* Whurr Publishers, London

Wyatt JP (2003) *Oxford Handbook of Accident and Emergency Medicine*. Oxford University Press, Oxford

Chapter 12

Fundamental aspects of skin care

Di Keeton

The skin is a multifunctional organ capable of fulfilling multiple roles. It is the largest organ of the body and plays an important role in both physical and psychological overall health. It is tough enough to act as a shield against injury, yet supple enough to permit movement. The external appearance of the skin is very important to how an individual feels about himself or herself. It tells stories to the outside world and can dictate how the individual is accepted and treated by outsiders. It is well documented that skin conditions such as eczema can cause considerable distress and disruption, not only to the day-to-day life of the sufferer, but also to other family members and family life in general (Lawson *et al,* 1998).

Skin functions

Barrier

Skin protects the body from the outside world and holds us together. It repels water and keeps out micro-organisms that could cause harm. It is naturally slightly acidic, helping to reduce the number of bacteria that live on the skin while protecting the normal bacteria that are essential for healthy skin to function. Skin is able to repair itself. It has special cells, the melanocytes, that produce melanin and afford some protection from ultraviolet radiation from the sun. When disease or external events alter this balance, the barrier function of the skin and the health of the individual is compromised.

Temperature regulation

The skin helps to control and regulate body temperature. Blood vessels in the dermis vasoconstrict in the cold to conserve heat and vasodilate in the heat to encourage heat loss. Sweating also helps because its evaporation from the skin surface aids cooling.

Sensation

There are millions of nerve endings in the skin that allow us to enjoy the sensation of touch as well as experience pain and itch.

Immunological

The dermis layer holds a number of immunological cells (Langerhans and mast cells) which go into action when a foreign body breaches the skin surface. This is a positive response to handling foreign proteins and it protects the body. However, in conditions such as eczema and psoriasis it is thought that these responses are triggered unnecessarily, in that the response is against itself, resulting in chronic disease.

Biochemical reactions

The skin has an important role in vitamin D metabolism which is vital for the natural absorption of calcium and phosphate, necessary for healthy bone structure.

Skin structure

Human skin is composed of three layers:

- Epidermis
- Dermis
- Subcutaneous tissue fat layer

The *epidermis* is the almost waterproof outer layer that acts as a barrier, and includes the 'dead layer' or stratum corneum, which contains special oils that prevent the evaporation of water. The ongoing cycle of growing and shedding of dead cells takes approximately 52–75 days (but can be quicker in some skin diseases such as eczema). The *dermis* is a connective tissue layer consisting mainly of collagen and blood vessels, mast cells, hair follicles, nerve cells, and provides nutritional and physical support to the epidermis. The skin on the face is 0.12 mm (thinnest on lips and round eyes) and on the body is 0.6 mm (palms and soles 1.2– 4.7 mm). Skin thickness, sensitivity and condition should be taken into account when choosing and applying topical treatments.

Eczema

Atopic dermatitis or eczema is a chronic skin disorder. It can be intensely dry, itchy, erythematous and inflamed and can affect any part of the body, especially the flexures and creases (Williams *et al,* 1994). The intense itching can be very distressing, causing some children to scratch themselves to bleeding point. The more they scratch the more they itch, resulting in sleepless nights and raw bleeding skin.

Current pharmacological treatments, including emollients and topical steroids, are largely effective. Emollients are the mainstay of controlling the symptoms of eczema. However, the effects of emollients are short-lived, so the frequency of use and how they are applied to the skin is pivotal to their effectiveness.

Application of emollients

Emollients are the mainstay of controlling eczema. They help to repair the skin's natural barrier function by gently cleansing the skin and providing a protective layer that reduces moisture loss and hydrates and moisturises the skin. They are available as lotions, gels, creams, ointments and pastes, and the type used depend on the age of the child and the site and severity of the eczema, as well as patient preference.

Reasons for the procedure

- To hydrate and soothe skin affected by eczema
- To improve lichenification (thickening) of the skin
- To reduce the itch
- To reduction the need for topical steroids
- To improve quality of life for the child and whole family
- To demonstrate the correct method of topical therapy for maximum effectiveness

Pre-procedure

Equipment required

- Prescribed emollients
- Spatula and dish (if emollient not in pump dispenser)
- Non-sterile gloves
- Clean towel or sheet
- Access to sink
- Protective clothing if required (such as tubular garments or bandages)

Specific patient preparation

- The environment should be warm and provide appropriate privacy
- Give a full explanation, appropriate to the child's age, with full rationale of proposed treatment
- To maximise the hydration effect, emollient should be applied to clean skin immediately (5–10 minutes) after daily bathing/washing with a bath emollient/appropriate soap substitute
- Applications should be repeated as often as possible, at least three times a day
- Effective emollient therapy requires application of at least 250 g per week, depending on severity
- Ensure regular soaps are not used because they dry and irritate the skin

During the procedure

- Emollients should be at room temperature
- Use a spatula (if not in a pump dispenser) to place emollient onto a clean dish and apply to the skin with a gloved hand from the dish to ensure the product stays sterile, so reducing infection risk (pump-dispenser products may be dispensed straight onto the hand or skin)
- If applying after a bath, the skin should be patted dry and not rubbed because this creates heat and irritation and can cause damage to delicate skin cells
- If applying to the face, treat that first
- Expose parts of the body or limb to be treated
- Work from top to bottom and cover as you go with a sheet or towel to prevent the child becoming cold
- Apply emollient liberally in downward strokes following the line of hair growth (to prevent folliculitis)
- Do not rub in – allowing emollient to soak into the skin will have a cooling and soothing effect, but rubbing creates heat, irritates the eczema and increases the itch
- Apply a single layer of protective clothing (such as wrap garments) directly over emollient to enhance effectiveness and protect the skin from scratching
- If topical steroids are being used, ideally, if possible, wait 30–60 minutes before applying the emollient as this will avoid diluting the steroid and allow maximum therapeutic effects
- Loose clothing may be worn during this time to keep child warm and comfortable
- Protective clothing may be worn over emollients for comfort and to enhance emollient therapy, but steroids should be used with caution as their potency may be increased up to ten-fold when applied under wet wraps. Protective wraps, wet or dry, should not be worn if the skin is infected and weeping because the garments my stick causing more skin damage on removal
- Repeat with other areas of the body

Post-procedure

- Ensure the child is comfortable
- Dispose of or clear away equipment, replacing any necessary items for ongoing applications
- Document in the patient's notes the state of the skin and the applications
- Re-apply emollients at least three or four times a day or whenever skin is dry and irritated

As a guide, emollient therapy should exceed steroid use approximately ten-fold.

Application of topical steroids

Topical steroids are anti-inflammatory so they reduce the itch and inflammation of the skin and can be very effective in the treatment of active troublesome eczema. They are applied either once or twice a day. To gain maximum benefit, once-a-day treatments are best at night. There are numerous steroid preparations, classified as mild, moderate, potent and very potent in strength. They come as creams, ointments, lotions and gels. The strength and type of steroid prescribed will depend on the child's age, the skin site, and the severity of the eczema. An ointment base provides better penetration and has a lower risk of causing irritation. Apply the preparation thinly in FTUs (fingertip units) as shown in see *Table 12.1* (Long and Finlay, 1991).

Table 12.1: Recommended prescribing quantities per age in fingertip units (FTU)

	Face	Arm	Leg	Trunk	Trunk (back) + neck + hand + foot (front) + buttocks
3–6 months	1	1	1.5	1	1.5
1–2 years	1.5	1.5	2	2	3
3–5 years	1.5	2	3	3	3.5
6–10 years	2	2.5	4.5	3.5	5

Reasons for the procedure

- To provide an important anti-inflammatory effect
- To improve (reduce) lichenification (thickening of the skin)
- To reduce itch

Pre-procedure

- As for emollient therapy (above)
- Steroids are always applied in conjunction with emollients (30–60 minutes before) therefore the same preparation applies

During the procedure

- Apply no more than twice daily. If once a day, night time is best
- The FTU (500 mg) rule is a guide only. For effective treatment, apply sufficient steroid to leave a light shiny film
- Apply gently in downward strokes over affected areas
- 1% hydrocortisone may be applied to the face or body. Stronger steroids are not generally recommended for the face
- Topical steroids should be used with extreme caution beneath occlusive bandages as the potency may be increased up to ten-fold

Application of wet or dry wraps

These occlusive dressings for the treatment of dry, itchy, poorly controlled eczema may be applied dry as a single layer or wet as a double layer. They allow a much greater quantity of emollient to be used. They are normally worn at night but may be used during the day as well. Care should be taken not to use wraps over weeping or infected eczema because they may stick as they dry, causing further damage when removed. Retention bandages should be light, elastic, tubular bandages that come in different colours for different ages and different parts of the body. They come in rolls of different lengths (1 m, 3 m, 5 m and 10 m) age-appropriate sizes (*Box 12.1*).

Full-body garments for ages 6 months to 14 years are now available for use in the community but not in the hospital setting.

Box 12.1: Tubular bandage sizes

The width size is identified by a coloured line that runs the length of the bandage.

Red line	Young babies	Arms
Green line	Under 5 years	Arms and legs
Green line	Over 5 years	Arms
Blue line	Over 5 years	Legs
Yellow line		Trunk

Reasons for the procedure

- To overdose the skin with moisturisers to prevent it drying too fast
- To allow deeper absorption of moisturisers
- To cool and comfort itchy skin
- To protect the skin from scratching
- To promote the healing process
- To enhance sleep patterns
- To reduce the need for topical steroids

Pre-procedure

- Wraps are usually applied after a bath so follow guidelines for bathing and applying emollients (as above)

Equipment required

- Prescribed emollients and topical steroids (as above)
- Select correct sizes, in sufficient quantities, before starting
- Measure and cut with scissors required lengths as shown in *Box 12.2*
- If applying as wet wraps remember to cut double for each area
- Bowl or sink for hot water
- Towel
- Clean garments or bandages should be used each day; they can be washed at 60°C several times and re-used
- When used in hospital they are one-use only

Box 12.2: Guide to measuring lengths of tubular bandages

Arms	Top of shoulder to tips of fingers + 8 cm
Legs	Top of thigh to the toes + 8 cm
Body	Top of neck to base of bottom + 5 cm. Cut small holes for arms (these will stretch once on)
Ties	8 × 2–3 cm strips for leftover bandages for tying garments together
Double arms/legs	To totally cover the hands and feet, measure one length for each limb but double it. Only half will be wetted, applied and then twisted at the toes and/ or fingers and pulled back up

Specific patient preparation

- To achieve maximum benefit, protective bandages or garments are best worn at night after bathing and application of topical emollients
- Some children also find them helpful and comfortable to wear during the day

During the procedure

- Place two arm strips, two leg strips and two body strips into very warm water (this should be as hot as adult bath water to prevent child getting too cold)
- Apply topical steroids as prescribed and liberal amounts of emollient to each area in turn
- Wring out one wet strip and apply over the top of a thick layer of emollient, followed directly by a dry layer, and repeat for rest of the body
- Make two small holes where each piece meets, to keep them in place, and use ties to hold arm and leg wraps to the bodysuit
- Cut holes for fingers and toes to prevent the wraps being pulled up the limbs
- If using just overnight, it may be sufficient to use a single dry layer following the same process
- The child's pants or nappy can be worn as normal, with loose, light pyjamas (it is important not to overheat the child once wraps are applied)

Post-procedure

- Ensure the child is comfortable
- Dispose of and clear up equipment, replacing any necessary items for ongoing applications
- Document in patient's notes the state of skin and applications applied

Factors to be considered when applying topical application

- State and severity of eczema
- Area of skin affected
- Signs of infection, weeping or crusting
- Wrap bandages should not be used on open, weeping skin
- Allergies or sensitivities to topical treatments
- Child's usual eczema treatment routine (so changes can be explained)
- Child, parent or carer's usual compliance and understanding of treatment
- The only emollient that works is the one that the child and carer like and are happy to use frequently
- Distress increases eczema irritation so distraction therapy may be needed to make the treatment enjoyable for the child and carer and improve its effectiveness

Student learning outcomes about use of emollient therapy and protective bandages

Emollient therapy:

- ✓ Improves the quality of life
- ✓ Is key to control and management of atopic eczema, used in a daily bath, as soap and as moisturiser
- ✓ Gives added protection against infection if one with antimicrobial properties is used
- ✓ Softens and rehydrates the skin while helping prevent infection
- ✓ Protects the skin from outside irritations
- ✓ Reduces the itch factor and improves sleep
- ✓ Should be used every day and not just when the skin 'looks' bad
- ✓ Reduces the need for topical steroid therapy

REMEMBER:

- ✓ The average quantity of emolient for a toddler to achieve adequate therapy is 250 g a week and for an older child it is 500 g a week
- ✓ Topical steroids should be used intermittently in conjunction with emollients (but emollient therapy should exceed steroid use ten-fold)
- ✓ Steroids are best applied about 30 minutes before the emollient
- ✓ You should understand the safe use of topical steroids, and understand the safe and appropriate use of protective garments

References

Lawson V, Lewis-Jones MS, Finlay AY, Reid P, Owens RG (1998) The family impact of childhood atopic dermatitis: the Dermatitis Family Impact questionnaire. *Br J Dermatol* **138:** 107–13

Long CC, Finlay AY (1991) The fingertip unit – a new practical measure. *Clin Exper Dermatol* **16:** 444–47. www.bad.org.uk

Weston T (1991) Atlas of Anatomy. Marshall Cavendish Books, London

Williams HC, Strachan DP, Hay RJ (1994) Childhood eczema: disease of the advantaged? *BMJ* **308**: 1132–35

Further reading

British Medical Association (2006) *BNF for Children*. BMJ Publishing, London

Goodyear HM, Spowart K, Harper JL (1991) 'Wet-wrap' dressings for the treatment of atopic eczema in children. *Br J Dermatol* **125:** 604

Useful websites

British Association of Dermatologists
www.bad.org.uk

Comfifast by Shiloh Healthcare Ltd
www.shiloh.co.uk/comfi

Guidelines for the Management of Atopic Eczema
www.eGuidelines.co.uk

Learning about Wet Wrapping with Thomas and the Happy Wrappers
www.wetwraps.co.uk

National Eczema Society website
www.eczema.org.uk

Skin Care World
www.skincareworld.co.uk

Tubifast by SSL International plc
www.sovereign-publications.com/tubifast.htm

Chapter 13

Fundamental aspects of neurological assessment and monitoring

Chrissie Ward

Neuroscience is a very daunting speciality, especially for newly qualified nurses. Many nurses shy away from it as they find the terminology complex. This chapter will give you a comprehensive guide to the commonly performed procedures, providing the detail required to understand the management of epilepsy and external ventricular drains, and an understanding of how to assist with a lumbar puncture and how to perform neurological observations using the Glasgow Coma Scale.

Neurological observations

The Glasgow Coma Scale (GCS) is an assessment tool that is often combined with the recording of vital signs under the umbrella term 'neurological observations'. The GCS consists of a set of observations that indicate how well the brain is functioning (Jennett and Teasdale, 1974). It is used in most neurological centres and the National Institute for Clinical Excellence (NICE, 2003) recommends that the GCS should be used to assess all brain-injured patients. In paediatric practice a *modification* of the original GCS has been made so that the assessment is more relevant to child development (Patterson *et al*, 1992).

The National Paediatric Neuroscience Benchmark Group (NPNBG) identified certain factors that are desirable when assessing the neurological status of infants and children (Warren, 2000):

- Factor 1: The coma scale should reflect stage of development or usual ability
- Factor 2: A suitably qualified nurse should carry out the assessment
- Factor 3: A teaching and education programme should be established
- Factor 4: Documentation should be suitable for use in children and infants
- Factor 5: Continuity of care is achieved by one assessor with bedside handover

The Glasgow Coma Scale assesses two aspects of consciousness:

- Arousal (being aware of the environment)
- Cognition (demonstrating an understanding of what the observer has said through an ability to perform tasks) (Shah, 1999)

Each activity the patient performs is given a score. The best score is 15 and the worst is 3. A reduction in the score should be urgently brought to the attention of the doctors in charge of the patient.

Assessment with the Glasgow Coma Scale

Reasons for the procedure

- To monitor level of consciousness
- To aid diagnosis
- To indicate the effectiveness of treatment
- To recognise early and prevent secondary injury

Pre-procedure

Equipment required

- Neurological observation chart appropriate to the age of the child
- Torch
- Pen
- Sphygmomanometer
- Thermometer
- Watch with a second hand
- For an infant or young child, a distraction toy or comforter

Specific patient preparation

- Initially observe the child from a distance; include observations of eye opening, appropriateness of vocalisation, motor activity and posture, interaction with family and any seizure activity (Ferguson-Clark and Williams, 1998)
- Conduct specific baseline observations in relation to individual development, including names of pets, toys and comforters

During the procedure

- Observe head size, for tense bulging fontanelle in infants, distended scalp veins, and sun-setting eyes
- Apply the categories shown in *Box 13.1* in the assessment of eye opening, verbal responses and motor responses (the criteria for scoring each parameter are given in *Box 13.2;* these provide information about responses in the brain)

Box 13.1: Modified Glasgow Coma Scale

		0–18 months (infant)	18 months–5 years (child)
EYE OPENING	4	Eye opening spontaneously	Eye opening spontaneously
	3	Eye opening to speech	Eye opening to speech
	2	Eye opening to pain	Eye opening to pain
	1	No response	No response
BEST VERBAL RESPONSE	5	Coos, babbles or cries	Orientated and appropriate
	4	Irritable cry	Confused
	3	Cries inappropriately	Inappropriate use of words
	2	Moans to pain	Inappropriate sounds
	1	No response	No response
BEST MOTOR RESPONSE	6	Spontaneous movements	Obeys commands
	5	Withdraws to touch	Localises to touch
	4	Withdraws from pain	Withdraws from pain
	3	Abnormal flexion to pain	Abnormal flexion to pain
	2	Extension to pain	Extension to pain
	1	No response to pain	No response to pain

Lowest possible score = 3
Highest possible score = 15
Modified from Jennett and Teasdale, 1974 (source Paterson *et al*, 1992)

Box 13.2: Criteria for scoring in the Glasgow Coma Scale

Eye opening

The assessment of eye opening shows that the arousal mechanisms located in the brainstem are functioning (Jannett and Teasdale, 1974). The best response is when the patient opens his or her eyes spontaneously and scores 4. Opening the eyes in response to speech scores 3. Opening the eyes to painful stimuli scores 2. No response – even to painful stimuli – scores 1. Painful stimuli should be applied as a means of safeguarding the patient's well-being and can be applied in three ways:

- *Trapezius pinch:* take approximately 5 cm of the trapezius muscle between the thumb and the forefinger and twist
- *Supraorbital pressure*: feel the orbital rim and apply pressure to the orbital ridge to stimulate the supraorbital nerve – but avoid this if a facial fracture is suspected
- *Sternal rub*: rub the centre of the sternum using the knuckles of a clenched fist

It is important to recognise that fear may influence the patient's response. Involvement of the parents may be necessary.

cont./..

Verbal response

The verbal response assesses consciousness by ascertaining whether the patient is aware of himself or herself and the environment.

- *Orientated coos/babbles:* for the patient to score 5 when assessing the child's verbal response, it must be related to the child's individual development using words that are familiar
- *Confused/irritable cry*: the child may be able to hold a conversation with the observer but not answer all questions accurately. Parents will be able to confirm if this is normal for them. Equally, if the baby is crying a high-pitched irritable cry, parents will be able to confirm this is not normal for them. In this case, the patient will score 4
- *Inappropriate words/cry*: only if the child replies in inappropriate words or cries only to pain, the child will score 3
- *Incomprehensible words/moans to pain*: the child is less aware of the environment, and his or her verbal response will be in the form of incomprehensible sounds. If the child responds only with sounds the score will be 2. Verbal and painful stimuli may be required
- *No response*: if there is no verbal response to either verbal or painful stimuli, the score is 1

Best motor response

- *Follows a command/spontaneous movement*: it is important to be aware of responses, which are normal in infancy but would be abnormal in an adult. If the child can follow a command, the score is 6. Painful stimuli may need to be used to determine a response
- *Localises to pain/withdraws to touch*: if the child responds to pain or light touch and attempts to remove the source, the score is 5
- *Withdraws from pain*: if the child withdraws from central painful stimuli, the score is 4
- *Abnormal flexion*: in response to a central painful stimuli, the patient will bend an arm and rotate the wrist, resulting in spastic posture. Abnormal flexion score is 3
- *Abnormal extension*: in response to a central painful stimulus, the child will extend his or her arms or may rotate an arm inwards. This scores 2
- *No response*: the child has no motor response to central painful stimuli and scores 1

Assessment of the papillary response

Examination of the pupils and their reaction to light is a vital additional assessment that indicates raised intracranial pressure (ICP) and may result in compression of the cranial nerves (occulomotor nerve).

- Inform and explain the procedure to the child, as appropriate
- Wash hands
- Darken the environment if possible
- Hold both of the child's eyes open and note the shape and size of both pupils. Pupils are normally round with an average size of 2–5 mm. Both pupils should be equal in size. Dilated pupils are a sign of raised intracranial pressure. Close the eyes in unconscious patients in order to prevent corneal damage

- Holding one eye open, move a bright light from the outer aspect of the eye towards the pupil – the pupils should constrict. Remove the light source and the pupils should dilate to their original size. Repeat for the other eye
- Record observation and report any changes
- Assessment of the pupil can be carried out in both conscious and unconscious patients. Assessment of pupil involves looking at:
  - The shape of both pupils
  - The size of both pupils
  - The reaction to light

The consensual light reflex

- Hold both eyelids open and shine a light as described above – the pupils in both eyes should constrict equally.

Vital signs

Vital signs form a part of the neurological assessment, as the centres for the vital signs are located in the brainstem. Damage to this area can affect their function.

- *Blood pressure and pulse* – as the ICP rises, the brain becomes hypoxic and ischaemic. To counteract this effect and to perfuse the brain, the body responds by increasing the arterial blood pressure, which results in the patient becoming bradycardic
- *Respiration* – if the brainstem is affected, there are changes in the rate and pattern of breathing. Apnoea and Cheyne–Stokes breathing are caused by the sudden rise in ICP
- *Temperature* – damage to the hypothalamus may result in alterations in temperature control

Power in limb movements

Arms and legs should be assessed for normal power, mild weakness, severe weakness, spastic flexion, extension and no response.

- In infants, assess the arms by offering them a toy to each hand, and the legs by pushing the limb from the foot to measure any resistance
- In older children, ask them to squeeze your hands, and to push your hand away with their foot

Post-procedure

- Document findings on a chart
- Inform medical staff of any significant changes

Lumbar puncture

A lumbar puncture (LP) is an invasive procedure that involves the removal of cerebrospinal fluid (CSF) through a puncture into the subarachnoid space of the spinal cord. It should be avoided if the patient demonstrates any of the following:

- Raised intracranial pressure
- Depressed consciousness
- Concomitant coagulopathy (associated problem with clotting)
- Tissue sepsis
- Congenital abnormalities of the lumbar region (Bassett, 1997).

The procedure is often a source of discomfort and stress to the child and the family because it involves the child remaining absolutely still for a prolonged period of time. Consequently, infants and young children may require a general anaesthetic. Entonox for pain relief can be used in most cases (see also *Chapter 7*). Each child should be assessed by the multidisciplinary team.

Reasons for the procedure

- To aid diagnosis
- To facilitate the administration of intrathecal medicine (Bassett, 1997; Blows, 2002)
- To relieve communicating hydrocephalus

Pre- procedure

Equipment required

- Trolley
- Lumbar puncture needle/spinal needle
- Dressing pack
- Antiseptic to clean skin
- 10 mL syringe
- Needles of various gauges
- Local anaesthetic
- Three sterile universal containers labelled 1,2 and 3
- Two glucose blood bottles
- Phlebotomy equipment
- Manometer
- Three-way tap
- Small dressing (establish if there are any allergies)

- Sterile gloves
- Gloves

Specific patient preparation

- A nurse should supervise the child if Entonox is to be used. The Entonox would be prescribed, and the nurse assessed and competent in giving the Entonox (see also *Chapter 7*). Parents may be helpful in reassuring and keeping the child still
- Offer the patient toilet facilities as necessary
- Establish a method of communication with the child to indicate that he or she wishes to move
- The child may wish to cuddle a favourite toy
- Obtain a sample of venous blood 30–60 minutes before the procedure being undertaken and place this in a blood glucose bottle. This can then be compared with CSF glucose level (Tate and Tasota, 2000)
- Position the patient as close to the edge of the bed as possible, for ease of access. Children are usually controlled best by lying on their side with their head flexed and knees drawn up towards the chest. Or the child can sit up and bend over a table with the back exposed. Such a position curves the spine, maximises spaces between the vertebrae, and facilitates entry of the lumbar puncture needle/spinal needle (Bassett, 1997; Tate and Tasota, 2000; Blows, 2002). Even cooperative children need to be held gently to prevent possible trauma from unexpected, involuntary movement (Wong, 1999)
- EMLA cream is placed under an occlusive dressing to decrease pain of the lumbar puncture

During the procedure

- Another nurse should be available to assist the doctor/practitioner
- Assist the doctor/practitioner in preparing for the aseptic procedure
- The lumbar puncture needle/spinal needle is introduced below the level of the spinal cord into the lumbar cisterna through the third or fourth lumbar vertebra (L3 or L4), passing via the dura and arachnoid maters into the subarachnoid space
- A manometer is attached to measure CSF pressure (60–160 mmH_2O) (a rise in pressure indicates raised ICP)
- Three samples are collected, in numerical order, because initially blood caused by the trauma may contaminate the sample. The CSF sample is taken for protein, glucose, lactate and lymphocytes (*Box 13.3*)
- Place a small dressing on the puncture site
- Note the colour of CSF; it is usually watery, clear liquid. However, if it is continuous fresh blood, this is indicative of a very recent bleeding into the subarachnoid space. A continuous yellow stain (xanthochromia) may be indicative of an older subarachnoid bleed

Box 13.3: Normal CSF values (Blows, 2002)

Protein	15–45 mg per 100 mL
Glucose	40–80 mg per 100 mL
Lactate	1.1–1.9 mmol per litre
Lymphocytes	0–5 cells per mm^3

Post procedure

- Post lumbar puncture headache may occur, related to postural changes in pressure. This is less severe if the child lies flat for 1–2 hours and fluid are encouraged
- Analgesia should be given as prescribed and the effect evaluated. The dressing site should be checked for signs of leakage, bleeding or inflammation, and the dressing changed as required
- Ensure that all CSF samples are secured, the bottle labelled and forwarded with the correct microbiology request form
- Dispose of equipment
- Record the date and time that the procedure was undertaken in the patient's documentation
- The findings may indicate a number of medical conditions (*Box 13.4*)

Box 13.4: Changes related to medical conditions (Bassett, 1997; Blows, 2002)

Rise in protein	Infection of the meninges or brain; brain tumour
Disturbance in lactate	Central nervous system infection
Reduction in glucose	Bacterial infection
Increase in lymphocytes	Infection

External ventricular drains (EVDs)

External ventricular drains (EVDs) are a temporary system that allow drainage of CSF from the lateral ventricles of the brain. EVDs are commonly used within neuroscience for the management of patients who require drainage of CSF in order to control raised intracranial pressure associated with head injury, subarachnoid haemorrhage, acute hydrocephalus secondary to cerebral aqueduct obstruction, posterior fossa tumours, or purulent meningitis.

Effects of CSF on intracranial pressure

The Monro Kellie hypothesis states that the skull is a rigid compartment filled to capacity essentially with substances such as blood, brain matter and CSF, which cannot be compressed. As such, an increase in one or more of the components will result in an increase in the overall pressure within the skull, unless another component decreases in volume (Lindsey *et al*, 1991). Intracranial pressure is therefore affected directly by any changes in volume of CSF within the brain. These changes in volume may be the result of:

- A change in the rate of production of CSF
- An obstruction to CSF flow within the ventricular system
- A change in the rate of absorption of CSF

Problems associated with production, flow or absorption of CSF can cause increased intracranial pressure and may be an indication for an EVD.

Positioning of the EVD and CSF drainage

The drainage of the CSF depends upon gravity. The level of the flow chamber will determine the amount of CSF drained. The zero point for the EVD system is the location of the foramen of Munro. The flow chamber should be positioned at a prescribed distance in cm above this zero point. This level will determine the amount of CSF drainage (for example, if the drain is set at 15 cm and the ICP is less than 15 cmH_20 then there will be no drainage; if however the level is 15 cm and the ICP is greater than 15 cmH_20 the system will drain to maintain the pressure). CSF flows from the lateral ventricles via the foreamen of Munro into the third ventricle.

- If the flow chamber is placed above the level of the foramen of Munro it will lead to insufficient drainage of CSF and an increase in ICP, with potentially devasting consequences relating to increased ICP
- If the flow chamber is placed below the level of the foramen of Munro it can lead to excessive drainage of CSF and subsequentcollapsing of the ventricle

The EVD system is suspended by an adjustable cord from the IV drip-stand and placed at the head of the bed, with the flow chamber facing the foot of the bed, so that it is visible at all times. The zero mark of the EVD scale must correspond to the level of the foramen of Munro and should be accurately measured using a spirit level. The flow chamber of the EVD system must be aligned at the level, prescibed in cm, by the neurosurgeon (eg. 10 cm).

Summary of nursing care

The flow chamber must be positioned at the prescribed distance in cm above 0 cm pressure level. Ensure this level is prescribed in the patient's notes and is clearly documented on the chart. The anatomical reference or zero point is the location of the foramen of Munro, which is estimated at the external auditory meatus in the supine patient.

- Ensure the EVD system is at the head of the bed with the drip chamber facing the foot of the bed
- Observe the tubing at regular intervals for patency or kinking and that the CSF level is oscillating
- Ensure that the tubing has not been clamped and that the three-way taps are open
- Record CSF drainage every 2 hours on daily fluid charts. Report excessive drainage to a neurosurgeon
- Observe CSF for colour and consistency. Report if cloudy, milky or xanthrochromic. Colour and consistency of CSF should be clearly documented.
- Monitor at least hourly the patient's neurological status and papillary responses and report any significant changes to a neurosurgeon (or as patient's condition dictates)
- Clamp the EVD for short periods if necessary (during transfer, for example). Unclamp the EVD as soon as possible or if the patient's neurological condition deteriorates. If the CSF is blood stained, caution not to block off the system must be exercised
- The EVD tubing must not be irrigated, changed or manipulated unless absolutely necessary
- A strict aseptic technique must be used during any sampling or maintenance procedures
- Report any CSF leakage, and observe site for signs of infection
- Change the collection bag when three-quarters full using an aseptic technique

Complications associated with EVD

Inadequate drainage of CSF may cause the ventricle to enlarge, with subsequent rises in intracranial pressure, and it may occur:

- If the EVD system is placed too high above the level of the foramen of Munro, minimising CSF drainage
- If CSF drainage is obstructed, as may occur when:
  - tubing is kinked or inadvertently clamped
  - the three-way tap is turned the wrong way
  - the drainage bag is full
  - the tissue or thick CSF blocks the system

Excessive drainage of CSF may also occur if the system is placed too far below the level of the foramen of Munro. It may cause the ventricles to collapse and pull the brain tissue away from the dura, and cause tearing of the blood vessels, resulting in a subdural or subarachnoid haemorrhage (Bracke *et al*, 1978).

CSF drainage

Drainage of more than 50 mL is considered excessive (each patient must be considered individually). CSF is normally clear and colourless. There are three ways to describe the colour of CSF, which should be documented in the patent's notes:

- Clear colourless
- Xanthochromic (discoloured usually yellow, orange or brown due to the breakdown of red cells from previous haemorrhage)
- Blood stained (as a result of recent haemorrhage or surgery)

CSF may also be described as turbid (cloudy) and this occurs if there are increased white blood cells as a result of Infection.

The drainage tubing must be checked for patency at the beginning of each shift and at regular intervals thereafter. If the level of CSF is not oscillating in the tubing, the flow chamber may be dropped to below the foramen of Munro for a brief period *only* to check whether CSF drains into the chamber; once this has been observed, the flow chamber must be re-aligned to prevent overdrainage of CSF. If at any time an EVD appears to be blocked, a neurosurgeon must be contacted immediately because it may be necessary to flush the system. The process of flushing an EVD must only be performed by a member of medical staff.

Clamping the EVD

Clamping an EVD may result in inadequate CSF drainage and a subsequent rise in intracranial. However, there are occasions when it may be necessary to clamp the system for short periods, such as when repositioning patients. The decision to clamp the EVD must be made following assessment of the patient's clinical condition and neurological status. *Never* clamp it for more than 30 minutes.

On occasions patients with EVDs are prescribed intrathecal antibiotics, like vancomycin. Following administration of the drug, the EVD must be clamped for 60 minutes to allow for absorption. It is the responsibility of the qualified nurse at the bedside to consult with a member of the medical team regarding this and to unclamp the EVD afterwards as instructed.

Epilepsy

The brain is like an electrical circuit, with impulses flowing from nerve to nerve. Epilepsy is clinically defined as the tendency to have repeated, usually spontaneous, seizures that originate in the brain (Lanfear, 2002). Seizures can take many forms, and the site of the seizure activity affects the initial symptoms and impairment of brain functions.

Types of seizures

Generalised seizures

In generalised seizures, the discharge spreads symmetrically throughout the brain from the beginning. These seizures can be classified as:

- Absence seizures (petit mal)
- Myoclonic seizures
- Clonic seizures
- Tonic seizures
- Tonic–clonic seizures (grand mal)
- Atonic seizures (drop attacks)

Partial seizures

In this type of seizure, the paroxysmal discharge spreads locally from a focus of abnormal cells in the cortex. They are classified as:

- Simple partial seizures
- Complex partial seizures
- Secondary generalised seizures

Management of a child experiencing a tonic–clonic (convulsive) seizure

What to do

- Stay calm and check the time to monitor how long the seizure lasts
- Make the child comfortable lying down (ease to the floor if sitting) and put something soft under the head; loosen any tight clothing, including jewellery around the neck, and remove glasses if worn
- Remove nearby objects that could be harmful and stop other people from crowding around
- Once the movements have stopped, roll the child on to his or her side and place in the recovery position, if possible
- Check the child's airway is clear
- Allow the child to recover in his or her own time (it might take some time)
- Provide privacy and offer assistance if there has been any incontinence
- Stay with the child, giving reassurance until he or she has fully recovered

What NOT to do

- Do not put anything into the child's mouth or attempt to force the teeth apart
- Do not attempt to constrain the child's convulsive movements
- Do not move the child, unless he or she is in a dangerous place
- Do not give the child anything to drink until he or she is fully awake (Russell and Wehrie, 1998)

When to call a doctor

- If this is a first unexplained seizure
- If injuries have occurred
- If the seizure shows no sign of stopping after 5–10 minutes (or 2 minutes longer than is usual for that child)
- If there is one seizure after another without stopping

Management of a child experiencing a minor seizure

Minor seizures take many forms so the response of the onlooker needs to vary. If a child falls abruptly, ensure that he or she has not sustained an injury that requires attention. If there is prolonged confusion, as with complex-partial seizures, take the following measures.

- Gently protect the child from obvious danger (a gentle touch to the arm can be reassuring and the child can be steered to a safe place)
- Keep other people from crowding around
- Speak gently and calmly to the child to help him or her to re-orientate more quickly
- It may be better to observe a child who is confused rather than repeatedly offer help and have it rejected (with what might be misunderstood as aggression)
- Stay with the child until he or she is able and safe to resume a normal routine

Sometimes a convulsive seizure occurs at the end of a minor attack, so be prepared for this (Russell and Wehrie, 1998).

Seizure assessment and documentation

During the seizure, observe the child's:

- Position before the seizure
- Respiration
- Colour

- Facial expressions eg. grimacing
- Vocalisations and movements (eg. screaming or crying, eye deviations, head turning, limb movements, stiffening)
- Incontinence

Post seizure document details of:

- Date and time of the seizure
- Duration of the seizure
- A description of the event
- Recovery time, length of time and behaviour
- Neurological assessment

References

Bassett C (1997) Medical investigations 1: Lumbar puncture. *Br J Nurs* **6:** 405–06

Blows W (2002) Diagnostic investigations. Part 1: Lumbar puncture. *Nurs Times* **98**(36): 25–26

Bracke M, Taylor AG, Kinney AB (1978) External drainage of cerebrospinal fluid. *Am J Nurs* **78**(8): 1355–58. Cited in: Terry D, Nesbit K (1991) Nursing care of the child with external ventricular drainage. *J Neurosci Nurs* 23(23), 345-47

Ferguson-Clark L, Williams C (1998) Neurological assessment in children. *Paediatr Nurs* **10**(4): 29–35

Jennett B, Teasdale G (1974) Assessment of coma and impaired consciousness. *Lancet* **2:** 81 –84

Lanfear J (2002) The individual with epilepsy. *Nurs Stand* **16**(46): 43–53

Lindsey KW, Bone I, Callender R (1991) Neurology and Neurosurgery Illustrated, 2nd edn. Churchill Livingstone, Edinburgh

National Institute for Clinical Excellence (2003) *Head Injury, Triage, Assessment, Investigations and Early Management of Head Injury in Infants, Children and Adults: Clinical Guidelines 4*. NICE, London

Paterson RJ, Brown GW, Salassi-Scotter M, Middaugh D (1992) Head injury in the conscious child. *Am J Nurs* **92**(8): 22–27

Russell A, Wehrie E (1998) *Health Care Assistant's Guide to Epilepsy.* Unison, London

Tate J, Tasota FJ (2000) Eye on diagnostics: Looking at lumbar puncture in adults. *Nursing* **30**(11): 91

Warren A (2000) Dissemination of a research study on the reliability of coma scoring influenced work by the National Paediatric Neurosciences Benchmarking Group to improve this practice in other paediatric centre. *Paediatr Nurs* **12**(2): 14–18

Wong D (1999) *Nursing Care of Infants and Children*, 7th edn. Mosby, Oxford

Further reading

Woodward S, Addison C, Shah S, Brennan F, Macleod A, Clements M (2002) Benchmarking best practice for external ventricular drainage. *Br J Nurs* **11**(1): 47–53

Chapter 14

Fundamental aspects of renal care

Marion Aylott and Helen Pearson

Urethral catheterisation

This is the introduction of a specifically designed tube through the urethra into the bladder. There are two types of urethral catheterisation:

- Short-term intermittent
- Indwelling

Short-term intermittent catheterisation is a procedure in which a catheter is inserted for long enough to drain the bladder of its contents and is then promptly removed. This catheter has one lumen and one port. The procedure is used for children with neuropathic bladder problems (for example, spina bifida). Intermittent self-catheterisation can be undertaken by people of all ages to empty their bladder of urine or by a nurse or doctor to measure residual urine after the patient has passed urine. Children who are unable to carry out the procedure themselves may have it undertaken by a parent at home to drain their bladder of urine. Modern-day intermittent catheters can be used almost anywhere when drainage of the urinary bladder is required (Robinson, 2006).

Indwelling catheterisation is a procedure in which a specialised catheter that can be left in the bladder for an extended period of time (days to weeks depending on the material it is made from and manufacturer's instructions) for continuous drainage of the bladder into a collection bag. This catheter has two ports and lumens; one to connect to the urine collection container and one for the attachment of a syringe to insufflate the balloon which keeps the catheter within the bladder.

A clean technique or an aseptic (sterile) technique?

A systematic review conducted by Dunn *et al,* (2000) noted the paucity of studies investigating catheterisation technique. A single study which met the COCHRANE criteria for randomised controlled trials demonstrated that the use of a surgical sterile catheterisation technique did not reduce the rate of catheter-associated urinary tract infections (Carapeti *et al* 1996). It is speculated that a clean, non-sterile technique involving hand washing with soap and water, wearing non-sterile gloves, cleansing genitalia with tap water, no catheter pack and the balloon filled with tap water are sufficient measures. It is arguable whether an aseptic technique is really ever achieved when catheterising children. But can the use of sterile instruments and a good aseptic technique be abandoned in favour of clean technique on this evidence, given the high incidence of catheter-associated nosocomial infections and resultant morbidity (Barber, 2002)? This chapter will present a non-touch aseptic technique that is child-centred, pragmatic, simple and applies methods to reduce the risk of cross infection.

Standard precautions

There is always the potential for contact with a child's blood and body fluids while inserting or delivering catheter care. Gloves and apron must be worn, not only to protect the user, but also to prevent infection in the child.

Reasons for the procedure

Diagnostic

- To collect accurately timed volumes of urine for renal function studies
- To monitor urine output in severely ill children
- To monitor urine output in children with suspected urinary obstruction or neurologic incontinence, or following urologic surgery (in these circumstances the surgeon will perform the catheterisation only)

Therapeutic

- To relieve obstruction to urine flow
- To instil medications into the urinary bladder
- To facilitate urethral repair of the urethra or surrounding structures (doctor)

In these circumstances the surgeon will perform the catheterisation only.

Complications of the procedure

- Trauma
- Tissue inflammation
- Encrustation
- Colonisation by micro-organisms
- Infection

Pre-procedure

Equipment

- Clean working surface or dressing trolley
- Dressing pack (check the in-date, the aseptic sterilisation indicator, and if intact and dry)
- Potable tap water (suitable for drinking) at room temperature in plastic container
- Two pairs of well-fitting gloves (in order to get a good fit may need to use sterile gloves)
- Apron
- Alcohol hand-rub
- Sterile single-patient use 10 mL syringe
- Anaesthetic aqueous lubricating gel (2% lidocaine gel) (British National Formulary [BNF], 2006)
- Catheter of appropriate size and type (see *Boxes 14.1* and *14.2*)
- Sterile drainage system for urine collection (use collection bag with paediatric urine meter if accurate measurement of hourly urine output is required)
- 5 mL or 10 mL syringe as appropriate for indwelling catheter (with balloon) only
- Manufacturer's instructions (Medical Devices Agency [MDA], 2000)

Specific patient preparation

- Informed child/parent consent must be obtained before the procedure is carried out (Department of Health, 2004)
- The child and the parents are entitled to request that the procedure is carried out by a specific gender of healthcare professional to fit in with their cultural or personal preferences. These issues should be addresses at the time of obtaining consent and information giving
- Genitalia should be washed by the child or parent (may be preferable) with soap and water or bath (if appropriate). Bacteria enter the bladder from periurethral contamination at the time of catheter insertion or later due to capillary action (Maki and Tambyah, 2001). Washing the perineal area thoroughly with soap and water before the sterile catheterisation procedure begins is not, in practice, routinely done unless the patient has faecal incontinence. If so, this important step should not be omitted (Barber, 2002)
- Children's memories of painful and frightening experiences can have long-term consequences for their reactions to later healthcare interventions. Distraction techniques and preparation have been shown to reduce anxiety and distress and improve coping (McGrath, 2006). Consider the child's age and developmental level when planning these activities
- Urethral catheterisation is a frightening procedure for children, and for many children, both boys and girls, it is also painful. A double-blind randomised study compared children who received either lubrication with either KY Jelly or 2% lidocaine. The results were stunning. The level of pain and distress reported by the children in the study was significantly lower in the lidocaine group (Gerard *et al*, 2003)

- Select the appropriate type and size of catheter. They come in three lengths: paediatric, female 250 mm, and male 450 mm. They should be comfortable (Robinson, 2006), easy to insert and remove, and must minimise secondary complications such as tissue inflammation, encrustation, colonisation by micro-organisms and infection (Department of Health/Hospital Infection Society, 2001). The appropriate size and material of catheter is determined by the age and sex (see *Box 14.1*) and intended function of the catheter (indwelling or intermittent) (see *Box 14.2*). Always use smallest diameter possible to reduce the risk of causing spasm and bypassing. Larger catheters can also lead to urethral erosion, and impair paraurethral gland function. The paraurethral glands produce mucous that protects against ascending bacteria; compression of these glands can result in urethritis or ascending infection (EPIC, 2001)
- A systematic review of research comparing latex versus silicone catheters found no significant difference in the incidence of bacteraemia (Johnson *et al*, 2006). However, the incidence of bacteraemia is significantly reduced when catheters coated with silver alloy or silver oxide are *in situ* for up to 28 days (Lai and Fontecchio, 2002)
- No evidence exists to support routine monthly catheter changes. Rather, nurses should monitor patients closely for signs of blockage or encrustation and should change the catheter based on specific patient needs (Department of Health/Hospital Infection Society, 2001)
- Assemble equipment on the bottom of a dressing trolley or on a flat surface nearby
- Read and follow the manufacturer's instructions (MDA, 2000)

Box 14.1: Catheter size and length of insertion according to age and weight

0–5 months (3–6 kg)	Boys: 6 Ch, insertion depth 4 cm ± 2 cm Girls: 6 Ch, insertion depth 1.5–2 cm
6–12 months (4–9 kg)	Boys: 6 Ch, insertion depth 6 cm ± 2 cm Girls: 6–8 Ch, insertion depth 1.5–2 cm
1–3 years (10–15 kg)	Boys: 8 Ch, insertion depth 8 cm ± 2 cm Girls: 8 Ch, insertion depth 1.5–3 cm
4–7 years (16–20 kg)	Boys: 10 Ch, insertion depth 10 cm ± 2 cm Girls: 10–12 Ch, insertion depth 2–4 cm ± 2 cm
8–12 years (21–40 kg)	Boys: 12 Ch, insertion depth 12 cm ± 2 cm Girls: 12 Ch, insertion depth 3–4 cm ± 2 cm
Over 13 years	Boys: 12–14 Ch, insertion depth 16–20 cm ± 2 cm Girls: 12–14 Ch, insertion depth 4–6 cm ± 2 cm

Box 14.2 Types of catheter and recommended uses

Type	Recommended use
Polyvinyl chloride (PVC)/PVC non-balloon	Short-term only Maximum 7 days Intermittent use only Can be re-used
Teflon-coated with latex core*	Short-term Up to 28 days
Silicone	Long-term Can be used for up to 12 weeks
Hydrogel-coated latex*	Long-term Can be used up to 12 weeks
Silicone-elastomer-coated latex*	Long-term Can be used up to 12 weeks
Hydrogel-coated silicone	Long-term Can be used up to 12 weeks
Silver-coated	Short-term or long-term in high-risk patients Expensive Reduces incidence of urinary tract infection by 40% (<14 days) (Neil Weis and Van Den Broek, 2004)

**Caution: unsuitable for those sensitive to latex; NHSE, 2003*

During the procedure

- Explain the procedure of urethral catheterisation to the child in an age- and developmentally appropriate manner, and to parents if they are present
- Screen the bed (NMC, 2004)
- Urethral catheterisation of a child requires two nurses, one of whom will perform the catheterisation, and one who will act as an 'assistant' (Jamieson *et al*, 2002)
- Ask the assistant to help the child into a semi-recumbent sitting position. For girls, legs must be abducted, with the feet resting about hip-width apart. For boys, legs must be flat and extended. Maintain the child's privacy with a suitable cover until ready to proceed
- Wash your hands and put on a disposable apron (Workman and Bennett, 2003). Hand washing is the single most important step in preventing the spread of infection
- Open the outer paper cover of the catheterisation pack and slide the inner pack onto the top shelf of the trolley or prepared surface
- Open the pack using finger tips to pull out all four corners of the package, taking care not to contaminate the 'sterile field' within

- Ask the assistant to open the other packs using a non-touch aseptic technique and drop them onto the centre of the sterile field
- Ask the assistant to run warm tap water into the plastic container and place it on the edge of the sterile field closest to the child
- Draw up the required amount of water with the syringe to inflate the balloon, according to manufacturer's instructions, and put to one side. More water than required will cause trauma to the bladder entrance and less water may mean that the catheter might fail to stay in place
- Decant a generous amount of the lidocaine gel (1–2 cm) onto a piece of sterile gauze (this will be smeared on the catheter later)
- Ask the assistant to remove the cover that is maintaining the child's privacy
- Take hold of the dressing towels and place the towel under the child's buttocks and thighs (*if the child is wriggling, leave the towel in place, wherever you manage to get it!*)
- If the child allows you, cleanse the genitalia
- *For girls* (in an ideal world, if the child allows you to follow best practice):
  - With your *non-dominant* hand, separate the labia minora so that the urethral meatus can be seen
  - With your *dominant* hand cleanse the external genital region with gauze swab soaked in warm tap water (it is as effective as antiseptic preparations for this purpose)
  - Cleanse anterior to posterior, inner to outer, one swipe per swab, and discard the swab away from sterile field (Hilton, 2004)
  - Put a generous blob of lidocaine gel onto a gauze swab and place it over urethra. Note the time – ideally you need a delay of 5 minutes for the lidocaine to work (BNF, 2006)
- *For boys* (in an ideal world, if the child allows you to follow best practice):
  - With your *non-dominant* hand, wrap a sterile gauze swab around the penis. Retract the foreskin if necessary
  - With your *dominant* hand, cleanse the glans penis with gauze swab soaked in warm tap water (it is as effective as antiseptic preparations for this purpose)
  - Insert the nozzle of the lidocaine gel into the urethra and squeeze the gel gently in
  - Remove the nozzle and discard the tube
  - Massage the gel along the urethra (note the time – ideally you need a delay of 5 minutes for the lidocaine to work)
- Change gloves
- Remove the catheter from the plastic sheath with the still sterile dominant hand and hold the end of the catheter loosely coiled in the palm
- Inject the balloon to check for patency – the catheter balloon should fill symmetrically (*Figure 14.1*). Discard and request another catheter if the balloon does not inflate or inflates asymmetrically. Deflate the balloon
- Wipe the sterile gauze swab with lidocaine generously over the tip of the catheter (approximately 3–4 cm) and place in receiver

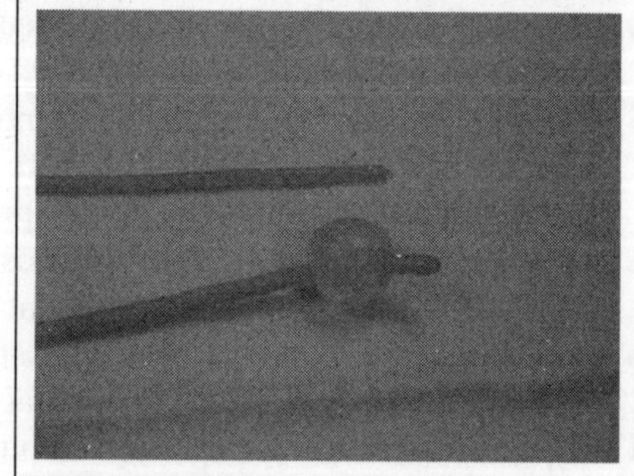

Figure 14.1: Inflation of catheter balloon

- *For girls:*
  - Place the receiver containing the catheter between the child's legs
  - Ask the assistant with gloves on to remove the gauze swab with lidocaine placed over urethra earlier
  - Slowly insert the catheter tip into the urethral orifice and angle downward to allow the catheter to follow the angle of the urethra
  - Advance the catheter usually about 1.5–8 cm, depending on the age of the child, until a flowback of urine appears in the tube
  - NEVER force the catheter against resistance – if you feel resistance STOP the procedure and inform the doctor
- *For boys:*
  - Place the receiver containing the catheter between the child's legs
  - Slowly insert the catheter tip into the urethral orifice and advance the catheter, usually about 6–25 cm, depending on the age of the child, until a flowback of urine appears in the tube
  - NEVER force the catheter against resistance – if you feel resistance STOP the procedure and inform the doctor
- If the catheter is designed to be indwelling (left *in situ*) inject the pre-determined (manufacturer's instructions) volume of water via the injection port in order to inflate the balloon. NEVER inflate the balloon unless you get flowback of urine into the catheter
- Gently pull the catheter until the inflation balloon is snug against the bladder neck to prevent leakage
- Connect the catheter drainage tube to the urine collection system
- Secure the catheter in place to prevent tension on the catheter. Unsecured urinary catheters can lead to bleeding, trauma, pressure sores around the meatus, and bladder spasms from pressure and traction (Hanchett, 2002). If the child desires, it is recommended that the catheter be secured to the thigh for girls and to the upper thigh or lower abdomen for boys. The lower abdomen position in boys decreases the potential for pressure necrosis and urethral erosion at the penile–scrotal junction (Smith, 2003a). Ambulatory boys may have problems with the abdominal position, so they can be instructed to secure the catheter to their upper thigh in the daytime and to change the position to the lower abdomen for sleeping. Ensure that the catheter will not become taught when the child moves
- If available, use a commercially designed support. Whatever product is selected, nurses should instruct the child and parents about the proper use and removal of the securement device
- Place the drainage bag below the level of the bladder and make sure the child is dry and comfortable
- Dispose of equipment in the clinical waste bag as instructed by trust policy (Duggall *et al*, 2002)
- Remove gloves and apron and wash hands
- Evaluate catheter function and the amount, colour, odour, and quality of the urine
- Record information in the patient's documentation including date and time of catheterisation, catheter type, batch number, manufacturer, size and amount of water instilled into the balloon

Post-procedure

- Catheter care should consist of maintaining good daily personal hygiene. Catheter manipulation should be avoided because it is thought to contribute to bacterial migration into the bladder around the catheter–meatal junction. Meatal cleansing is necessary only if there is bleeding, discharge or encrustation, usually with *Proteus microbilis* (Pratt *et al*, 2001)
- Although drainage bags are designed with either an anti-reflux valve or an anti-reflux chamber to prevent reflux of contaminated urine from the bag into the tubing they should still be positioned below the level of the child's bladder (Maki and Tambyah, 2001)
- Keep drainage bags off the floor. Studies have shown that retrograde bacterial migration from the outlet tube is a major source of bacterial contamination (Cravens and Zweig, 2000)
- Ideally, drainage bags should be hung on a stand with the tubing in a straight line, avoiding looping or kinking to promote unobstructed urine flow
- Transporting children with drainage bags positioned on their abdomens or between their legs should be avoided
- Do not allow the outlet tube to touch the collection container or floor when emptying (Cravens and Zweig, 2000)
- Empty the drainage bag when more than half full but less than two-thirds full to avoid opening the closed drainage system too frequently and avoid traction on the catheter from the weight of the drainage bag
- Catheters should be removed as soon as possible or not required (Department of Health, 2003)
- Catheter irrigation is not recommended unless obstruction with clots or mucous is anticipated and is a medical responsibility (Getliffe, 2003)
- If appropriate, encourage oral fluids; *adequate fluid intake is necessary*. 30 mL/kg of body weight is currently recommended as adequate intake. This should allow for a daily urinary output of 1–4 mL/kg per 24 hours. This output serves to keep urine dilute and will help decrease catheter encrustations and urinary tract infections. Encourage the child and the parents to avoid fluids that irritate the bladder, such as caffeine, citrus, and carbonated drinks (Getliffe, 2003)
- *Maintain a closed system whenever possible*. If the patient changes from a leg bag to a larger overnight bag, careful hand-washing is required, and cleaning the contact ports with an antiseptic such as Steret is recommended (Getliffe, 2003)

This internet site provides a free link to a 12-minute video on minimising the trauma of paediatric urethral catheterisation: www.uihealthcare.com/topics/medicaldepartments/urology/catheterization/index.html/.

Student skill laboratory activity

✓ Assemble the equipment you would require to undertake a catheterisation.
✓ Practice male and female catheterisation on a mannequin.

Obtaining a catheter urine specimen

A catheter specimen of urine (CSU) is the collection of a clean, fresh, uncontaminated sample of urine via an indwelling urethral catheter.

Catheter-associated urinary tract infection is the most frequently reported complication of urinary catheterisation. More than 40% of all nosocomial infections are catheter-associated (Filetoth, 2002). Diagnosis of urinary tract infection can be difficult in a patient with a long-term indwelling catheter, especially because patients may be asymptomatic (Breathnach, 2005). Ideally, urine for a culture and sensitivity should be obtained from a newly inserted catheter to avoid culturing the system (catheter) rather than the urine.

Reasons for the procedure

- To determine infection (National Institute for Clinical Excellence [NICE], 2003)
- To obtain urine for electrolyte analysis for children with renal impairment (Postlethwaite and Webb, 2002)
- To obtain a fresh specimen of urine for ward analysis

Pre-procedure

Equipment

- Two 70% alcohol-impregnated wipes
- Sterile specimen pot
- Apron
- Non-sterile gloves
- Appropriate request form
- 22 G needle, if required (see manufacturer's instructions)
- 10 mL syringe
- Cardboard receiver
- Sharps container

Specific patient preparation

- Explain the procedure to the child and parents as appropriate (Department of Health, 2004)
- Ensure privacy for the child (Department of Health, 2004)
- Check the identity of the child against the request form (Higgins, 2000)
- Read the manufacturer's instructions (MDA, 2000)

During the procedure

- Wash your hands (the single most important step in preventing the spread of infection)
- Put on gloves and apron
- Drainage bags now come with a special 'safe sampling' port which is designed to obtain urine specimens while maintaining a closed system. It is recommended that urine specimens are obtained directly through this port using an aseptic technique (McGillivray, 2005)
- Occlude the drainage tubing just below the port temporarily using forceps. This allows the urine to collect in the tubing
- Once sufficient urine has accumulated above the clamped tubing, swab the port with an alcohol-impregnated wipe and allow to dry (30 seconds)
- Withdraw the urine following the manufacturer's instructions using a needle, blunt cannula and syringe or Luer lock syringe. If using a needle, insert it a at 45° angle
- Withdraw the needle, decant carefully into a specimen pot, secure the lid and dispose of the needle and syringe directly into a sharps container
- Wipe the port with alcohol-impregnated wipe
- Discard of clinical waste including gloves and apron according to trust policy
- Wash your hands

Post-procedure

- Document the date and time of the specimen taken on the request form and label according to trust requirements
- Dispatch for analysis to the appropriate laboratory
- Record the procedure in the child's nursing records (NMC, 2004)
- NB: *Bacterial colonisation of the urethra and the bladder is inevitable.* This will result in expected 'urine dip' reactivity for nitrite and possibly white blood cell reactivity. Treatment of a urinary tract infection is not indicated based on the 'urine dipstick' reactivity. Studies state that unless there are >10 white blood cells per high-power-field (HPF) or the child is having clinical symptoms of a catheter-associated infection, he or she should not be treated (Simpson, 2001)

Student skill laboratory activity

- ✓ Assemble equipment required for CSU.
- ✓ Practise the skill of inserting a needle into a catheter port.
- ✓ Withdraw a mock sample and transfer into a sterile container.

Emptying a catheter bag

The drainage bag should be emptied when more than half full but less than two-thirds full using standard precautions and a non-touch technique.

Reasons for the procedure

- To avoid opening the closed drainage system too frequently and introducing infection
- To avoid traction on the catheter leading to trauma of urethra and bladder neck from the weight of the drainage bag

Pre-procedure

Equipment

- Non-sterile gloves
- Apron
- Receptacle (sterile jug, cardboard urine bottle, bedpan, bowl)
- Paper towel to cover receptacle
- 70% alcohol-impregnated wipes

Specific patient preparation

- Inform child and parents of what you are about to do
- A play specialist might be of assistance here

During the procedure

- Wash hands
- Put on gloves and apron as standard precautions

- Clean catheter bag outlet with an alcohol wipe
- Empty urine into receptacle, taking care not to touch the exit port with the container (to avoid contamination of the exit port which might lead to ascending infection)
- Close the valve!
- Clean the outlet with a second alcohol wipe to minimise the risk of ascending infection
- Transport the urine container to the dirty utility room covered by a paper towel
- Measure urine in a jug
- Discard urine in the sluice
- Place a cardboard urine receptacle in the bedpan macerator or decontaminate, the plastic jug in the bedpan washer, and place in CSSD (central sterile supplies department) returns crate
- Remove gloves and apron and dispose of in clinical waste bin
- Wash hands

Post-procedure

- Record urine volume as required

Catheter removal

This is the removal of a specifically designed tube from the bladder through the urethra.

Reasons for the procedure

- To minimise infection – early removal of a catheter effectively minimises infection (NICE, 2003)

Pre-procedure

Equipment required

- Select syringe recommended by manufacturer (Luer lock or Luer tip)
- Non-sterile gloves
- Apron

Specific patient preparation

- Explain the procedure to the child and parents as appropriate (Department of Health, 2004)
- Ensure privacy (Department of Health, 2004)

- Read the manufacturer's instructions (MDA, 2000)

During the procedure

- Wash your hands, the single most important step in preventing the spread of infection
- Put on non-sterile gloves and apron
- Loosen the syringe plunger by moving it up and down in the syringe barrel
- Withdraw the syringe plunger 0.5 mL from the end of the barrel
- Attach the syringe:
  - Luer lock – insert and twist to lock
  - Luer tip – seat firmly, do not twist or force
- Allow water to come back by gravity. DO NOT aspirate the plunger. DO NOT cut off inflation port. Studies have demonstrated that aspiration by pulling on the syringe plunger may result in collapse of the inflation lumen, may encourage formation of creases, ridges, or cuffing at the balloon area, and may increase the catheter balloon diameter size on deflation (Robinson, 2003). This enlargement of the balloon area can result in difficult removal and urethral trauma
- Due to the small diameter of the inflation lumen, allow at least 30 seconds for the balloon to deflate
- If water does not return:
  - Re-position the child, upright, with legs dependent if possible
  - Ensure that the catheter is not in traction (balloon compresses at bladder neck)
  - Check to see if urine is free flowing in the tubing
  - Re-attach the syringe to the inflation port and wait for 5–30 minutes
  - Apply very gentle aspiration (forceful aspiration can collapse the inflation lumen)
  - Attempt to add 3–5 mL to the balloon
  - Cut inflation port valve. Catheter should start to fall out under gravity
  - If still unsuccessful, notify the doctor
- Once the expected amount has been removed from the balloon, slowly and smoothly remover the catheter
- Check the catheter tip for pus, encrustation or damage. If present, report to the doctor
- Make the child comfortable
- Empty urine from the collection bag into the sluice toilet, dispose of the urine bag and catheter followed by gloves and apron into the clinical waste bin
- Wash your hands

Post-procedure

- Inform the child and parent that it is not unusual to experience urgency, frequency and discomfort for 24 hours
- Request that the child uses a urine bottle, a bedpan in the toilet, or that the parents save the next three nappies for you to weigh (1 g = 1 mL)

- Record urine output, colour and nature of the first three urinations following removal of the catheter (Smith, 2003b)
- Also ask the child or parent to inform you if the child fails to void or develops abdominal pain immediately, as these measures assist in the early detection of urinary retention and/or infection

Obtaining a midstream specimen of urine

A midstream specimen of urine (MSU) is often taken following the detection of abnormalities from a ward urinalysis or when the child is exhibiting the signs and symptoms of a urinary tract infection. It is the most reliable non-invasive method but it may not be possible in very young children or those with special needs as it requires coordination and the ability to hold a urine stream mid-point once started. Theoretically, the specimen is less likely to be contaminated as the urethral area will have flushed through from the initial stream of urine (Higgins, 2000). If you are unable to obtain an MSU, discuss with doctors the risks and benefits of invasiveness and reliability of a suprapubic bladder aspiration (gold standard with 99% specificity) (Higgins, 2000) or a 'clean catch' specimen.

Reasons for the procedure

- To collect an uncontaminated urine specimen from a single void

Pre-procedure

Equipment required

- Sterile jug or cardboard receiver
- Sterile specimen pot
- Gloves
- Apron
- Microbiology form

Specific patient preparation

- Discuss with the child in an age/developmentally appropriate manner that it is important to catch the middle part of the urine flow from a single void

During the procedure

- Wash your hands
- Ask the child to wash his or her hands thoroughly with soap and hand-hot water first (it may be necessary to supervise this)
- Ask the child to cleanse his or her genitalia with soap and water and dry thoroughly (the same as they do when they wash normally) in order to minimise the risk of contamination prior to the collection of the specimen (Higgins, 2000)
- In order to prevent meatal contamination, ask girls to separate their labia while passing urine and ask boys to retract their foreskin
- Ask the child to pass urine into the toilet initially and then to hold it, then pass urine into the sterile jug or receiver, and then to hold it, and then complete voiding into the toilet
- Put on gloves and apron and decant urine from sterile container into the sterile specimen pot
- Discard the clinical waste, and gloves and apron into clinical waste receptacle
- Label the specimen container, dispatch to the microbiology laboratory immediately according to policy

Post-procedure

- Document the date and time of the specimen taken on the request form and label according to trust requirements
- Dispatch for analysis to the appropriate laboratory
- Record the procedure in the child's nursing records (NMC, 2004)

Student skill laboratory activity

✓ Identify the equipment that you would require to collect a midstream specimen of urine.
✓ Discuss strategies that you might suggest a child use to obtain the specimen accurately.

Obtaining a 'bag' specimen of urine

This is a method for getting a urine sample from an infant or child with special needs, who still requires a nappy, and with good skin integrity for testing purposes. Urine collection methods alter the diagnostic validity of urinalysis and these differences have important implications for the diagnostic and therapeutic management of children with suspected urinary tract infections. A suprapubic aspiration should be conducted by the doctor to secure a more reliable sample for microbiology: 99% specificity (McGillivray *et al,* 2005). A 'bag' collection is preferable to using an Ontex pad or cotton-wool balls in the nappy as the anti-flowback valve prevents skin irritation from urine and minimises contamination of the specimen (Rao *et al*, 2004).

Reasons for the procedure

- To collect urine specimen non-invasively
- To detect abnormalities using ward urinalysis
- To obtain a sample when an infant exhibits signs and symptoms of a urinary tract infection

Pre-procedure

- Assess skin integrity in the groin area – do not proceed if there is any evidence of potential or actual skin breakdown

Equipment required

- Appropriate size U-Bag (pre-term, infant, or paediatric) to avoid leakage or contamination with faeces (*Figure 14.2*)
- Nappy bowl with warm water
- Wipes
- Clean nappy
- Two pairs of non-sterile gloves
- Two aprons
- Waste bag
- Appropriate specimen container

Specific patient preparation

- Explain all procedures and care as in an appropriate way to the family and encourage parental participation to promote cooperation and understanding (NPSA, 2004)
- Consent should be obtained prior to the procedure from the infant's parent(s) (British Medical Association, 2001; Department of Health, 2001)

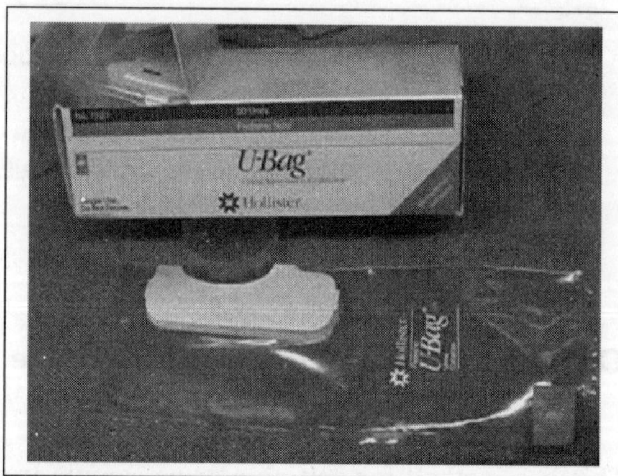

Figure 14.2: Urine collection device

During the procedure

- Wash hands
- Put on non-sterile gloves and apron
- Lay the infant on their back and socially wash, with warm tap water, each skinfold in the genital area. Wash around the anus last. The skin must be clean and dry: do NOT use oils, powders and lotions as these will leave a residue on the skin leading to sample contamination and interfere with the adhesives ability to stick
- Ensure that the skin surface is thoroughly dry before proceeding
- Remove the protective backing from the bottom half of the adhesive patch (It is easier to leave the top half of the adhesive covered until the bottom section has been applied to the skin)
- *For girls (Figure 14.3):*
  - Stretch the perineum to separate the skinfolds and expose the vagina
  - Apply the adhesive to the skin, starting at the narrow bridge of skin that separates the vagina from the anus (perineum), and working outward
- *For boys (Figure 14.4):*
  - Place the bag over the penis
  - Apply the adhesive to the skin starting at the narrow bridge of between the anus and the base of the scrotum (perineum) and work outward
- Press the adhesive firmly against the skin, avoiding wrinkles
- Once the bottom portion of the adhesive patch is in place, remove the paper backing from the upper portion
- Work upward to complete secure application
- For active infants, this procedure may take a couple of attempts (lively infants can displace the bag)
- Place a nappy securely over the bag

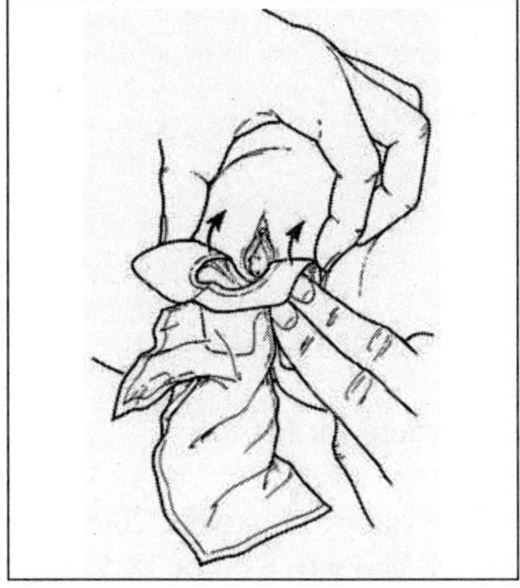

Figure 14.3: Applying a urine bag to a female infant

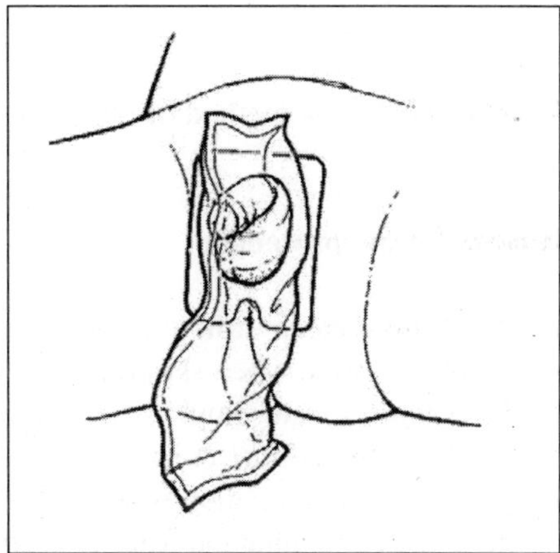

Figure 14.4: Applying a urine bag to a male infant

- Dispose of clinical waste appropriately and remove gloves and apron and discard in the clinical waste bin
- Wash hands
- Check nappies every 15 minutes so that the bag can be removed soon after the infant has urinated
- IMPORTANT! Do not leave a U-Bag on an for more than 1 hour (as per manufacturer's guidance regarding skin integrity)
- Apply gloves and apron
- Carefully and gently remove the bag by pressing the skin away from the adhesive, bit by bit
- Wash the genitalia and surrounding skin thoroughly to ensure removal of adhesive residue (may irritate the skin), dry and apply a clean nappy
- Tilt the bag to draw the urine away from the bottom corner and tear off the plastic cover over the port
- Pour the urine carefully into the specimen container
- Dispose of clinical waste, then gloves and apron appropriately
- Wash your hands

Post-procedure

- Document the date and time of the specimen taken on the request form and label according to trust requirements
- Dispatch for analysis to the appropriate laboratory
- Record the procedure in the child's nursing records (NMC, 2004)

Obtaining a 'clean catch' specimen of urine

A 'clean catch' is a method of obtaining a urine sample for urinalysis.

Reasons for the procedure

- To obtain a clean urine sample if the child does not require application of U-Bag
- To obtain urine when skin integrity precludes use of U-Bag
- To obtain a clean sample when suprapubic aspiration is not indicated for MC&S (microscopy, culture & sensitivity) (Bayer, 2002)
- To avoid contamination when cotton-wool balls are placed in the nappy (Boxwell, 2000)
- To avoid contamination from collection pads and because pads are bulky (6.5 cm × 18.5 cm) and should NOT be cut (Rao *et al*, 2004)

Pre-procedure

Equipment required

- Suitable receptacle
- Thumb or finger from a sterile, non-powdered glove (secured to the skin with yellow soft paraffin for a baby or infant)
- Cardboard receiver placed at end of the child's urethra to obtain a 'clean catch' of urine
- Cardboard urine bottle (for boys)
- Cardboard bedpan placed over the toilet (for girls)

Specific patient preparation

- Parental collaboration is essential for proper urine collection from their child
- Determine an collection method that is age/developmentally appropriate

During the procedure

- Carry out approximately 10 minutes after a feed or drink
- Wash hands
- Put on non-sterile gloves and apron
- Ask the child or parent to wash, with warm tap water, each skinfold in the genital area. Wash around the anus last. The skin must be clean and dry. Do NOT allow them to use oils, powders and lotions as these will leave a residue on the skin leading to sample contamination
- Either apply the glove finger, as above, or hold the receptacle in place, or ask the child to use the urine bottle or bedpan when ready
- You might need to use psychological aides if developmentally appropriate (running taps, blowing bubbles, music, or guided imagery)
- Check the receptacle every 15 minutes to remove the container soon after the child has urinated into it, so a fresh sample is obtained (Chon *et al*, 2001)
- Once a sample is obtained, congratulate the child and/or thank the parents for their assistance, make the child comfortable and transport the sample to the dirty utility room
- Test urine by the urinalysis procedure described below or decant into the specimen container as required
- Dispose of urine into the sluice toilet and the cardboard receptacle into the macerator
- Remove gloves and apron and dispose of in clinical waste bin
- Wash hands

Post-procedure

- Document the date and time of the specimen taken on the request form and label according to trust requirements
- Dispatch for analysis to the appropriate laboratory
- Record the procedure in the child's nursing records (NMC, 2004)

Urinalysis

This is testing of the physical characteristics and composition of freshly voided urine for abnormalities with reagent strips. The normal composition of urine (Higgins, 2000; Graham, 2002; Layton, 2003) is:

- 96% water
- 2% salt
- 2% urea (metabolic waste produced in liver)
- pH 4.6–8.0

This is an important non-invasive investigation. As urine culture results are not usually available before 24 hours after collection, empiric therapy is frequently started on the basis of urine screening tests (McGillivray *et al,* 2005).

Reasons for the procedure

- To screen for ill health (early indicator in children) (Liaw *et al*, 2000)
- To monitor the effectiveness of treatment (eg. glycosuria in diabetes mellitus)
- To establish a baseline

Pre-procedure

Equipment required

- Bottle of reagent strips (in date)
- Non-sterile gloves
- Apron

Specific patient preparation

- Obtain urine sample by an appropriate method and take to dirty utility room

During the procedure

- Wash hands (the single most important step in preventing the spread of infection)
- Put on gloves and apron
- Aspirate urine from cotton balls when wet with a syringe (0.1 mL is sufficient) and place on test stick or dip test stick in urine briefly
- Read the test stick after designated time (manufacturer's instructions) (*Figure 14.5*)

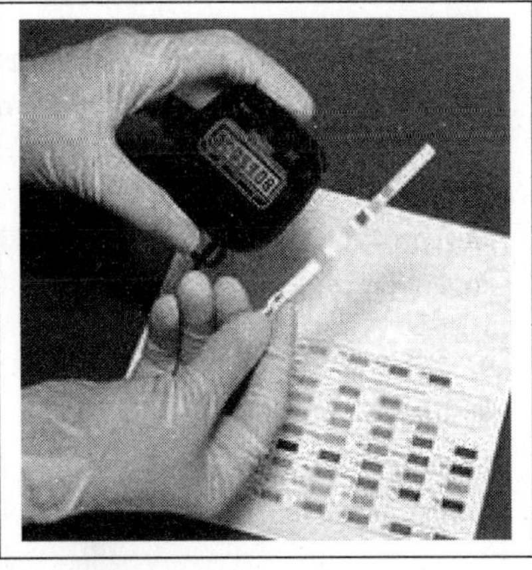

Figure 14.5: Urine testing: timing exposure of chemstick

Post-procedure

- Record the procedure and the analysis results and any pertinent observations of the urine for example odour in the child's nursing records (NMC, 2004) and be knowledgeable about the relevance of findings (see *Boxes 14.3* and *14.4*)

Box 14.3: Appearance and odour of urine and their common causes

Appearance

Colourless to slightly yellow, no sediment – Normal
Dark yellow – Metronidazole excretion
Dark yellow (froths when shaken) – Conjugated bilirubin
Red to brown – May contain haemoglobin or myoglobin
Red–orange – Rifampicin excretion
Amber – Carrots
Brown – Paracetamol poisoning
Smokey red – Intact red cells
Red – Beetroot
Brown to black – Inborn error of metabolism
Sediment – Presence of bacteria or blood cells

Odour

Odourless – Normal
Ammonia – Urinary tract infection
Acetone – Ketoacidosis

Box 14.4: Substances screened for during routine urinalysis, terminology of results and indications

Glucose	
Negative	Normal
Positive (glycosuria)	Diabetes mellitus Renal tubular disease (if absence of hyperglycaemia) Inadvertant IV dextrose overdose (neonate)
Blood	
Negative	Normal
Positive (haematuria)	infection Septicaemia Trauma post catheterisation Suprapubic bladder aspiration
Haemoglobin (Hb)	
Negative	Normal
Positive	Blood transfusion reaction Haemolytic anaemia
Ketones	
Negative	Normal
Positive (ketonuria)	Abnormal and increased breakdown of fatty acids Acute gastrointestinal disorders (eg. pyloric stenosis) Febrile illness (neonates) Inability to utilise insulin Excessive dieting/starvation
Bilirubin and urobilinogen	
Normal	0.1–1.0 EU/dL
Positive	>1.0 EU/dL Physiological jaundice (in days 4–7 of life) Pathological jaundice (liver disease, bile duct obstruction, excessive destruction of red blood cells)
False positive	Phenothiazides
White cells	
Negative	Normal
Positive	Bladder or renal tract infection Sepsis
Nitrates	
Negative	Normal
Positive	Presence of gram-positive bacteria (urinary tract infection) Indirectly (renal, bladder or genital abnormalities)

Proteins	
Negative	Normal
1 g/L (++)	Normal in first 48 hours of life
Positive (proteinuria)	Pregnancy
	Urinary tract infection, sepsis
	Cardiac failure
	Renal disease
Specific gravity	
1.005–1.020	Normal
<1.005	Intact renal function with high fluid intake, *or*
	– diabetes insipidus
	– acute tubular necrosis
	– pyelonephritis
1.010 (fixed, regardless of input or output)	Acute glomerulonephritis
	Severe renal damage
1.020	Nephrotic syndrome
	Dehydration
	Heart failure
	Shock
	Acute glomerulonephritis
	Liver failure
pH	
4.6–8	Normal
<4 (strong acid)	Dehydration
	Potassium depletion
	Ketoacidosis
>8 (strong alkali)	Alkalaemia due to vomiting
	Renal tubular necrosis
	Stale urine

References

Barber LA (2002) Clean technique or sterile technique? Let's take a moment to think. *J Wound Ostomy Continence* **29:** 29–32

Bayer PLG (2002) *Urine Analysis*. Bayer, Berkshire

Boxwell G (2000) *Neonatal Intensive Care Nursing*. Routledge, London

Breathnach AS (2005) Nosocomial infections. *Medicine* **33**(3): 22–26

British Medical Association (2001) *Consent, Rights and Choices in Health Care for Children and Young People*. BMJ Books, London

British National Formulary (2006) *British National Formulary for Children*. BMJ PublishingCompany, London

Carapeti EA, Andrews SM, Bentley PG (1996) Randomised study of sterile *versus* non-sterile urethral catheterisation. *Ann Roy Coll Surg Engl* **78:** 59–60

Chon DH, Frank CL, Shortliffe LM (2001) Pediatric urinary tract infections. *Pediatr Clin North Am* **48:** 1441–59

Cravens DD, Zweig S (2000) Urinary catheter management. *Am Fam Physic* **61**(2): 369–76

Department of Health (2003) *Winning Ways: Working Together to Reduce Healthcare-Associated Infection in England*. DH, London

Department of Health (2004) *National Service Framework for Children, Young People and Maternity Services*. DH, London

Department of Health and Hospital Infection Society (2001) Guidelines for preventing infections associated with the insertion of and maintenance of short-term indwelling urethral catheters in acute care. *J Hosp Infect* **47**(Suppl 1): S39–S46

Duggall H, Beaumont M, Jenkinson M (2002) *Infection Control: A Handbook for Community Nurses*. Whurr Publishing, London

Dunn S, Pretty L, Reid H, Evans D (2000) *Management of short-term indwelling urethral catheters to prevent urinary tract infections No. 6*. The Joanna Briggs Institute, Adelaide

EPIC (2001) Guidelines for prevention of infections associated with the insertion and maintenance of short term indwelling urethral catheters in acute care. *J Hosp Infect* **32**(3): 175–90

Filetoth Z (2002) *Hospital-Acquired Infection*. Whurr Publishing, London

Gerard LL, Cooper CS, Duethman KS, Gordley BM, Kleiber CM (2003) Effectiveness of lidocaine lubricant for discomfort during pediatric urethral catheterisation. *J Urol* **170**(2): 564– 67

Getliffe K (2003) Managing recurrent urinary catheter blockage: problems, promises and practicalities. *Wound Ostomy Continence* **30**(3): 146–51

Graham H (2002) Urine analysis in the neonate: An important diagnostic aid. *J Neonat Nurs* **8**(5): 151–54

Hanchett M (2002) Techniques for stabilizing urinary catheters. *Am J Nursing* **102**(3): 44–48

Higgins C (2000) *Understanding Laboratory Investigations: A Text for Nurses and Healthcare Professionals*. Blackwell Science, Oxford

Hilton P (2004) *Fundamental Nursing Skills*. Whurr Publishing, London

Jamieson EM, McCall JM, Whyte LA (2002) *Clinical Nursing Practice, 4th edn. Churchill Livingstone, Edinburgh*

Johnson JR, Kuskowski MA, Wilt TJ (2006) Systematic review: antimicrobial urinary catheters to prevent catheter-associated urinary tract infection in hospitalized patients. Ann Int Med **144**(2): 116–26

Lai K, Fontecchio S (2002) Use of silver-hydrogel urinary catheters on the incidence of catheter-associated urinary tract infections in hospital patients. *Am J Infect Cont* **30**(4): 221–25

Layton KL (2003) Diagnosis and management of pediatric urinary tract infections. *Clin Fam Pract* **5:** 2

Liaw LCT, Nayar DM, Pedler SJ, Coulthard MG (2000) Home collection of urine from infants by three methods: survey of parents' preferences and bacterial contamination rates. *BMJ* **320:** 1312–13

Maki DG, Tambyah PA (2001) Engineering out the risk of infection with urinary catheters. *Emerg Infect Dis* **7**(2): 342–47

McGillivray E, Mok E, Mulrooney M, Kramer A (2005) Head-to-head comparison: 'clean-void' bag versus catheter urinalysis in the diagnosis of urinary tract infection in young children. *J Pediatr* **147**(4): 451–56

McGrath JM (2006) Family presence during procedures: Breathing life into policy and everyday practices. *Newborn Infant Nurs Rev* **6**(4): 242–45

Medical Devices Agency (2000) *Single Use Medical Devices: Implications and Consequences of Reuse, DB2000(04)*. MDA, London

National Health and Safety Executive (2003) *Latex and You*. INDG320 C100 06/03. HSE, London

National Institute for Clinical Excellence (2003) *Prevention of Health-Associated Infection in Primary and Community Care*. NICE, London

Neil Weis BS, Van den Broek PJ (2004) Urinary catheter policies for long-term bladder drainage. *Cochrane Database* Syst Rev CD004201. Cochrane Library http://www.cochrane.org/reviews/en/ab004201.html

National Health and Safety Executive (2003) *Latex and You*. INDG320 C100 06/03. HSE, London

National Patient Safety Agency (2004) *Right Patient- Right Care*. NPSA, London

Nursing and Midwifery Council (2004) *Code of Professional Conduct*. NMC, London

Postlethwaite R, Webb N (2002) *Clinical Paediatric Nephrology*, 3rd edn. Oxford University Press, Oxford

Pratt RJ, Pellowe CM, Loveday HP, Robinson N, Smith GW (2001) Guidelines for preventing infections associated with the insertion and maintenance of short-term indwelling urethral catheters in acute care. *J Hosp Infect* **47**(Suppl): S39–S46

Rao S, Bhatt J, Houghton C, Macfarlane P (2004) An improved urine collection pad method: a randomised clinical trial. *Arch Dis Child* **89**(8): 773–75

Robinson J (2003) Deflation of a foley catheter balloon. *Nurs Stand* **17**(27): 33–38

Robinson J (2006) Intermittent self-catheterisation: principles and practice. *Br J Commun Nurs* **11:** 144–52

Simpson L (2001) Indwelling urethral catheters. *Nurs Stand* **15**(46): 47–55

Smith J (2003a) Indwelling catheter management: From habit-based to evidence-based practice. *Ostomy Wound Manag* **49**(12): 34–45

Smith L (2003b) Which catheter? Criteria for selection of urinary catheters for children *Paed Nurs* **15**(3): 14–18

Workman BA, Bennett CL (2003) *Key Nursing Skills*. Whurr Publishers, London

Useful websites

Minimizing the Trauma of Pediatric Urethral Catheterization Using Lidocaine Gel
www.uihealthcare.com/topics/medicaldepartments/urology/catheterization/index.html

University of Ottawa
intermed.med.uottawa.ca/procedures/ucath/images/perineum_of_female2.html
intermed.med.uottawa.ca/procedures/ucath/images/perineum_of_male_en.html

Chapter 15

Fundamental aspects of wound prevention and care

Marion Aylott and Helen Pearson

Wound prevention

Individualised wound prevention management begins with the process of a child-specific skin-risk assessment and preventive and therapeutic strategies to prevent wounds, such as pressure sores and epidermal stripping, and, if necessary, includes liaison with specialists in tissue viability, dermatology or infection control (National Institute for Clinical Excellence [NICE], 2001; 2003). Supracapillary pressures cause occlusion of the capillary bed. This pressure leads to the development of localised tissue ischaemia, leading to cellular death and tissue necrosis (Butler, 2006).

Skin integrity

Skin integrity is an established quality indicator of nursing care as part of clinical governance (Wilson, 1999). Breakdown in skin integrity represent a serious and often preventable problem in the paediatric acute care environment (Butler, 2006). The negative effect of immobility and physiological instability on a patient's skin does not discriminate with regard to age or developmental level (Diegelmann and Evans, 2004), and epidermal disruptions from medical devices, incontinence, wounds and therapies can leave the child susceptible to infection (Noonan *et al,* 2006).

Unique challenges present in the infant and child population due to their skin immaturity. In the adult population perinasal and peristomal skin compromise is not common (Ratcliffe *et al,* 2005; Robertson *et al,* 2005), but 27% of children with nasogastric tubes and ostomies had altered skin integrity (Carr *et al,* 2001, Noonan *et al,* 2006). The prevalence of epidermal stripping is between 8% and 17% (McLane *et al,* 2004). The prevalence of pressure ulcers in children ranges from 4% to 13% (Groenevald *et al,* 2004; McLane *et al,* 2004) as compared to a rate of up to 29.2% in adults (Curley *et al,* 2003), and different areas are susceptible to pressure ulcers in children. In infants and children, they are often found on the occiput, ears, sacrum and scapula (Amlung *et al,* 2001). Medical devices contribute to pressure-related injury in infants and young children (Curley *et al,* 2003) including a 9% incidence of pressure-related skin injury with the saturation probe. Further evidence of injury is reported relating to the following medical devices:

- Spinal immobilisation boards (Murdoch, 2002)
- Spinal braces (Hampton and Collins, 2003)
- Body casts (Wukich and Motko, 2004)
- Continuous positive airway pressure devices (Dixon and Ratcliffe, 2005)

Risk assessment and care

Research has demonstrated that children differ from adults in the anatomical sites of skin breakdown; however, treatment remains the same (Butler, 2006). Accurate assessment, documentation, prevention, and treatment are all key factors (White and Denyer, 2006). An abundance of nursing research exists in relation to skin breakdown prevention and management in adults, but little relates to children. The available literature on paediatric skin care has been based on adult research in an attempt to meet the special needs of the paediatric population.

Although there is a newly emerging awareness that acutely ill and immobilised infants and children are at risk for skin disruption due to pressure injury, there is a paucity of research data upon which to guide practice. Most prevention and treatment protocols are extrapolated from adult research findings and recommendations. Given the anatomical and physiological differences between adults and children, serious concerns arise regarding the safety, efficacy and effectiveness of adult studies. This guideline uses general principles arising from adult data and relates specifics that are underpinned by child-based evidence only.

Early intervention can be an effective preventative measure if patients at increased risk for pressure ulcer development are identified.

Reasons for the procedure

- To identify at-risk individuals
- To maintain and improve tissue tolerance to injury
- To protect against the adverse effects of pressure, friction, and shear

Identify at-risk individuals

- Limited information exists regarding the identification of risk factors associated with skin breakdown in the sick child in comparison to those found in the adult literature. However, risk factors that have been identified in the adult population include:
  - immobility
  - neurological impairment
  - impaired perfusion
  - decreased oxygenation

  - poor nutritional status
  - presence of infection
  - moisture
  - acidaemia
  - vasopressin therapy
  - surgery
  - hypovolaemia
  - weight
- Various tools exist for assessing adults, and the Braden scale (frequently used in adults) has been adapted into the Braden Q scale for paediatrics (Bedi, 1993) but it has not yet been validated
- The Paediatric Pressure Risk Assessment tool (*Box 15.1*) will help you to determine tolerance of the skin and supporting surfaces (including soft tissue) to endure the effects of pressure without incidence. It will also help you to identify factors that place a child at risk for pressure ulcer development (Barnes, 2004)
- Adequate involvement of the child, if possible, and the parents in treatment and prevention strategies is highly recommended; involving the child and parents can provide a sense of autonomy and empowerment in care

Maintain and improve tissue tolerance to injury

- Children must be given adequate nutrients to reduce the risk of developing pressure ulcers and to support healing. To achieve this, nutritional support should be designed to prevent or correct nutritional deficits, maintain or achieve positive nitrogen balance, and restore or maintain serum albumin levels. Nutrients that have received primary attention in the prevention and treatment of pressure ulcers include protein, arginine, vitamin C, vitamin A, and zinc (Novartis Nutrition Corporation, 2006)
- Maintain/assist the child in maintaining a good standard of personal hygiene. Moisture macerates the surrounding skin, causing superficial erosion of the epidermis. Primary sources of skin moisture include perspiration, urine, faeces, and drainage from wounds or fistulas

Protect against adverse effects of pressure, friction, and shear

- A turning schedule must be instituted immobile and unconscious children. Interventions to reduce pressure over bony prominences are of primary importance. A significant decrease in the incidence of occipital pressure ulcers was observed (16.9% to 4.8%) by instituting a prevention protocol of repositioning the head at least every 2 hours (Baldwin, 2002)
- Heels should be suspended off the bed using pillows or use heel-lift devices (Samaniego, 2003)
- The head of the bed should not be elevated for more than 2 hours to avoid shearing injury to the sacral area (Suddaby, 2005). A rolled-up blanket is always useful under the child's upper thighs, or the bottom of the bed can be elevated to reduce the chances of sliding down in the bed

- Airflow through the surface of a mattress reduces moisture and pressure for those at high risk (Bryant, 2000)
- Practice safe moving and handling (Smith, 2005) as skin is injured by friction
- Manual handling aids and devices such as hoists, transfer boards, or slide sheets may be useful adjuncts for minimising tissue injury
- The head of the bed must be lowered as much as can be tolerated before repositioning, to help minimise friction and shear (Smith, 2005)
- Mechanical injury from friction can be reduced by application of a barrier dressing, such as transparent films or hydrocolloids, over at-risk areas (Suddaby, 2005)
- Superficial skin damage can occur when adhesive products are used with any paediatric patient (the chronically ill and critically ill are at higher risk). A skin tear or epidermal stripping is a partial-thickness wound, with loss of the epidermis and possibly the dermis (Bryant, 2000), resulting from inadvertent removal of these layers by mechanical means (eg. tape removal). Use skin barrier protective films and pectin-based 'anchors' (like Granuflex dressing) to eliminate direct tape-to-skin contact when securing nasogastric tubes (Baharestani, 2007)
- Pressure injury can be caused by probes and blood-pressure cuffs applied tightly and/or left *in situ* for long periods; change probe and cuff sites at least every 4 hours (Baharestani, 2007)

Post-procedure

- Document assessment and care to aid consistency of care and communication between carers (Nursing and Midwifery Council [NMC], 2004)
- Carry out evaluation and audit in discussion with the child and parents to review wound-prevention approaches, including outcomes, the effectiveness of skin integrity management, and satisfaction of the child and parents (Tendra, 2005; White and Denyer, 2006)

Box 15.1 Paediatric pressure risk assessment tool (adapted from Bedi, 1993)

Build and weight for age (*average according to age*)	Above average	1
	Overweight	2
	Below average	3
Skin condition	Healthy	0
	Clammy (poor perfusion/pyrexial)	1
	Cannulation (intravenous/arterial)	1
	Dehydrated (dry skin/poor turgor)	2
	Poor perfusion	2
	Oedematous/discoloured	2
	Broken skin	3
Mobility	Full, normal for age	0
	Restless, wriggly	1
	Needs limited assistance	2
	Skeletal traction/plaster of Paris/splint	2
	Dependent on others	3
Appetite/nutrition	Normal for child	0
	Insufficient/gastric feeding	2
	Poor (eg. drinks little/IV fluids)	2
	No enteral nutrition	3
Elimination/nappy area	Completely continent	0
	Occasional incontinent/catheterised	1
	Frequently incontinent/nappy rash	2
	Fully incontinent	3
Drugs	IV antibiotics	1
	IV analgesia/sedation	2
	Cytotoxic drug therapy	3
	High-dose steroids/NSAIDs	3
Thermal injury	Lower body <2% ± upper body <8%	0
	General distribution 10–24%	1
	Lower body 3–24%	2
	Mainly upper body 25–35%	2
	Lower body >25% or generally >35%	3

TOTAL RISK SCORE:		**ACTION:**
Low risk 0–5	Assess every 3–5 days	Change child's position regularly; consider dietary intake
Medium risk 6–10	Assess daily	Consider position 2-hourly; diet; fluids; soft foam/airwave mattress
High risk 11–14	Assess 4-hourly/daily	Consider position 2-hourly; diet; fluids; airwave mattress; tissue viability specialist nurse
Very high risk >14	2-hourly pressure-area care	Diet; fluids; airwave mattress; tissue viability specialist nurse

Wound management

The recommendations within this procedure are based on the best available research evidence. However, research in this area is limited, based on single studies with limited sample size, largely of the adult population.

The wound management procedure includes:

- Wound assessment and documentation
- Taking a wound swab
- Wound cleansing
- Wound dressing

The goals of wound management in children are to:

- Promote healing
- Alleviate pain
- Lessen emotional distress
- Minimise scarring
- Decrease the risk of infection

Principles of asepsis and antisepsis

Antisepsis is the use of chemical solutions for disinfection; antisepsis does not imply sterility. The use of antiseptic solutions in wound cleansing is contraindicated as these solutions within a wound are carcinogenic (Humes and Lobo, 2005). Aseptic techniques are those aimed at the minimisation of cross infection during procedures. Infection control experts stress the importance of 'strict aseptic technique' for wound care. However, the concept of what is 'essential' for asepsis remains controversial (Barber, 2002). This finding reflects the paucity of research evidence currently available to support or refute the efficacy of these aseptic precautions. There is a real concern about using what is described as a 'clean' technique unless there is sufficient reliable data to show that it did not put the child at increased risk of infection. Currently, the best available evidence supports the use of hand-washing together with the practise of an aseptic non-touch technique (ANTT) as effective in reducing the incidence of healthcare associated wound infections (Breathnach, 2005).

Wound assessment and documentation

Most wounds, irrespective of the underlying cause, heal without difficulty. Normal wound healing is a well-orchestrated and complex series of events consisting of overlapping phases of inflammation, granulation, epithelialisation and remodelling (Leaper *et al,* 2002). Wound healing can be defined as 'the physiological process by which the body replaces and restores the function of damaged tissue' (Flanagan, 1996). The process of wound healing is a continuum and can take up to 2 years. However, the healing process can be impaired by many factors including infection or ischaemia, systemic factors such as malnutrition and diabetes, and factors specific to chronic wounds such as impaired growth-factor production and enzyme imbalance (Harding *et al,* 2002).

Nursing care must address both intrinsic and extrinsic factors contributing to wound healing; holism is the key (Casey, 1999; Russell, 2000). In order to make a decision about wound care, the nurse must consider the condition of the child, including their physical condition, age, all pertinent medical treatments, the location and characteristics of the wound (Worley, 2004).

Reasons for the procedure

Taking a wound swab

A sample of exudate is taken from a wound, placed in a medium, and sent to the microbiology laboratory with an appropriate form requesting 'microscopy, culture and sensitivity' (MC&S) (Hilton, 2004):

- To identify pathogenic bacteria within a wound
- To determine prescription and administration of appropriate antibiotics
- To assist in the choice and prescription of dressing

Wound cleansing

Fluids are used to remove loosely adherent debris and necrotic tissue from a wound surface:

- To create an optimal environment for wound healing
- To facilitate rapid wound healing

Wound dressing

A material covering is used that provides an optimal environment:

- To create an optimal environment for wound healing
- To promote rapid wound healing

Pre-procedure

In order to deliver wound management holistically the children and young peoples' nurse must draw on the principles of evidence-based practice, asepsis, integrated child-centred and family-centred care, pain assessment, respect and choice, maintaining a safe physical and psychological environment, and communication including the provision of information (Casey, 1999). Furthermore, parental involvement should be encouraged as wound care does not necessarily mean a hospital stay or an extended hospital stay (Duggall *et al,* 2002).

Atraumatic wound management

- Pain arising from wounds is multidimensional in nature. Nurses must consider a broad holistic approach to its management including good child-friendly psycho-emotional preparation, type of wound/skin condition, care setting, appropriate choice of dressing materials and adequate analgesia (Young, 2006)
- Administer adequate analgesia with sufficient time to reach a therapeutic level prior to wound care (Department of Health, 2004)
- If appropriate, consider the use of Entonox (Laterjet, 2002) (for more on administration of Entonox see *Chapter 7*)
- Avoid any unnecessary stimulus to the wound that is likely to cause pain (such as a draught from an open window)
- Read the manufacturer's instructions (and follow them) about techniques for removal of dressing *in situ* to avoid unnecessary manipulation of the wound and damage to delicate healing tissue (Hampton and Collins, 2003)
- Position the infant or negotiate with the child a position of comfort that enables the wound to be exposed at the same time as maintaining dignity
- Invite the child and/or parent to be involved as much as he or she wishes, perhaps removing the dressing themselves (Bale and Jones, 2006)
- Reassure the child that they will be given time to pace the procedure according to their preference. Inform them that if they are 'worried' they can stop the procedure for 'time out' either verbally or by clapping their hands or raising a finger. Enrol the assistance of a play specialist if appropriate (Department of Health, 2004)
- Select a dressing that you anticipate will address the most important factors for healing the wound concerned, while also considering the general health of the child (Casey, 2001)

Integrated child and family-centred care

Family presence during procedures is an emotionally charged topic. Research evidence advocates family-centred care and family presence during invasive or painful procedures has been found to be beneficial in alleviating distress in the child (McGrath, 2006). When parents choose to be partners in care-giving procedures, several steps are needed to be taken to ease their anxieties and provide them with opportunities to help the child overcome the procedure. Steps can be taken to facilitate parental participation in procedures:

- Before a procedure, give the parents information about what will happen during the procedure, what the child's likely responses will be and what their role should be
- Provide parents with ways to participate actively that make the process easier for all involved (talking, touching, comforting, soothing the child) while facilitating the procedure by holding the child still in an appropriate position. Encourage questions during this discussion

- Assess the parents' stability in being able to cope and be present for their child. Parental presence should not be forced; parents must also have an option to decline being present and to back-out without guilt. If parents decide not to be with their child during the procedure, they should still be fully informed about it. When the procedure is completed, they should be invited back to the bedside or treatment room to comfort their child. If parents decline to be present for a procedure, do not assume that this sets precedence; they must always be given the choice prior to each procedure
- Parents know their child best, and they should be asked to use this knowledge to participate in their child's distress and intervene appropriately
- Explain the procedure of wound care to the child in an age/developmentally appropriate manner. Discuss issues openly with the child and offer choices (the child might prefer a waterproof dressing to allow bathing or swimming). For adolescents, cosmetic acceptability of dressings will be important. However, consider younger children who may interfere with dressings; keeping them covered, under clothing or disguised, may help 'little pickers' to forget about the wound
- If available and appropriate utilise the help of the play specialist for preparatory play and distraction during the procedure

Informed assessment

Collect information prior to the procedure to limit unnecessary exposure of the wound regarding the following (Kumar and Leaper, 2005):

- History of the wound (cause, duration, overall health, ill health)
- Current medication (antibiotics, steroids, chemotherapy)
- Physical condition of the child (temperature, pulse, respirations)
- Type of wound (acute or chronic)
- Skin sensitivities or allergies
- Pain assessment

Equipment required

- Wound assessment chart or appropriate documentation
- Cleaned dressing trolley according to trust policy, usually hand-hot water and detergent and thorough drying (hospital setting), or other suitable clean and stable surface (such as a plastic tray placed on bedside table) (Workman and Bennett, 2003)
- Sterile wound pack containing gauze squares, plastic container, sterile towel (check in-date, aseptic sterilisation indicator, and if intact and dry)
- Appropriate dressing(s) if required (primary and secondary)
- Materials for securing dressing (tape, bandages)
- Clinical waste bag
- Warm (body temperature) potable water (suitable for drinking) or normal saline
- Sterile gloves (two pairs)
- Apron

- 10 mL syringe
- 22 G needle
- Sharps container
- Sterile wound swab and medium (for wound swab)
- Ampoule of sterile water (for wound swab)
- Sterile wound swab (for wound swab)
- Microbiology request form (for wound swab)

During the procedure

- If possible adjust the height of the bed, sit on a chair, or kneel on the floor to ensure a safe working environment (Smith, 2005)
- Wash hands and put on apron
- Set out equipment on trolley or other suitable surface
- Prepare a sterile field
- Hand your assistant the waste bag and ask them to attach this to the side of your trolley, nearest to the child, to avoid taking soiled material across the sterile field
- Put on gloves, invite the child and/or parent to remove the dressing themselves or remove dressings yourself and discard into a clinical waste bag
- Remove gloves and discard into clinical waste bag
- Wash hands and re-glove
- Using your Trust's wound assessment document or *Box 15.2* as a framework, assess the:
  - position of wound and dimensions (length, width, depth)
  - nature of wound (epidermal, dermal, subcutaneous)
  - appearance of wound tissue (*Box 15.3*)
  - condition of surrounding skin
  - nature of exudates (colour, consistency, amount, odour)
  - presence of infection
- Ask your assistant to check and document your assessment (NMC, 2004)

Box 15.2: Wound assessment

Appearance	1 – Necrotic (black) 2 – Slough (yellow) 3 – Infected (green) 4 – Granulating (red) 5 – Epithelialising (pink)
Size	Widest length Widest width Deepest depth

Exudate	Colour Consistency Amount
Infection	Surrounding skin hot to touch Inflammation of surrounding skin (redness, pain, swelling around the wound margin, evidence of pus, sometimes offensive odour) (Benbow, 2005) Swab taken Microbiology result
Pain	Score Analgesia given
Additional information	Parental information Distraction techniques Diagram in notes Photograph taken
Care given	Cleansing irrigation Choice of dressing

Box 15.3: Describing wound appearances

COLOUR	INDICATION
Black	Necrotic tissue which is dehydrated and needs to be debrided in theatre by a surgeon or by autolysis
Yellow	Can suggest infection if the yellow exudate is pus; or the yellow exudate may be slough which is composed of neutrophils that naturally infiltrate the wound to cleanse it of foreign particles before being phagocytosed by macrophages
Green	Infected pus often with offensive odour
Red	Presence of invading capillaries, giving the wound-bed a granular appearance; if traumatised they will bleed, indicating the presence of healing
Pink	Epithelisation of tissue growing in from the wound margins towards the centre of the wound

If a wound swab is indicated

- Ask your assistant to use an aseptic non-touch technique (ANTT) to open the swab packaging for you to retrieve the contents without contaminating your hands (Workman and Bennett, 2003)

- Identify where you will take the wound swab from; this should be an area of viable (pink) tissue where there are signs of infection
- Open the top of the swab packaging carefully
- Hold the swab packet in your non-dominant hand and undo the lid from the container holding the culture medium by twisting the top anticlockwise. Discard the lid with your dominant hand. Keep hold of the medium container ready to receive the swab
- Carefully remove the cotton-tipped swab from the swab packaging with you dominant hand
- Avoid accidentally contaminating the swab
- If the surface of the wound appears to be dry, first moisten the swab with sterile water to ensure sufficient organisms are obtained for culture (Irving, 2006)
- With the swab between your fingers, roll it with a rotating action gently across the surface of the wound
- Carefully and immediately place the wound swab in the medium container

If cleansing is required

- Place the sterile drape beside the wound, at its lowest point (irrigation fluid will drain to lowest point with gravity)
- Draw up 10 mL warm (body temperature) potable tap water or normal saline into the syringe (Fernandez *et al*, 2006). Use of cold fluid will suspend cell division until the wound has re-established body temperature (Jamieson *et al*, 2002)
- Attach a 22-G needle (this will give a pressure of 13 p.s.i. recommended for wound irrigation) (De Smet, 2006)
- Irrigate the wound starting in the cleanest area and ending in the dirtiest area, if possible (Dulecki and Pieper, 2005). Take care if the child is wriggly while you are armed with an unsheathed needle!
- Re-fill the syringe and continue irrigating until loosely adherent debris and necrotic tissue are removed from the surface of the wound
- Discard needle and syringe into sharps container immediately after use
- Apply an appropriate primary and secondary dressing if required (*Table 15.1*) that should maintain a moist environment, not cause maceration, maintain an optimum wound-bed temperature and pH (to allow healing to take place), be impermeable to pathogens, allow trauma-free removal, be contaminant free, require infrequent changes (to prevent tissue damage) and be cost-effective (Watson and Hodgkin, 2005; Krishnan, 2006)
- Remember to consider the site of the wound (a wound in the nappy region needs an impermeable dressing to prevent contamination by urine and faeces, and wounds across joints need a dressing that allows flexibility)
- Secure the dressing with tape or bandage as preferred

Post-procedure

- If appropriate, return the bed to a safe height (Smith, 2005)
- Make the child comfortable (NMC, 2004)

- Wrap all used disposable items in the sterile field and place them in disposable bag. Discard in the clinical waste receptacle (Hilton, 2004)
- Remove apron and gloves and wash hands (Hilton, 2004)
- Clean trolley or chosen home surface with hand-hot water and detergent
- If taken, label the wound swab and microbiology form, including date and time it was taken, and send to microbiology laboratory according to local procedure (Filetoth, 2002)
- Document assessment and care to aid consistency of care and communication between carers (Benbow, 2005)
- Perform evaluation and audit in discussion with the child and parents to review wound management approaches, including outcomes, effectiveness of pain management, and child and parent satisfaction (White and Denyer, 2006; Tendra, 2005)

Wound dressing

Primary wound dressings for different wound types are shown in *Figure 15.1* and *Table 15.1* describes the pros and cons of different types of wound dressings.

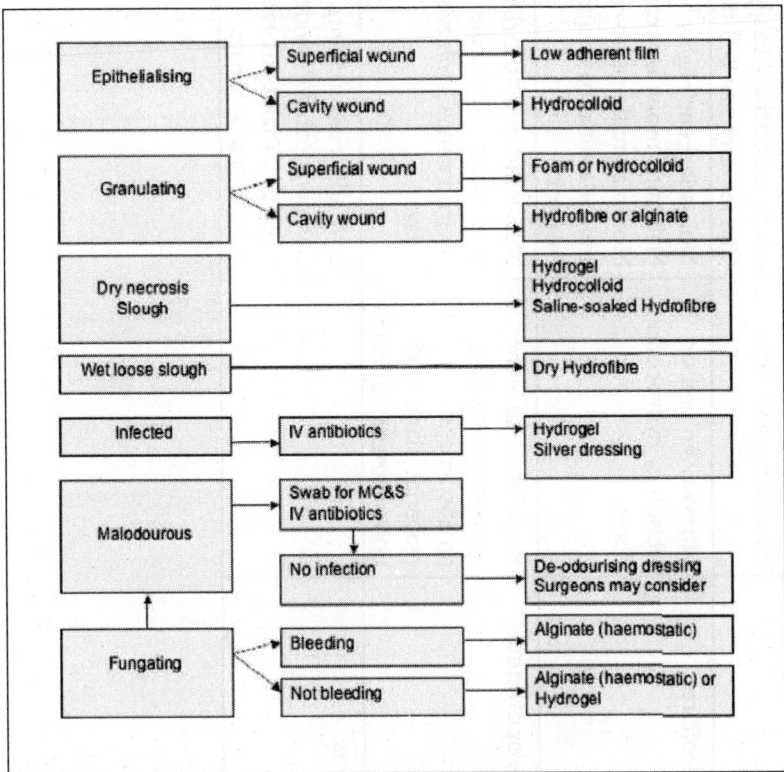

Figure 15.1: Primary wound dressing for different wound types

Table 15.1 Wound dressing selection

Wound dressing	Description	Advantages	Limitations
Hydrocolloid	Wafer dressing with microgranular suspension of pectin or gelatine polymers	Absorb exudate/Waterproof outer layer/Gas permeable/Permeable to moisture and micro-organisms	Over-use may lead to over-granulation
Hydrogels	Sheet or gel of insoluble polymers	Rehydrates/Debrides/Absorbs exudate/Soothing/Easily removed/Can leave *in situ* 2–3 days	Not for massively exudative wounds/Watch out for maceration to surrounding skin
Hydrofibres	Non-woven pad or ribbon of hydrocolloid fibres	Non-adherent/Highly absorbent/Maintains moist environment/Non-traumatic removal/Debrides and cleans necrotic and infected wounds	Not for infected wounds/Watch out for maceration to surrounding tissue
Hydropolymers	Perforated ethylene acrylate enveloping an absorbent material island with polyurethane backing	Non-adherent/Absorbs low-level exudate/Provides moist environment/Can leave *in situ* up to 7 days	Not for clinically infected wounds/Not for shallow granulating wounds/Not for light to moderately exudative wounds
Foams		Low adherence/Highly absorbent/Gas permeable/Provides thermal insulation/Maintains moisture/Can leave *in situ* 3–5 days	Not for highly exudative cavities/Not for hard black necrotic wounds

Wound dressing	Description	Advantages	Limitations
Films	Thin polyurethane membrane with either vinyl or acrylic adhesive backing	Vapour permeable/Hypoallergenic/Transparent (permits constant observation)/Non-absorbent/Impermeable to water and micro-organisms/Provides warm and moist environment/Suitable for superficial clean wounds/Can provide prophylaxis of friction damage/Can provide intravenous or intra-arterial catheter fixation/Can Leave *in situ* up to 7 days	Not for shallow wounds/Not for superficial skin loss (eg. intravenous cannula sites)/Not for exudate or infected wounds/Requires waterproof secondary dressing
Alginate	Flat sheet, ribbon, strip or rope manufactured from seaweed	Highly absorbent/Conforms to shape of wound/Haemostatic/Provides warmth and moisture/Easily removed by irrigation with saline/Can leave *in situ* 3–5 days/Recommended for infected wounds	Not for full-thickness burns/Not for pre-term neonates (absorbs calcium)/Little benefit for dry wounds and black eschar (activity depends on presence of wound exudate/fluid)/Requires secondary dressing to keep in place
Collagen	Gel, paste, powder or pad derived from bovine, porcine or avian collagen	Accelerates wound repair/Good for recalcitrant wounds (those not responding to treatment or that appear to have stalled in the wound-healing process)	Not for full-thickness burns/Bovine collagen contraindicated in persons with sensitivities/Requires a secondary dressing/Unpleasant odour

Wound dressing	Description	Advantages	Limitations
Silicone	Flexible polyamide net coated with soft silicone	Porous/Semi-transparent/Low adherence/Slightly tacky silicone coating facilitates application and retention of dressing to peri-wound area/Prevents maceration by inhibiting lateral movement of exudates onto surrounding skin/Current preferred burn-injury dressing because non-adherent and prevents cell invasion while allowing exudate through to a secondary dressing (like a one-way nappy liner)/Removed with minimal discomfort	Expensive!
Paraffin impregnated	Cotton or viscose gauze impregnated with paraffin	Low adherence (as long as dressing does not dry out)/Provides moisture/Can leave *in situ* up to 7 days	Not for shallow granulating wounds/Not for mild to moderate exudative wounds/Not for infected wounds
Antiseptic dressings	Cotton gauze impregnated with antiseptics	Was a popular adjunct to systemic antibiotic therapy for infected wounds	Iodine products contraindicated (retard healing due to cytotoxic effects on fibrocytes and inhibit epithelialisation) (Gilchrist, 1997)/Chlorhexidine products contraindicated (carcinogenic when used directly on wound surface) (Leaper *et al*, 2002)
Odour-reducing dressings	Cotton bandages impregnated with charcoal between the layers	Good for fungating, infected and gangrenous wounds where mal-odour is a problem	Should NOT be cut into because charcoal fibres may shed into the wound
Simple dry dressings	Knitted viscose and polyester fabric	Semi-adherent due to built-in perforations/Good for Superficial clean wounds/Good for dry wounds usually over joints that require padded protection (elbows and knees)	Not for even slightly exudative wounds due to adherence/Does not provide a moist healing environment

Wound dressing	Description	Advantages	Limitations
Simple dry gauze	Knitted cotton fabric	Adherent/Absorbent	Suitable as secondary dressing/NOT to be used as primary dressing due to adherence/Does not provide a moist healing environment
Biological dressings	Larvae of the common green bottle fly (*Lucilia sericata*) bred in sterile conditions	Larvae are necrophagus (avoid healthy, viable tissues)/Larvae have direct antibacterial activity/Can leave *in situ* 3 days/Effective for sloughing and necrotic wounds	Causes physical discomfort, transient pyrexia, and bleeding (rare)/ Contraindicated in wounds that connect with body cavities
Silver-containing dressings	Cotton bandage impregnated with silver	Absorbs and interacts with wound exudate to form soft, hydrophilic, gas-permeable gel that traps bacteria and conforms to wound contours/Broad antibacterial spectrum/Good for exuding lesions including infected wounds, heavily colonised wounds partial-thickness burns, and most other granulating wounds/Good for ribbon packing of deeper cavity wounds and sinuses/ Successful treatment of methicillin-resistant *Staphylococcus aureus* (MRSA)/Easy to apply/Easy to remove (no pain or trauma)/Leaves minimal residue on wound	Causes hypersensitivity reaction in some (although supposedly designed to be hypoallergenic)/Expensive/No known contraindications to use of Aquacel Ag, but dressing of little value if applied to wounds that are very dry or covered with hard black necrotic tissue

Student skill laboratory activity

- ✓ Prepare a trolley ready to undertake an aseptic wound dressing change and wound swab.
- ✓ Identify the equipment required to take a wound swab.
- ✓ Practice taking a wound swab on a mannequin.
- ✓ Perform a simple dressing change on a mannequin.

Intravenous cannula-site assessment

An intravenous (IV) cannula is a small plastic tube inserted into a vein for the direct administration of continuous or intermittent intravenous fluids and medications by a registered nurse who has undergone additional training. However, it is the responsibility of the nurse caring for the child to observe and monitor the intravenous fluid delivery and skin integrity.

> *It is recommended that IV cannula sites with continuous infusions are assessed at least every hour in children (4 hourly for adults) (RCN, 2003) and that IV cannula sites being used for administration of intermittent medications is assessed at least 8 hourly (Smith* et al, *2004).*

Reasons for the procedure

Intravenous cannulae offer direct access to the vascular system, but they also provide a route of entry for microorganisms – a potential cause of serious illness. Although intravenous cannulae are a necessary part of treatment, the cannulae is introduced through a break in the skin, one of the body's natural defences against infection. Other cannula-related complications that can occur, with or without fever or bacteraemia, are described below:

- **Cellulitis** is warm, erythematous and often tender skin that surrounds the site of cannula insertion
- **Phlebitis** is indicated by the presence of acute inflammation of the vein wall and characterised by proximal skin redness (erythema), heat, swelling and pain around the cannula entry site. It causes discomfort, and often precedes or is associated with more severe infections. It is most commonly caused by mechanical trauma resulting from the cannula rubbing against the lumen of the vein, or by chemical irritation brought on by the infusion fluid
- **Thrombophlebitis** is inflammation of the vein with accompanying clot formation. Early detection is essential as the clot can detach, become mobile emboli and travel around the body. The vein is often turgid and feels 'corded' when palpated. Tracking may be evident (red lines running away from the infusion site)

- **Purulent thrombophlebitis** is seen as warm, erythematous skin over an indurated or tender vein with purulent drainage from the cannula wound. Pus may drain spontaneously or may be expressed with pressure. This infection is dangerous and frequently leads to bacteraemia
- **Extravasation/infiltration** results when the tube is accidentally dislodged from the vein into the tissues (due sometimes to 'fiddling fingers') and causes the leakage of infusion fluid into the surrounding tissues. It occurs when the cannula punctures the vein wall. This *extravasation* (more commonly known as *infiltration*) is painful and is commonly referred to as 'tissuing'. It may also occur as a result of venospasm caused by chemical irritation. Swelling at the insertion site is the most obvious effect, but other signs include blanching and cooling of the skin, limited movement and discomfort
- **Leakage** results when connections between the cannula hub and intravenous giving set become loose, causing leakage and loss of fluid or medication

Complications

- Cellulitis
- Phlebitis
- Extravasation
- Disconnection
- Pain/discomfort
- Trauma
- Thrombophlebitis
- Purulent thrombophlebitis

Pre-procedure

Equipment required

- Non-sterile gloves

Specific patient preparation

- Inform the child and/or parents in an age/developmentally appropriate way what you are intending to do and why, to gain consent and assistance (NMC, 2004)
- Plan distraction therapy and/or play ahead of task if deemed necessary (2004 National Service Frameworks)
- Swaddle infants aged less than 1 year with limb with IC cannula device accessible as this helps the infant to self-soothe (Lissauer and Fanaroff, 2006)

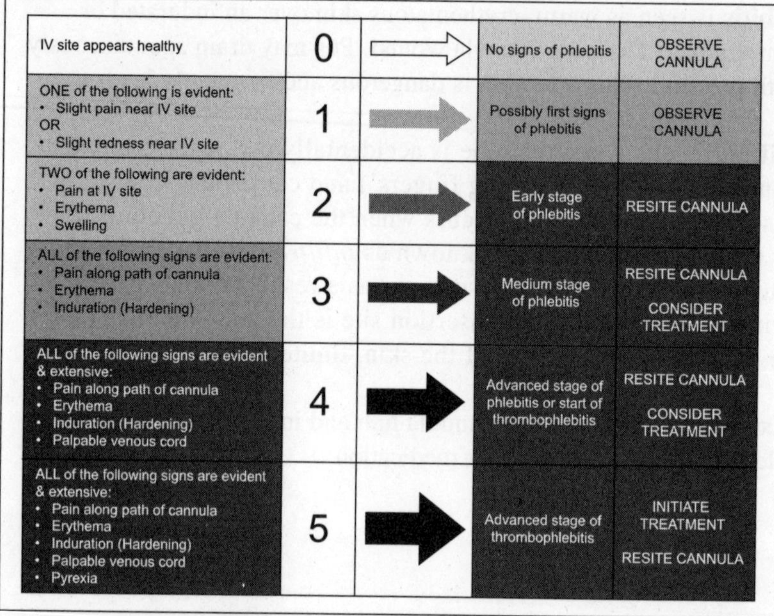

IV site appears healthy	0	→	No signs of phlebitis	OBSERVE CANNULA
ONE of the following is evident: • Slight pain near IV site OR • Slight redness near IV site	1	→	Possibly first signs of phlebitis	OBSERVE CANNULA
TWO of the following are evident: • Pain at IV site • Erythema • Swelling	2	→	Early stage of phlebitis	RESITE CANNULA
ALL of the following signs are evident: • Pain along path of cannula • Erythema • Induration (Hardening)	3	→	Medium stage of phlebitis	RESITE CANNULA CONSIDER TREATMENT
ALL of the following signs are evident & extensive: • Pain along path of cannula • Erythema • Induration (Hardening) • Palpable venous cord	4	→	Advanced stage of phlebitis or start of thrombophlebitis	RESITE CANNULA CONSIDER TREATMENT
ALL of the following signs are evident & extensive: • Pain along path of cannula • Erythema • Induration (Hardening) • Palpable venous cord • Pyrexia	5	→	Advanced stage of thrombophlebitis	INITIATE TREATMENT RESITE CANNULA

Figure 15.2: Visual infusion phlebitis (VIP) score (reprinted with the permission of Southampton University Hospital Trust)

During the procedure

- If possible, adjust the height of the bed, or sit on a chair or kneel on the floor to ensure a safe working environment (Smith, 2005)
- Wash hands and put on gloves
- Remove any bandages or clothes obscuring vision of the cannula site
- At the interval recommended, or when indicated by the patient's complaints or behaviour, check the cannula site for infiltration (extravasation), phlebitis (*Figure 15.2*), or signs of infection, and equipment integrity
- Assess the cannula site from its entry point (break in the skin) upwards; this evaluation should include gentle palpation of the insertion site through the intact dressing and visual inspection through the transparent dressing for the following signs (Clark, 2007):
  - appropriateness of dressing
  - integrity and cleanliness of dressing
  - leakage of fluid
  - redness
  - induration of vein
  - warmth
  - tenderness
  - itching or other irritation
  - oedema (due to extravasation of fluid)

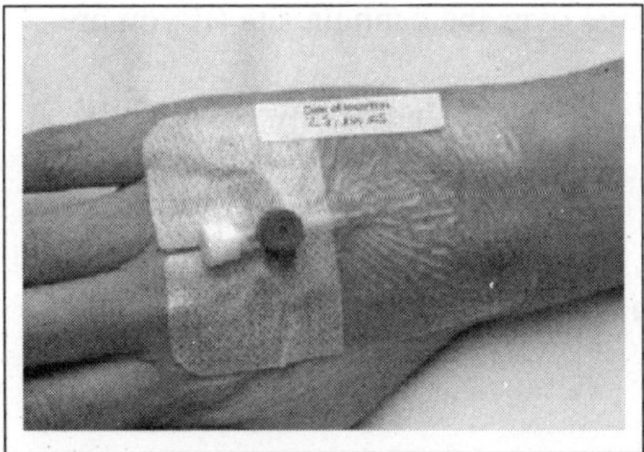

Figure 15.3: Label showing age of cannula

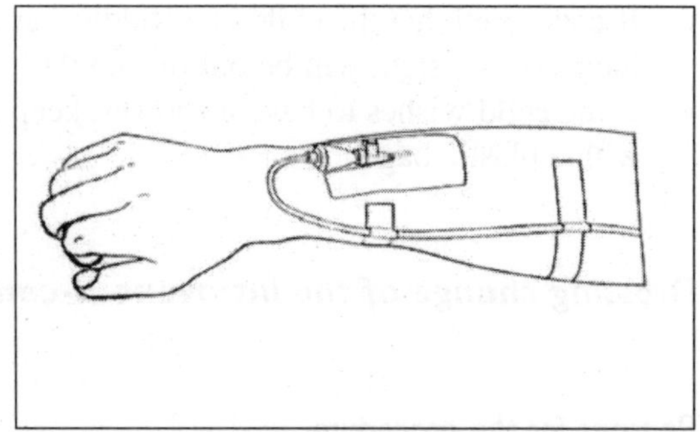

Figure 15.4: Securing IV administration tubing

- Some units use a scoring system to help evaluate the cannula site (*Box 15.2*)
- Consider the above in the light of the child's systemic temperature
- If you are unable to observe the site reliably inform a registered nurse who is 'IV trained' or a doctor who will need to re-dress the cannula site with an appropriate transparent dressing
- If the dressing is damp, loose or dirty, or there are signs of inflammation or extravasation, or the pump is alarming or the child is complaining of disproportionate pain (cannulae can be uncomfortable) inform a registered nurse who is 'IV trained' or a doctor immediately
- Check the date and time of insertion on the paper label secured to the edge of the IV dressing (*Figure 15.3*). If, according to the label, the cannula has been *in situ* for 72 hours inform a registered nurse who is 'IV trained' or a doctor that the cannula is 72 hours old and needs replacing
- If an infusion is running, secure the tubing of the administration set to prevent pulling and accidental dislodgement of the cannula (*Figure 15.4*). If this has already been done, check the skin integrity around the tape for inflammation or irritation
- You may consider, by observing the child's behaviour, that there is a risk of trauma to the vein caused by traction on the cannula. Application of a secondary dressing such a gauze padding and/or a bandage can significantly reduce this risk
- If appropriate, return the bed to a safe height (Smith, 2005)
- Make the child comfortable (NMC, 2004)
- Remove gloves and wash hands (Hilton, 2004)

Post-procedure

- Document assessment and care to aid consistency of care and communication between carers (Benbow, 2005)
- If appropriate, and using age-appropriate language, ask the child to let you know straight away if they feel any burning or pain sensation at the site
- Inform the child (if appropriate) in an age/developmentally appropriate manner not to fiddle with the cannula as this will get germs in it and make it sore

- If concerned that the child is a 'fiddler' apply a bandage over the cannula site (if you are lucky, out of sight will be out of mind!)
- If the child wishes to have a shower, keep the cannula site clean and dry by covering it with a plastic bag

Dressing change of the intravenous-cannula site

Reasons for the procedure

Complete site care should be performed when an IV device dressing is not dry, clean and securely intact. This is an aseptic non-touch technique (Barber, 2002).

Complications

- Introduction of infection
- Accidental dislodgement of the cannula

Pre-procedure

Equipment required

- Disposable towel or Incontinence pad
- Cleansing agent such as Steret (aqueous chlorhexidine for pre-term neonates; Boxwell, 2001)
- Transparent IV dressing
- Gloves (two pairs)
- Disposable apron
- Alcohol hand gel
- A 'second pair of hands'
- Clinical waste bag (small)

Specific patient preparation

- Inform the child and/or parents in an age/developmentally appropriate way as to what you are intending to do and why, to gain consent and assistance (NMC, 2004)
- It is best if this is a two-nurse procedure with mobile children (preferably where one nurse has performed this procedure before)
- Plan distraction therapy and/or play ahead of task (NSF, 2004)
- Swaddle infants under 1 year of age with limb with IV cannula accessible as this helps the infant to self-soothe (Lissauer and Fanaroff, 2006)

During the procedure

- Gather equipment and supplies to avoid unnecessary interruptions in the procedure (Millam, 2000)
- Wash hands (both nurses)
- Put on gloves and apron (both nurses)
- Explain the procedure again to the child and emphasise the importance of remaining still throughout to prevent dislodgement of the cannula
- Protect the area under the arm with a disposable towel or Inco-Pad to collect any spillage
- Ask your 'helper' to hold the cannula securely in place while you remove the old dressing carefully and dispose of into clinical waste bag
- Remove gloves, cleanse hands with alcohol hand-rub and put on new gloves (Breathnach, 2005)
- Cleanse the insertion site and surrounding area with a cleansing agent (as advised by local policy) and allow time to dry (Barber, 2002). If pus or exudate is present, the cannula should be removed (see next procedure)
- Apply the new dressing, taking care not to touch the part that will be directly over the insertion site (Barber, 2002)
- If an infusion is running, secure the tubing of the administration set to prevent pulling and accidental dislodgement of the cannula (Hampton and Collins, 2003)
- Dispose of soiled dressing and other waste correctly
- Remove gloves and wash hands

Post-procedure

- Make the child comfortable
- Document the care and report any abnormalities

Removing an IV cannula

Reasons for the procedure

- To discontinue therapy
- To remove because of complication such as phlebitis or extravasation

Complications

- Trauma
- Introduction of infection

Pre-procedure

Equipment required

- Sterile gauze pads (2 × 2 inches)
- Tape
- Gloves
- Disposable apron

Specific patient preparation

- Inform the child and parents in an age/developmentally appropriate way as to what you are intending to do and why, to gain consent and assistance (NMC, 2004)
- Plan distraction therapy and/or play ahead of task
- Swaddle infants under 1 year of age with limb with IV cannula accessible as this helps the infant to self-soothe (Lissauer and Fanaroff, 2006)

During the procedure

- Gather equipment and supplies to avoid unnecessary interruptions in procedure (Millam, 2000)
- Wash your hands
- Put on gloves and apron
- Explain the procedure again to the child and emphasise the importance of remaining still to prevent discomfort/pain
- Protect the area under the arm with a disposable towel or Incontinence pad to collect any spillage
- Turn off IV extension clamp, if present, to prevent fluid running out onto the child and you
- Loosen the dressing and tape, by peeling the edges back toward the puncture site to minimise trauma to the puncture site (Benbow, 2005)
- Stabilise the cannula while removing the dressing and tape to prevent unnecessary movement that could injure the vein (Hampton and Collins, 2003)
- Hold sterile gauze over the site and remove the cannula carefully and smoothly, keeping it almost flush with the skin. CAUTION! Do not press down on top of the cannula point while it is still in the vein (Diegelmann and Evans, 2004)
- Quickly press a sterile pad over the puncture site, and hold firmly until the bleeding stops (usually 1–2 minutes)
- If, for example, the cannula site is in the back of the hand or arm, elevate the arm to reduce venous pressure and help collapse the vein to facilitate clot formation. Do not bend the arm at the elbow as this causes haematoma formation (Diegelmann and Evans, 2004)
- Observe site for redness, swelling or haematoma
- Dispose of equipment, apron and gloves according to trust policy
- Apply clean pad with tape or a plaster as required
- Wash your hands

Post-procedure

- Check the site for bleeding, redness, swelling or haematoma 15 minutes after removal and report any abnormalities (Smith *et al*, 2004)
- Document care (NMC, 2004)

Student skill laboratory activity

✓ Familiarise yourself with different IV cannula and the IV dressings available.
✓ Place a cannula in a 'wound sponge' and apply the IV dressing so that you can observe the tip of the cannula site.

References

Amlung SR, Miller WL, Bosley LM (2001) The 1999 National Pressure Ulcer Prevalence Survey: A benchmarking approach. *Adv Skin Wound Care* **14:** 297–301

Baharestani MM (2007) Pressure ulcers in neonates and children: An investigation of the problem. *Adv Skin Wound Care*. www.medworm.com/rss/medicalfeeds/conditions/Pressure-Sores.xml

Baldwin KM (2002) Incidence and prevalence of pressure ulcers in children. *Adv Skin Wound Care* **15**(3): 121–24

Bale S, Jones V (2006) *Wound Care Nursing: A Patient-Centred Approach*, 2nd edn. Elsevier, London

Barber LA (2002) Clean technique or sterile technique? Let's take a moment to think. *J Wound Ostomy Continence Nurs* **29:** 29–32

Barnes S (2004) The use of a pressure ulcer risk assessment tool for children. *Nurs Times* **100**(14): 56–58

Bedi A (1993) A tool to fill the gap: Developing a wound risk assessment chart for children. *Prof Nurs* **9**(2): 112–20

Benbow M (2005) *Evidence-Based Wound Management*. Whurr Publishing, London

Boxwell G (2001) *Neonatal Intensive Care Nursing*. Routledge, London

Breathnach AS (2005) Nosocomial infections. *Medicine* **33**(3): 22–26

Bryant RA (2000) *Acute and Chronic Wounds: Nursing Management*, 2nd edn. Elsevier, Basingstoke

Butler TC (2006) Pediatric skin care: Guidelines for assessment, prevention and treatment. *Pediatr Nurs* **32** (5): 443–50

Carr M, Poje C, Kingstone L, Kielma D, Heard C (2001) Complications of pediatric tracheostomy. *Laryngoscope* **111:** 1925–28

Casey G (1999) Wound management in children. *Paediatr Nurs* **11**(5): 39–44

Casey G (2001) Wound dressings. *Paediatr Nurs* **13**(4): 39–42

Clark A (2007) *The Nursing Management of Intravenous Drug Therapy*. www.internursecom/cgi-bin/gopl/library/articlecgi?uid=5963;article=BJN_6

Curley MAQ, Quigley SM, Lin M (2003) Pressure ulcers in pediatric intensive care: Incidence and associated factors. *Pediatr Crit Care Med* **4:** 284–90

Curley MA, Razmus IS, Roberts KE, Wypij D (2003) Predicting pressure ulcer risk in pediatric patients: the Braden Q scale. *Nurs Res* **52:** 22–33

De Smet K, van den Plas D, van Hoomissen C, Jansens H, Sollie P (2006) Study of the environmental effect of a commercial wound cleanser used with different mechanical forces. *J Hosp Infect* **64:** 264–70

Diegelmann RF, Evans MC (2004) Wound healing: an overview of acute, fibrotic and delayed healing. *Front Biosci* **9:** 283–89

Dixon M, Ratcliffe C (2005) Pediatric pressure ulcers: One hospital's experience. *Ostomy Wound Manag* **51:** 44–46;48–50

Department of Health (2004) *National Service Framework for Children Young People and Maternity Services*. DH, London

Duggall H, Beaumont M, Jenkinson M (2002) *Infection Control: A Handbook for Community Nurses*. Whurr Publishing, London

Dulecki M, Pieper B (2005) Irrigating simple acute traumatic wounds: a review of the current literature. *J Emerg Nurs* **31**(2): 156–60

Fernandez R, Griffiths R, Ussia C (2006) Water for wound cleansing. *Cochrane Database for Systematic Reviews,* Issue 4, Art. No. CD003861. DOI: 10.1002/14651858.CD003861.

Filetoth Z (2002) *Hospital-Acquired Infection*. Whurr Publishing, London

Flanagan M (1996) A practical framework for wound assessment 1. Physiology. *Br J Nurs* **5**(22): 139–47

Gilchrist B (1997) Should iodine be reconsidered in wound management? *J Wound Care* **7:** 10–20

Groenevald A, Anderson M, Allen S, Bressmer S, Goldberg M, Magee B (2004) The prevalence of pressure ulcers in a tertiary care pediatric and adult hospital. *J Wound Ostomy Continence Nurs* **31:** 108–20

Hampton S, Collins F (2003) *Tissue Viability: A Comprehensive Guide*. Whurr Publishing, London

Harding KG, Morris HI, Patel GK (2002) Healing chronic wounds. *BMJ* **324:** 160–63

Hilton P (2004) *Fundamental Nursing Skills*. Whurr Publishing, London

Humes D, Lobo DN (2005) Asepsis, antisepsis and skin preparation. *Surgery* **23**(8): 297–98

Irving V (2006) Wound care for preterm neonates. *Infant* **2**(3): 102–06

Jamieson EM, McCall JM, Whyte LA (2002) *Clinical Nursing Practice,* 4th edn. Churchill Livingstone, Edinburgh

Jones I, Tweed C, Marron M (2001) Pressure-area care in infants and children: Nimbus Paediatric System. *Br J Nurs* **10**(12): 789–95

Krishnan P (2006) The scientific study of herbal wound healing therapies: current state of play. *Curr Anaesth Crit Care* **17:** 21–27

Kumar S, Leaper DJ (2005) Classification and management of acute wounds. *Surgery* **23**(2): 47–51

Laterjet J (2002) The management of pain associated with dressing changes in patients with burns. *World Wide Wounds.* www.worldwidewoundscom/2002/november/Latarjet/Burn-Pain-At-Dressing-Changes/html

Leaper D, Paggi B, Compton GA, Orsted H, Teot L, Ockenfeis HM (2002) Growth factors and interactive dressings in wound repair. *Eur Wound Manag Assoc J* **2**(2): 17–23

Lissauer T, Fanaroff A (2006) *Neonatology at a Glance.* Blackwell Publishing, Oxford

McGrath JM (2006) Family presence during procedures: Breathing life into policy and everyday practices. *Newborn Infant Nurs Rev* **6**(4): 242–45

McLane KM, Bookout K, McCord S, McCain J, Jefferson LS (2004) The 2003 national paediatric pressure ulcer and skin breakdown prevalence survey: A multi-site survey. *J Wound Ostomy Continence Nurs* **31:** 168–78

Millam DA (2000) On the road to successful IV. *Nursing* **30**(4): 34–48

Murdoch V (2002) Pressure care in the paediatric intensive care unit. *Nurs Stand* **17:** 71–74; 76

National Institute for Clinical Excellence (2001) *Pressure Ulcer Risk Assessment.* NICE, London

National Institute for Clinical Excellence (2003) *Pressure Ulcer Prevention.* NICE, London

Nursing and Midwifery Council (2004) *Code of Professional Conduct.* NMC, London

Noonan C, Quigley S, Curley MAQ (2006) Skin integrity in hospitalised infants and children: A prevalence survey. *J Pediatr Nurs* **21**(6): 445–53

Novartis Nutrition Corporation (2006). An overview of the role of nutritional support in wound care. *Nutr Dietet* **63**(2): 5–32

Ratcliffe C, Scarano K, Donovan A (2005) Descriptive study of periostomal complications. *J Wound Ostomy Continence Nurs* **32:** 33–37

Robertson I, Leung E, Hughes D, Spiers M, Donnelly L, Mackenzie I (2005) Prospective analysis of stoma-related complications. *Colorect Dis* **7:** 279–85

Russell L (2000) Understanding physiology of wound healing and how dressings help. *Br J Nurs* **9**(1): 10–20

Samaniego IA (2003) A sore spot in pediatrics: risk factors for pressure ulcers. *Pediatr Nurs* **29**(4): 278–82

Smith SF, Duell DG, Martin BC (2004) *Clinical Nursing Skills*, 6th edn. Prentice Hall, New Jersey

Smith J (2005) *The Guide to The Manual Handling of People*, 5th edn. Backcare, Middlesex

Suddaby EC (2005) Skin breakdown in acute care pediatrics. *Pediatr Nurs* **31**(2): 132–48

Tendra (2005) *Issues in Neonatal Wound Care: Minimising Pain and Trauma*. Report of an Independent Advisory Group. www.tendra.com/item.asp?id=333&si=3

Watson NFS, Hodgkin W (2005) Wound dressings. *Surgery* **23**(2): 52–55

White R, Denyer J (2006) *Paediatric Skin and Wound Care*. Wounds UK, Aberdeen

Wilson J (1999) Clinical governance and the potential implications for tissue viability. *J Tissue Viability* **9**(3): 95–98

Worley C (2004) Quality of life. Part 1: Using the holistic caring praxis in skin and wound care. *Dermatol Nurs* **16**(6): 527–28

Workman BA, Bennett CL (2003) *Key Nursing Skills*. Whurr Publishers, London

Wukich DK, Motko J (2004) Safety of total contact casting in high-risk patients with neuropathic foot ulcers. *Foot Ankle Int* **25**: 556–60

Young T (2006) Principles of paediatric wound management. In: White R, Denyer J, eds. *Paediatric Skin and Wound Care*. Wounds UK, Aberdeen

Further reading

Royal College of Nursing (2005) *The Management of Pressure Ulcers in Primary and Secondary Care: A Clinical Practice Guideline*. RCN, London

Royal College of Nursing (2003) *Standards for Infusion Therapy*. RCN, London

Useful websites

Dressings.org
www.dressings.org/Dressings

Chapter 16

Fundamental aspects of end-of-life care

Helen Pearson and Marion Aylott

Nursing the dying child and supporting the family means using theory as the framework and your heart as the guide. There are no formulas. The child or young person is an observant patient who requires you to be honest and act as a companion in times of great life-altering changes. Most of all you must be prepared to be surprised. Indeed research with children informs us of three things:

- Children understand more than they are often given credit for
- Adults are one of their biggest barriers
- Dying children do not want to be 'fixed'

But most importantly, just like adults, children need and want and deserve honesty, truth and choices. Assessment is the foundation to all nursing care, including that of a terminally ill child, and the Nursing and Midwifery Council (NMC, 2004) states that nurses must:

> *"... undertake ... assessment of physical, psychological, social and spiritual needs of patients."*

Historically, bereavement researchers in the western world have developed models of grief in an attempt to help us to understand the process of dying. These are represented in different ways, as:

- A linear process
- A series of stages
- Tasks to be completed
- The re-investing of emotional energy
- A process of 'letting-go'

These approaches appear to mitigate against individualised care and, in essence, every death has a life of its own. This chapter will consider the care of the dying child in relation to the child's final wishes, and the support for the parents and extended family. It is written in the belief that the child concerned is always the expert. All children are different and their view of the world is unique and dynamic, being continually shaped and re-shaped by different experiences. When nursing a dying child we are witness to a profound journey. Therefore, we must endeavour to support the child as the expert storyteller of their own knowledge and loss experiences. Additionally, political, social, cultural, spiritual and other considerations must be considered in the light of a family-centred philosophy which, according to Kenyon and Barnett, (2001):

"... establishes a partnership with the child and the family receiving care, to promote the maintenance of the family functioning as a unit."

Communication between healthcare professionals

Areas shown to cause difficulty when engaging with the child about their illness and perception of their health include:

- Talking too much (Chatters, 2000)
- Failing to explore the child's values and attitudes (Puchalski and Larson, 1998)
- A tendency for discussing uncertainty using vague language (Tulsky *et al*, 1998)
- Avoiding the child's affective (emotional) concerns (Parle *et al*, 1997)
- Failing to assess the child's cognitive (intellectual) understanding (Black, 1998)
- Failing to assess the level of communication needed for each individual child (Chatters, 2000)

The language of loss

Bereavement	This is a state of experiencing or having experienced loss
Grief	This encompasses the subjective, personal feelings and reactions to loss
Mourning	This describes the private and public processes, rituals and practice of loss
Palliative care	This is defined by the World Health Organization (WHO, 2007) as the active total care of patients whose disease is not responsive to curative treatment. Control of pain, of other symptoms, and psychological, social and spiritual problems is paramount. The goal of palliative care is the achievement of the best quality of life for patients and their families. In addition, palliative care affirms life and regards dying as a normal process
Spirituality	According to Puchalski (1998), spirituality refers to whomever or whatever gives one a transcendent meaning in life
Religion	This can be expressed as the observable aspects of an individuals' spirituality

Children and death

What may seem normal or abnormal to adults may be quite the opposite to children (Erickson, 1963). Children may not express their concerns and spirituality in a direct way (Dixon and Stein,

2006); the use of music or art therapy can be vital. Children's expressions of grief and spirituality are both similar and different from those of adults (Fowler, 1995).

Adjusting to the reality of death and loss is complicated by:

- Developing conceptual understanding (not age) of death and dying (Dixon and Stein, 2006)
- Lack of or distortion of information received (Fowler, 1995)

The child's perspectives are important. Their grief experiences are influenced over time and are embedded not only in their development but also are dynamically inter-related with social and cultural contexts in which all experiences and learning exists. These are impacted upon by the duration and or complexity of illness (Davies *et al*, 2002). Children require developmentally appropriate spaces to see, experience, accept, reject and try out feelings and reactions (Hinds *et al*, 2005).

Table 16.1 explores children's perspectives of death more thoroughly.

Therapeutic intervention is aimed at restoring the fit between the world 'that is' and the world 'that should be'. Research has shown that the child needs to find meaning (at an age-appropriate cognitive level), to experience unconditional love, to feel they have a place in the family, and a need for hope which is an important source of spiritual strength (James and James, 2004). It is essential to consider a child's decision-making capacity with regard to developmental versus cognitive clarity. This relates to the child's legal competence, which is especially important if the child's needs are in conflict with the parent(s). The degree of information sharing (how much or how little regarding diagnosis, prognosis and hope) needs to be considered in close collaboration with the child and the family (Kenyon and Barnett, 2001. Partnership is a vital aspect of development of the treatment plan as the child's parents are the final arbiters (Ellershaw and Ward, 2003).

Table 16.1: Children's perceptions of death

	Aged 0–2	Aged 2–6	Aged 7–12	Aged over 12
Cognitive and emotional ability	*These children:* – have no concept of illness or death – are aware of parent's, family member's, and caregiver's stress and tension	*Children of this age*: – display magical thinking – believe that thoughts and behaviours are causes of events – see death as reversible – start to think in connected ways – live in the moment – are repetitive and physical in their grief	*Children of this age:* – understand death as irreversible, but unpredictable – may have many questions and a need for detailed information (may request details about disease, death, burial) – fear abandonment, body changes, and being different from their peers – have better understanding of cause and effect – can detect the feelings of others – have increasing capacity for expressive language	*Older children:* – are undergoing a time of dramatic physiological, cognitive, emotional, spiritual and social change – have increased sense of self – quest for knowledge, understanding, and awareness of place in the world – search for meaning and purpose – have increased understanding about significance, realities, finality and universality of death and the dying experience – may wish to speak about unrealised plans, their future, and causes of what they are going through – may express anger

	Aged 0–2	Aged 2–6	Aged 7–12	Aged over 12
Spirituality	*Trust versus mistrust* Faith has its roots in infancy and evolves as the child develops trust with their parents. In these early years the child develops a prototype for future relationships and experiences (truth relates to trust)	*Autonomy versus shame (age 2–3)* The child learns to assert independence (restraint can lead to the development of shame and doubt). The child's faith is influenced by images, teaching and stories. Meanings are interpreted literally *Initiative versus guilt (age 4–5)* There is development of purpose. The child learns to balance his or her desires with those of others, to develop obedience, and to abide by parental and religious rules. If introduced, the child verbalises perceptions of religion and awareness of prayer	*Industry versus inferiority* The child's sense of worth develops through competence. Failure leads to a feeling of inferiority, poor perception of self and can affect the ability to form relationships. The child can think in terms of natural and supernatural	*Identity versus identity confusion* The adolescent attempts to establish a clear identity. Thinking and emotions are complex. There is potential for conflict against parental values and rebellion. Fundamental questions are asked about relationship with a religion and the universe

	Aged 0–2	Aged 2–6	Aged 7–12	Aged over 12
Therapeutic intervention	*Offer comfort through sensory means such as:* – suckling – holding – singing	*Work with this age group to:* – dispel misconceptions about death as a punishment for bad thoughts or actions – provide concrete answers – offer limited choices – minimise separation from parent, familiar people, objects, and routines – arrange play time and developmental activities (school)	*These children:* – want honest concrete answers – like to be offered choices to promote a sense of control – need to be reassured that their illness or expected death is not a punishment – need to maintain access to peers	*Work with this age group to:* – provide them with privacy – respect their wishes and choices – support reasonable attempts to maintain/attain their independence – help them maintain access to peers – consider the benefit of peer support groups

Types of emotionally laden questions that children may ask

Am I going to die?
Is there life after death?
What is death?
What is it like to die?
Did I cause it?
Who am I now?
Who will be there?
Does it hurt?

Social and cultural considerations

There are a vast number of external factors which need to be considered aside from the child's age and gender. These include:

- Financial implications (time off work for the parents/care givers)
- Their family position
- The parents' child-rearing practices
- The nature of their relationships and attachments
- The roles of the child's key people during illness
- The child's ideas about rites of passage and norms for 'appropriate' grief
- The child's previous loss experiences
- How the child acquired their understanding of death
- The cause and nature of their imminent death (may involve stigmatisation)
- What the child knows about the rituals surrounding death, bereavement and mourning

Religious and spiritual considerations

Everyone has a spiritual dimension, a personal belief to the meaning of life. It is a unique and individual search for meaning about the infinite that is often – but not inextricably – linked with religion. The concepts of spirituality and religion are explored further in *Box 16.1*.

Box 16.1: Religion versus spirituality

Religion	Spirituality
From Latin *religio*	From Latin *spiritus*
Formalised system of beliefs and practices	A dynamic process
Influenced by historical, social, and cultural circumstances	Gives meaning and purpose to life events and relationships
It represents a *map*	Is often expressed through religion
It revolves around the community	It represents a *journey*
	It revolves around the individual

Three dimensions of spiritual need have been identified by Murray and Zentner (1989):

- The need for relationships with others and maybe a religious figure (this includes feelings of acceptance and love)
- The search for meaning – a need to feel life is worthwhile in the face of death
- The need to understand the relationship between one's own values and morals and own spiritual dimension

In any situation the hospital chaplaincy may be called to see the family, and may if appropriate contact the family's preferred religious or spiritual leader.

The end-of-life care program

The three-step end-of-life care programme (NHS, 2004) is illustrated in *Figure 16.1*. The steps are to:

- IDENTIFY – Identify the needs of the child and the family through discussion
- ASSESS – Assess what realistically can be put in place to aid the child by assessing their needs
- PLAN – Plan the child's care accordingly around previously identified needs. Allow for changes in the planned care depending on the his or her condition, which may deteriorate more quickly than anticipated

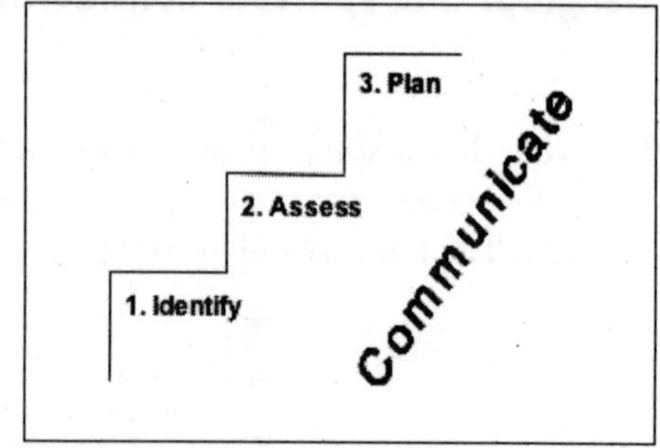

Figure 16.1: The three-step end-of-life care program (NHS, 2004)

The circle of care

What the child can expect

As a nurse you need to establish a relationship with the child and gain information either consciously or subconsciously to access the situation of the following:

- What does the child already know?
- What are the cultural, religious and social practices of the family?
- How have rituals been practiced, if any?
- What are the relationships in the family?

Identify your role:

- Act as a facilitator
- Encourage the child to identify their own needs with support
- Select interventions on a unique basis

Misconceptions of the nurse

It is important at all times to avoid misconceptions based on your own cultural or religious expectations, or ideas about what particular age group is capable of. You can get around this in a number of ways:

- Invite conversation with the child ('What would be helpful?')
- Never force your own beliefs on a child
- Do not presume anything. In an age/developmentally appropriate manner, conduct a spiritual assessment of the child (Stoll, 1979) covering the child's:
- Concept of a deity
- Sources of hope and strength
- Religious and spiritual practices
- Perceptions about the relationship between spiritual beliefs and health

McEvoy's BELIEF model (McEvoy, 2000) can help you to further evaluate the spiritual and religious needs of the child and family (*Box 16.2*).

Box 16.2: The BELIEF model (McEvoy, 2000)

B	Belief system
E	Ethics and values
L	Lifestyle
I	Involvement in a spiritual community
E	Education
F	Future events

Student skill laboratory activity

We enter conversations with our own knowledge, experiences and beliefs about death, grief and bereavement. Seizing opportunities for reflection, asking questions, exploring and creating dialogue with colleagues is a useful vehicle for continuing professional development in everyday practice. Take this opportunity to reflect on and discuss with colleagues issues relating to grief and bereavement.

Consider the following:
- ✓ What are my beliefs about death and dying?
- ✓ What are my beliefs about how children should be involved in end-of-life-care conversations?
- ✓ What do I need to know about an individual child and family?
- ✓ What are my comfort levels in sharing information and talking with children?
- ✓ Who in the healthcare team could assist in this process?

Expression of the child's emotions

It is important to ensure that the child can freely express their emotions and this can be aided by:

- Building a trusting relationship with child and family and spend time with them (Drake *et al*, 2003)
- Developing good listening skills and awareness of your own, and the child's and family members' verbal and non-verbal expressions (Lugton, 2002)
- Answering any questions openly and honestly (an approach to answering difficult questions is given in *Figure 16.2*)
- Touch must be used sensitively but it can provide great emotional comfort (Govier, 2000)
- Provide access to support from a spiritual group or the chaplaincy as appropriate (see *The role of the chaplaincy* below)

Promoting developmentally appropriate communication

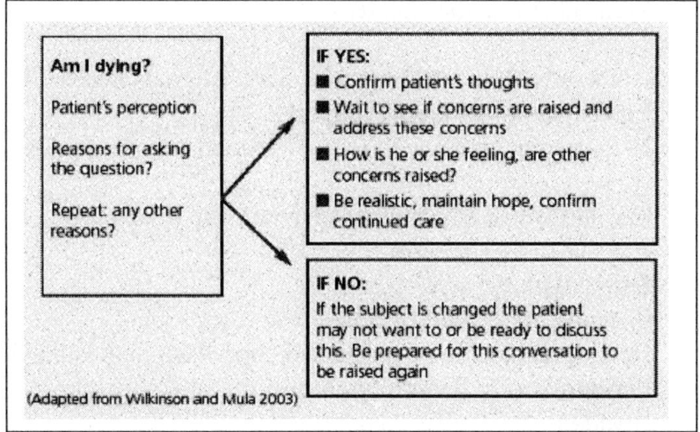

Figure 16.2: Approach to answering difficult questions (Wilkinson and Mula, (2003)

You can empower the child if you include him or her in any decision-making, and in this way help to reduce feelings of helplessness, provide choices and instil hope. You may find that the child wishes to plan his or her own death, including such things as where they die and who they have with them, perhaps making their own funeral arrangements. Explore appropriate ways to broach these matters with children of different ages and different levels of development, so that you can reassure them and provide continuing support. Ask yourself whether this level of information is acceptable to the family? Ask the child what he or she understands and how they are making sense of what is happening? Ensure you have communicated fully with the parents so that they are involved. How much does the child already know? What role do the parents want you to play? This can be seen as a three-way partnership in child, involving with child, parents and the nurse.

You can explore the child's level of understanding in many ways, including through play. Remember that play is the window into the child's unconsciousness. It may be appropriate to incorporate these methods:

- Drawing (a natural means of expression for children; Malchiodi, 1998)
- Using symbolism through guided imagery
- Using role play/drama
- Writing poetry
- Writing a journal
- Creating a memory box (a place for important things; Wolfe and Grier, 2005)
- Compiling a wish list of activities they want to do before they die

The role of the chaplaincy

It is best practice when considering the support needs of children and their parents and carers, for the healthcare professional to ask the family whether they would like some support from the trust's chaplaincy service (NHS, 2004). It is important that the nurse fully recognises the role of the chaplaincy and is able to explain how it works.

Remember that the chaplaincy:

- Is not only there for those who have religious needs
- Encompasses emotional support
- Helps people to come to terms with and make sense of what is happening

The support of a healthcare chaplain can involve:

- Sitting with the sick child
- Listening to the child's needs
- Helping the child to express and cope with what is happening to them
- Listening to the parents, grandparents and other care givers who are struggling with the situation
- Facilitating a collaborative/shared understanding between the various parties as they each cope in different ways

Having support from someone who is not clinically involved in the child's care, who is a trained listener and who can be an objective support is a great comfort to the parents. In terms of specific religious care, healthcare chaplains may be able to:

- Pray with the family
- Arrange for an appropriate faith representative to attend if the family wishes
- Arrange or provide sacramental care (eg. baptism)

Each healthcare trust has a procedure for referring to the chaplaincy department and there is usually 24-hour on-call provision. Healthcare chaplains have a code of conduct for their practice and will assess spiritual needs of the child and family on arrival. Chaplains get as involved as much as is wanted by the parents or child. It is vitally important not to make assumptions about anyone's faith needs when their faith group has been identified. The individuals involved should always be asked about their specific requirements. Individuals of the same faith have different ways of showing their faith and these differences should be respected. *Box 16.3* summarises the beliefs surrounding death of various faiths.

Once contact has been made with a child or family, the healthcare chaplain will assess, after discussion with all concerned, the nature and frequency of that support; it could start with daily visits and then be renegotiated as the situation progresses.

In a situation where a child is terminally ill, the healthcare chaplain will ascertain with the parents how much they want their child to know about their illness. Children may ask difficult questions and a healthcare chaplain's role can be tremendously important in helping to explore these issues with the child and, indeed, with the adults concerned.

Support for siblings is also necessary, particularly with long-term patients, because their own daily routines are likely to be significantly altered. Parents facing the loss of a child often lose perspective and concentrate on that one issue, sometimes forgetting the wider picture and other family members (Boot and Mackinnon, 2007).

Box 16.3: Religious and spiritual considerations immediately before and after death

This box gives an overview of several different faiths. By no means are these descriptions set in stone. Never assume that families of a particular faith will want to carry out these rituals. Rituals vary widely according to specific beliefs and personal feelings of the patient and family, and the child and family should always be consulted on an individual basis.

Buddhism

Buddhists believe in reincarnation of the soul and that the last thoughts before death contribute to rebirth. The family may pray silently or chant *daimoku* (to promote absolute happiness) and recite mantras (*gongyo*) rhythmically with the dying child. When the child dies, the parents might want his or her body to be bathed and dressed in new clothes. Buddhists generally prefer cremation to burial and there are no time constraints to convey to the coroner.

Christianity

Some Roman Catholics wish their child to be baptised prior to death if it has not been done before. Prayers for the dying child may be offered. In the event of sudden death, a priest may be called to anointing the child with oil and viaticum, administer final communion, and lead the family in prayers. Among non-Catholic Christians, rituals vary according to the specific faith and personal feelings, but may involve last sacraments and prayers, such as anointing the child's body with oil to symbolise the Holy Spirit and healing, and saying prayers of courage and acceptance into God's hands. Pentecostalists may pray and sing at the child's bedside with a priest, but there is no ritual anointing. Jehovah's Witnesses have no formal rituals, but congregational support is highly important. Either burial or cremation is acceptable and there are no time constraints.

Hinduism

Prayers from holy readings or hymns may be recited by the dying child. A *pandit* may perform holy rites by tying a thread around the child's neck or wrist to bless them, or sprinkle blessed water over the child or in his or her mouth. Hindus view death as mortality of the body but not of the soul. After death the parents may want to bathe, anoint and dress the body. Cremation is the thought to be best way for the soul to begin its journey. There is no time constraint on when this takes place.

Islamism

Muslims prefer to die in their own homes and it is a religious duty for all family members to visit the dying child. Prays may be said and the *Qur'an* read from. Ideally the child should be turned towards Mecca (*ka'bah*) (south-east). When the child dies, only other Muslims should touch the body; non-Muslims should put gloves on. The family may bathe the body and wrap it in white cotton. They believe the body belongs to God and post mortems are prohibited, so this issue must be handled with great sensitivity. Burial should take place within 24 hours. The coroner will endeavour to respect the family's wishes.

cont./..

Judaism

Jews normally recite prayers, and may invite a rabbi to lead the praying. Sometimes silence is preferred. The dying person (called a *goses*) is treated differently from living people: being touched may hasten their departure, and they must not be left alone, especially when their soul departs. After death, the eyes and mouth are closed and the body is washed and dressed. Orthodox Jews may not want the body to be touched until the rabbi has performed final rites. Non-Jewish people should wear gloves to touch the body. Post-mortems are a sensitive issue as they are regarded as a desecration of the body. The funeral should take place within 48 hours, and the coroner will try to respect this.

Rastafarism

When a child is dying, Rastafarians may carry out a ceremony involving prayers, but after death there are no particular requirements. Some Rastafarians accept death easily because they believe God is eternal, that people live forever, and it is more significant to focus on the living rather than the dead. Therefore the body of the deceased child may be seen as irrelevant. No lock of hair should be taken from the deceased. Generally burial is preferred to cremation and there are no time constraints.

Sikhism

Hymns from the *Guru Granth Sahib* may be recited by those with strong faith to the dying child. Other prayers and readings with family members may be said. Sikhs are normally cremated wearing the five signs of Sikhism. Cremation is preferred and should be carried out within 24 hours of death. The coroner will endeavour to respect the family's wishes.

Specific religious care

The chaplaincy service is invaluable to many parents and it is important that it is incorporated into the care pathways of children in hospital. It can bring meaning, hope and comfort in times of chaos and amidst uncertainty that people are experiencing (Boot and Mackinnon, 2007). The chaplain can undertake the following rites for people of the Christian and other faiths.

Baptism

Some families might want their child to be baptised before he or she dies, if this has not been done. A child of any age can be baptised; this act symbolises initiation into the family of the church. Parents sometimes believe that having their child baptised means he or she will automatically go to Heaven, and this belief can bring great comfort. In extreme cases, when the child is likely to die before a chaplain arrives, any other person who is already baptised and who is a practising Christian can carry out a baptism. The family may be given a certificate to remember the occasion.

Blessing

A short blessing service can provide some comfort when baptism is not an option. This service can be provided by and for people of all faiths and for those with none. It usually involves prayers for the child and the family and may involve naming a newborn baby. A certificate may be given in commemoration.

Commending

When a child is terminally ill the family may want the chaplain to 'commend' their child into God's care. Prayers will be recited at what can be a very emotional time because this is when some parents begin to face the reality of what is happening.

Spiritual space

Many hospitals provide a hospital chapel or multi-faith space where anyone can go to say a prayer or have some time alone to reflect. Healthcare professionals should inform families of such a place because this is another valuable part of the support network.

Neonatal death

If a baby dies in neonatal or maternity care, many hospital trusts provide a contract funeral service. Chaplains may take the service if the family wishes. This can be tremendously helpful for providing continuity of care, especially where the chaplain has been involved in support of the family around the time of death.

Staff support

Not only do healthcare chaplains support children and their families, but they also give vital support to the healthcare professionals who are affected by caring for a sick child or by a child's death. Such support may be provided by chaplain informally or more formally in a one-to-one or group setting.

The dying process

Physiological changes during the dying process

During the last hours or minutes of a child's life there will be signs of deterioration. It is important to consider the emotional impact on the child and the family as they may feel loss of control of the situation. Below is a list of stages which may occur dependent of the dying process that the child is in:

- Weakness and fatigue
- Decreased appetite and fluid intake
- Decreased blood perfusion
- Neurologic dysfunction
- Terminal delirium
- Changed respiration
- Reduction in ability swallow and sphincter control
- Pain
- Inability to close eyes

Weakness and fatigue

The child might demonstrate a decreased ability to move and joint position fatigue (tiredness/lethargy). As a consequence the child is at increased risk of pressure ulcers, and has a greater need for care. Consider how the child's activities of daily living are affected. You might be able to help the child by turning him or her, encouraging movement, and giving massage.

Appetite

The loss of appetite may reveal specific fears about 'giving in' or starvation. Reassure the family that for some children food may be nauseating, and that anorexia may be protective due to a risk of aspiration of food. Clenched teeth express desires/control. Your role will be to help the family find alternative ways of caring (eg. nasogastric feeding if appropriate).

Fluid intake

As the need for fluids decreases, you can supply oral re-hydration fluids and moisten the child's mouth with ice-chips or moistened mouth sponges. The child and parents may fear dehydration and thirst. Remind the family that dehydration does not cause distress, and that dehydration can be protective because of the risk of aspiration. Parenteral fluids may be harmful to the child, perhaps causing fluid overload, breathlessness, coughing and secretions.

Blood perfusion

Decreasing blood perfusion is another physiological sign of approaching death (Tortora and Derrickson, 2006). Signs include tachycardia, hypotension, peripheral cooling, cyanosis, mottling of the skin, and diminished urine output. Parenteral fluids will not reverse this process.

Neurologic dysfunction

According to Tortora and Derrickson (2006)3 the child may exhibit decreasing levels of consciousness. Communicating with the unconscious patient therefore will become more difficult, and this is particularly distressing for the family. Explain to them that the child's awareness is usually greater than his or her ability to respond, and always assume the child can hear *everything*. Work with the parents to maintain a familiar environment for the child, including him or her in all conversations, and giving constant assurance of your presence and his or her safety. Maintain physical contact and touching. Parents can give their child permission to die.

Terminal delirium

When terminal delirium sets in (Tortora and Derrickson, 2006) medical management can be provided with benzodiazepines such as lorazepam and midazolam. Seizures may occur. At this time the family needs a greater level of support and may need more education about what is happening to their child.

Respiration

Altered breathing patterns will occur, and symptoms can include breathlessness, diminishing tidal volume, apnoea, Cheyne–Stokes respirations, and increased use of accessory muscles (Tortora and Derrickson, 2006). The dying child may struggle for last reflex breaths. Management here involves increased family support. It should be explained that oxygen therapy may simply prolong the dying process.

Swallowing reflex

As death approaches, the ability to swallow will decrease (Tortora and Derrickson, 2006). The loss of the gag reflex will result in a build-up of saliva and secretions. Scopolamine may be administered to dry secretions. Other management options include postural drainage, positioning, and suctioning.

Sphincter control

The loss of sphincter control may lead to incontinence of urine and stools. The family needs knowledge and support to understand what their child is going through. The child can be made more comfortable by an increase in cleaning and skin care, and by the use of urinary catheters, absorbent pads and surfaces.

Pain management

Drake *et al* (2003) studied symptoms in dying children, observing that they and their families sometimes become fearful of increased pain. Pain management should be delivered in collaboration with regular re-assessment. If the child is unconscious, pain assessment can be made by observations of persistent versus fleeting expressions, grimacing or physiologic signs, and incidental versus resting pain. Distinction should be made from terminal delirium. Management changes when there is no urine output. Discontinue routine dosing and morphine infusions, giving breakthrough doses as needed (p.r.n.) and use the least invasive route of administration.

Eye closing

There is a loss of the retro-orbital fat pads resulting in insufficient eyelid length so that the eyes cannot be closed properly. This means there is increased conjunctival exposure which can cause dryness and pain. Help the child by maintaining conjunctival moisture.

As expected death approaches

As death becomes imminent, limit medications to essential ones only (Drake *et al*, 2003). Choose less invasive routes of administration – first choose the buccal mucosa or oral route, then rectal, then subcutaneous. Administer intravenously only rarely and intramuscularly almost never. Discuss with the family the status of the child, realistic care goals, and the role of the doctor and multidisciplinary team; discuss with them the symptoms that the family see and what the child experiences. Give the family support throughout the process (Rushton, 2005).

Care after death

The major roles of the nurse in caring for a body after death are carrying out legal requirements, protecting body tissues and discharging the body to an appropriate area for claim. In assuring the child and the family of a peaceful transition, the nurse's role importantly includes caring for the body with reverence to the religious, spiritual and cultural concerns that the child (and family) hold sacred (see *The role of the chaplaincy* above).

Care after death is often referred to as 'laying out' or 'last offices' and is the final process undertaken prior to the body being transferred to the mortuary. The last offices not only involves the legal requirements but also the specific cultural and religious beliefs (Dougherty and Lister, 2004). It is important to encourage involvement of the bereaved parents in this process as often this empowers them and gives them ownership of the child's death (Riches and Dawson, 2000).

When a child dies, a number of practical and legal procedures need to be undertaken. The process varies according to religious, cultural and spiritual beliefs (*Box 16.3*) but the general protocol is described below.

Practical procedures

A patient is not legally dead until certified that death has occurred. Verification of the death is usually undertaken by the doctor, and a death certificate is usually issued at this point. The nurse should know the requirements of their local trust regarding care of the body after death and should follow local procedure. Common to all procedures are cleanliness of the body and proper identification. If this is an anticipated death there is rarely any need for a coroner and organ donation is not suitable (check this with doctor certifying the death). The need for a post mortem should be determined and discussed with the parents by a doctor. If a post mortem is required all invasive lines (for example, intravenous cannulae, central lines, catheters, chest drains and nasogastric tubes) should be kept *in situ* and capped off.

The body of the deceased must be treated in a way that respects the sanctity of the human body. Nursing care includes maintaining privacy and preventing damage to the body (Department of Health, 2001). There is no need to rush the family at this point (consider the physiological changes that occur after death, as described in *Box 16.4*). After death, care shifts from the child to family, caregivers, and the nurse should support them in their traditions, rites, and rituals as appropriate (Department of Health *et al*, 2006) (see *Box 16.3*.) and remember:

- That the loss is different for everyone
- To invite those not present to bedside as appropriate
- To allow family time to witness what has happened
- To create a peaceful, accessible environment

Box 16.4: Physiological changes after death (McChance and Huether, 2006)

Algor mortis In algor mortis the lack of skin elasticity due to decreased body temperature, mandates that nurses take care when removing tapes to avoid skin breakdown. Wounds are best re-dressed and wrapped with bandage

Liver mortis This relates to the bluish discolouration seen as a by-product of red cell destruction which occurs in pooled blood. It is avoided through proper positioning of the body. Placing pillows under the head decreases the colouring of liver mortis to the face and head

Rigor mortis During this stage the body stiffens due to contracture of the skeletal and smooth muscles. It occurs 2–4 hours after death, so before this time the body must be laid flat and limbs positioned in natural alignment with the trunk, and eyes and mouth closed. Positioning of the limbs, jaw and eyelids increases the chance of a natural and comfortable appearance of the body after death

Depending on the family's religious beliefs, the body maybe washed and dressed according to the family or child's wishes as were discussed before death. Remember that a child's body weight increases by 15%. Consider the use of slides, slide sheets and hoists to move the body (Pike, 2004). Do warn the parents that when their child's body is moved, air may be forced out of the lungs so a sigh may be heard, and that all the muscles in the body relax after death which can cause the bladder, bowel or any open wounds to leak – without prior warning such things can be very distressing.

Anything that is left on or with the body, such as pieces of jewellery or a favourite teddy bear (*only* at the parents' request) will need to be documented. The child's other belongings should be given to the parents to take home with them.

Complete all the nursing and medical documentation (Department of Health, 1998). Correct ID bands must be secured to the child's body; usually there are two, one around the wrist and one around the ankle, preferably on opposite sides of the body. Write on each band the child's name, hospital number, ward, date of birth, and date of death. Attach a completed 'Notification of Death' form to the body, and hand the duplicate copy to the porter for the mortician. Then the body is transferred to the mortuary.

There are a few other tasks for the nurse to perform at this time:

- Notify other doctors and caregivers about the death
- Stop relevant community-based services
- Arrange to remove equipment and supplies from the bedside
- Secure valuables with executor
- Dispose of medications and biological waste

Taking the deceased home

Provided that there is no requirement for a post mortem, some parents may wish to take their child's body home. This request must be respected. Transferring the child's body back to the home can help the family accept the death and it also gives them an opportunity to say goodbye in private (Sloan *et al*, 1999). Aside from this, parents may feel that they are continuing their parental role and reconstructing their relationship with the deceased child (Culliford, 2002). There are no legal limitations here, but the parents would need to organise the transfer of the body, and the relevant healthcare professionals would need to authorise this.

Post mortem examination

Questions parents might ask if a post mortem is necessary

This is to give background information on what a post mortem entails, but when informing parents remember that they may not understand certain terminology.

What is the role of the coroner?

Individual coroners have jurisdiction over a specific geographical area, as laid down by statute. There are, for example, five coroners cover the county of Hampshire and the Isle of Wight. In total there are over one hundred coroners in the UK, each with their own way of working and dealing with issues that arise. The whole system operates under the Lord Chancellor's Department. In the case of the death of a child, the coroner and the coroner's officers are accustomed to dealing with issues that arise with particular sensitivity.

What happens about the death certificate?

Once any death has taken place, either in hospital or in the community generally, the hospital doctor or a general practitioner will be asked if they are prepared to sign the relevant form describing the cause of death so that registration of the death can take place and a death certificate can be issued to the family. There are a significant number of cases where the relevant doctor will not be prepared to sign the form in question because of uncertainty as to the cause of death; this does not mean there is anything suspicious about the death in question, simply lack of clarity as to how it came about. This will usually mean that a post mortem is necessary and only the coroner has power to order this.

What is a post mortem?

A post mortem involves examination of the main organs in the body. It includes conducting relevant tests to investigate possible illnesses or conditions, or involvement of alcohol or drugs as the cause of death.

How long does the post mortem take?

The body is removed on behalf of the coroner from the place where death has occurred and taken initially to the mortuary at the local hospital, where the post mortem examination usually takes place. A post mortem will normally take place within 48 hours of death. Once the cause of death has been clearly established, the body can be released back to the family's chosen undertaker for funeral arrangements to be made.

Is a post mortem normal?

Not many deaths of young children are from unnatural causes. However, there will always be a proportion that involve accidents of one kind or another. The coroner's officers will stay in constant contact with the family to provide whatever information is needed. Nurses are not directly involved with these events, but they should be aware that when a child's body undergoes a post mortem (or indeed an inquest) then the family's nightmare continues, and their grieving is even harder to bear. All families need considerable support during this period.

Why is a post mortem necessary?

Post mortems are carried out to establish a cause of death in all cases where this is not clear, as well as allowing careful investigation of any death that is suspicious. The funeral of even a very young child cannot take place without a known cause of death; if the treating doctor has not done this, then a post mortem examination will. Of course this is a very distressing time for parents in particular, even when there are no suspicious circumstances. In the case of children who suffered from a longstanding condition or illness, the doctor is usually prepared to sign for a specific cause of death, but a post mortem will often be needed in the case of sudden and unexpected deaths. The process of a post mortem and why it is necessary is explained by a coroner's officer to the parents thoroughly and carefully – the coroner alone decides whether it is necessary. Parents do not have the right to oppose this decision even if their reason is (understandably) that they find it difficult or distasteful to contemplate.

What happens during the post mortem?

The pathologists examines the body externally and internally. During the internal examination all the organs are removed and investigated, unless the coroner has asked only for specific organs. A post mortem is like a mini operation on the body's head, chest and abdomen. Tissue sample are taken for further analysis before the organs are returned to the body (but they are not usually returned to their original positions).

Can the parents say no to the post mortem?

The short answer is no. As stated above, parents do not have the right to oppose the coroner's decision. In all cases, immediate legal ownership of the body of any deceased person rests with the coroner, rather than the family or anyone else. Obviously it is important to be clear about this in case of family dispute or anything suspicious circumstances in the death.

What happens after the post mortem?

Various forms signed by the coroner during this process are taken by the family to the registrar who can then issue a death certificate. This must be done before the funeral can take place. As most families want the funeral to take place within 7 to 10 days, there is considerable pressure to produce everything that is necessary within a short period of time.

Follow-up bereavement care

After the death, and usually when an adequate time has passed, the family is normally offered a bereavement follow-up meeting with the consultant in charge of their child's care. This is perceived as a valuable aid in helping the family's journey of coming to terms with their loss (Nussbaumer and Russell, 2003). In this process the family may ask questions about whether they were to blame or could have done anything differently to prevent their child's death. It is an opportunity for them to ask any questions they may have thought of after the death, and time should be given to respond to these.

Caring for the professional carer

Research has shown that the death of a child has a major emotional impact on all those involved (Costello and Trinder-Brook, 2000). It is a time for the child's family to grieve as well as healthcare professionals. Nurses often develop close therapeutic relationships with the child and the family in the hospital and often represent the majority affected by a child's death. Therefore multidisciplinary and interprofessional de-briefing sessions are important for those involved to gain insight about what is sometimes an extremely complex situation (Ellershaw and Ward, 2003).

Acknowledgements

This chapter would not contain such detailed explanations in certain areas without assistance and guidance from Reverend Felicity Boot and Reverend Karen Mackinnon from Southampton General Hospital Chaplaincy, and Keith Wiseman, HM Coroner for Southampton and New Forest District. Finally, and most importantly, special thanks to the children and families who taught me so much – you are always in my thoughts.

References

Black D (1998) Coping with loss: The dying child. *BMJ* **316**: 1376–78

Boot F, McKinnon K (2007) *The role of the healthcare chaplaincy.* Professional conversation Jan/Feb 2007. Southampton University Hospital Trust, Hampshire

Chatters L (2000) Religion and health: public health research and practice. *Ann Rev Publ Hlth* **21**: 335–67

Costello J, Trinder-Brook A (2000) Children's nurses' experiences of caring for dying children in hospital. *Paediatr Nurs* **12**(6): 28–32

Culliford L (2002) Spirituality and clinical care. *BMJ*. **325:** 1434–35

Davies B, Brenner P, Orloff S, Sumner L, Worden W (2002) Addressing spirituality in pediatric hospice and palliative care. *J Palliat Care* **18**: 59–67

Department of Health (2001) *Essence of Care: Patient-Focused Benchmarking for Health Care Practitioners*. Department of Health, London

Department of Health IE, Melia KM, Boyd KM, Horsburgh D (2006) *Nursing Ethics,* 5th edn. Edinburgh, Churchill Livingstone

Department of Health/NHS Executive (1998) *For the Record: Managing Records in NHS Trusts and Health Authorities*. Department of Health, London

Dixon SD, Stein MT (2006) *Encounters with Children: Pediatric Behavior and Development.* Mosby Elsevier, Philadelphia

Dougherty L, Lister S (2004) *The Royal Marsden Hospital Manual of Clinical Nursing Procedures*. Blackwell Publishing, Oxford

Drake R, Frost J, Collins JJ (2003) The symptoms of dying children. *J Pain Symp Manag* **26**(1): 594–603

Ellershaw J, Ward C (2003) Care of the dying patient: the last hours or days of life. *BMJ* **326:** 30–34

Erickson E (1963) *Childhood and Society*, 2nd edn. WW Norton & Company, New York

Fowler J (1995) *Stages of Faith*. Harper Collins, London

Govier I (2000) Spiritual care in nursing: a systematic approach. *Nurs Stand* **14**(17): 32–36

Hinds PS, Oakes LL, Hicks J, Anghelescu DL (2005) End-of-life care for children and adolescents. *Sem Oncol Nurs* **21**(1): 63–62

James A, James AL (2004) *Constructing Childhood: Theory Policy and Social Practice.* Palgrave Macmillan, London

Kenyon E, Barnett N (2001) Partnership in nursing care (PINC): The Blackburn Model. *J Child Hlth Care* **5**(1): 36–38

Lugton J (2002) *Communicating with Dying People and their Relatives*. Radcliffe Medical, Oxford

Malchiodi CA (1998) *Understanding Children's drawings*. Jessica Kingsley, London

McChance KL, Huether SE (2006) *Pathophysiology: The Biologic Basis for Disease in Adults and Children*, 5th edn. Elsevier Mosby, St Louis

McEvoy M (2000) An added dimension to the pediatric health maintenance visit: The spiritual history. *J Pediatr Hlth Care* **14:** 216–20

Murray R, Zentner J (1989) *Nursing Concepts for Health Promotion*. Prentice Hall, London

National Health Service (2005) *The Gold Standards Framework: End of Life Care Programme.* NHS, London

Parle M, Maguire P, Heaven C (1997) The development of a training model to improve health professionals' skills, self-efficacy and outcome expectancies when communicating with cancer patients. *Soc Sci Med* **44:** 231–40

Pike AM (2004) Manual handling the deceased child in a children's hospice. *J Child Hlth Care* **8**(3): 198–209

Puchalski CM, Larson DB (1998) Developing curricula in spirituality and medicine. *Acad Med* **73**(9): 970–74

Riches G, Dawson P (2000) *An Intimate Loneliness, Supporting Bereaved Parents and Siblings.* Open University Press, Buckingham

Rushton CH (2005) A framework for integrated pediatric palliative care: Being with dying. *J Pediatr Nurs* **20**(5): 311–25

Sloan RP, Bagiella E, Powell T (1999) Religion, spirituality, and medicine. *Lancet* **353:** 664–67

Stoll RL (1979) Guidelines for spiritual assessment. *Am J Nurs* **1**(9): 574–77

Tortora GJ, Derrickson B (2006) *Principles of Anatomy and Physiology*, 11th edn. Wiley, Danvers

Tulsky JA, Fischer GS, Rose MR, Arnold RM (1998) Opening the black box: how do physicians communicate about advance directives? *Ann Intern Med* **129:** 441–49

Wolfe J, Grier HE (2005) Care of the dying child. In: Pizzo PA, Poplack DG, eds. *Principles and Practice of Pediatric Oncology*, 5th edn. Williams & Wilkins, New York

World Health Organization (2007) *Palliative Care.* www.who.int/cancer/palliative/definition/en/

Further reading

Heming D, Colmer A (2003) Care of dying patients. *Nurs Stand* **18**(10): 47–54

Ikeda D (2003) *Unlocking the Mysteries of Birth and Death: A Buddhist View of Life*, 2nd edn. Middleway Press, Santa Monica

Kawn C (2002) Families' experiences of the last office of deceased family members in the hospice setting. *Int J Palliat Nurs* **8**(6): 266–75

Klass D (1996) *Continuing Bonds: New Understanding of Grief.* Taylor & Francis, London

Koenig HG, McCullough M, Larson DB (2001) *Handbook of Religion and Health.* Oxford University Press, Oxford

Levesque R (2002) *Not by Faith Alone.* Oxford University Press, Oxford

Matthews DA, McCullough ME, Larson DB, Koenig HG, Swyers JP, Milano MG (1998) Religious commitment and health status. *Arch Fam Med* **7:** 118–24

Mc Neilly P, Price J, Surgenor M (2006) Breaking bad news to parents: the children's nurse's role. *Int J Palliat Nurs* **12**(3): 115–20

Mc Sherry W (2004) The language of spirituality: an emerging taxonomy. *Int J Nurs Stud* **41**(2): 151–61

McCallum DE, Byrne P, Bruera E (2000) How children die in hospital. *J Pain Symp Manag* **20**(6): 417–23

McGeehin Heilferty C (2004) Spiritual development and the dying child: The pediatric nurse practitioner's role. *J Pediatr Hlth Care* **18**(6): 271–75

National Institute for Clinical Excellence (2004) *Supportive and Palliative Care: The Manual.* NICE, London

Norouzieh K (2005) Case management of the dying child. *Case Manag* **16**(1): 54–57

Nursing and Midwifery Council (2004) *Code of Professional Conduct.* NMC, London

Nussbaumer A, Russell R (2003) Bereavement support following sudden and unexpected death in children. *Curr Paediatr* **13**: 555–59

Park Ridge Center (2000) *Religion, Sexuality, and Public Policy: Overview of World Religions.* www.parkridgecenter.org/Page658.html

Peate I, Whiting L (2006) *Caring for Children and Families.* John Wiley & Sons, Chichester

Penson J (1990) *Bereavement: A Guide for Nurses.* Harper & Row, London

Price J, McNeilly P, McFarlane M (2005) Paediatric palliative care in the UK: past, present and future. *Int J Palliat Nurs* **11**(3): 124–26

Schott J, Henley A (2002) *Culture, Religion and Childbearing in a Multiracial Society: A Handbook for Health Professionals.* Butterworth-Heinemann, Edinburgh

White G (2000) An inquiry into the concepts of spirituality and spiritual care. *Int J Palliat Nurs* **6**(10): 479–84

Whittle M, Cutts S (2002) Time to go home: assisting families to take their child home following a planned hospital or hospice death. *Paediatr Nurs* **14**(10): 24–28

Wilkinson S, Mula C (2003) *Communication in care of the dying.* In: Ellershaw J, Wilkinson S, eds. *Care of the Dying: A Pathway to Excellence.* Oxford University Press, Oxford

Willis E (2007) Symptom care flow charts: a case study. *Paediatr Nurs* **19**(1): 14–17

Index

Note: All procedures relate to children, but aspects that are specific to young people (puberty to adulthood) and infants (neonates to 1 year) are indicated under those entries. Italic page numbers refer to boxes, tables and figures, and figures are distinguished further by the suffix'f'.

B

C

H

I

Q

R

S